Calcium in Drug Action

Calcium in Drug Action

Edited by
George B. Weiss

University of Texas Health Science Center
Southwestern Medical School
Dallas, Texas

Plenum Press · New York and London

Library of Congress Cataloging in Publication Data

Main entry under title:

Calcium in drug action.
   "Originated from a more limited Symposium on 'Importance of Calcium as a Primary
Locus of Drug Action'... at the April, 1977 FASEB meeting in Chicago."
   Includes index.
   1. Calcium—Physiological effect—Congresses. 2. Drugs—Physiological effect—Con-
gresses. I. Weiss, George B. [DNLM: 1. Calcium—Pharmacodynamics—Congresses. 2.
Calcium—Physiology—Congresses. 3. Drug interactions—Congresses. QV276 S989c
1977]
QP913.C2C34   615'.7   78-8517
ISBN-13: 978-1-4684-3356-2   e-ISBN-13: 978-1-4684-3354-8
DOI: 10.1007/978-1-4684-3354-8

© 1978 Plenum Press, New York
Softcover reprint of the hardcover 1st edition 1978
A Division of Plenum Publishing Corporation
227 West 17th Street, New York, N.Y. 10011

PREFACE

Anyone surveying physiological and pharmacological journals can readily see that the biological actions of calcium ion are of increasingly widespread current interest. The scope of investigated actions and reactions in which a role for calcium ion is of some importance is so numerous as to convey the impression that calcium ion is everywhere and interacts with everything. This being so, the challenge in contemporary research is to focus on investigation of those actions of calcium ion which, in some manner, influence either significant physiological parameters or the manner in which pharmacological agents act.

This multi-authored book originated from a more limited Symposium on "Importance of Calcium as a Primary Locus of Drug Action" co-chaired by myself and Dr. Frank R. Goodman at the April, 1977 FASEB meeting in Chicago. This Symposium was organized in response to a perceived need for increased communication among workers in different areas of Ca^{2+}-related research. In the process of selecting the maximum of six areas for presentation within the format provided, it soon became apparent that this would result in only a limited sampling of current research efforts. Expansion of the number of areas to fourteen within a book format appeared to be the most logical mechanism to provide a more coherent interdisciplinary approach to consideration of various aspects of the roles of Ca^{2+} in drug action. This is not to imply that all relevant Ca^{2+}-related areas are surveyed within this volume. Rather, the fourteen chapters represent a sampling of the current status of our knowledge of Ca^{2+} as an essential component of the basic mechanisms by which various types of drugs exert their actions.

The specific goal of this volume is to foster an interdisciplinary approach to consideration of calcium in drug action. By this, I mean that Ca^{2+}-related research is usually system-oriented and included in sessions devoted to aspects of, for example, smooth muscle or secretory mechanisms. In contrast, there is no clearly delineated constituency for Ca^{2+} as a unitary field of research. However, there is a recognized need to compare and contrast the differing techniques and approaches employed to investigate the roles of Ca^{2+} as a basis for and a modifier of drug action. Hopefully, presentation of the varied cellular and subcellular actions of Ca^{2+} in different systems within the context of a single volume will encourage more widespread application of relevant techniques and approaches as well as increased communication within this general research area.

The organization of this book is intended to facilitate use by all investigators and students interested in any aspect of the cellular and subcellular basis of the roles of calcium in drug action. The fourteen areas considered have been arranged into three distinct sections emphasizing approaches to qualitative and quantitative analysis of Ca^{2+} distribution and movements (Chapters 1-4), subcellular sites and interactions of Ca^{2+} and drugs (Chapters 5-8), and the varied roles of Ca^{2+} in drug action in specific biological systems (Chapters 9-14). This separation is one based primarily on degree of emphasis and orientation. In all chapters, the objective is a definitive understanding of the cellular and molecular roles of Ca^{2+} in drug action.

As editor, I wish to convey my deepest appreciation to all of the contributors to this volume. The manner in which this volume was prepared necessitated a particularly high degree of coordination with respect to deadlines, preciseness of manuscript preparation and copy editing. The exceptional level of responsiveness and capability on the part of all of the authors made my job as editor a far less burdensome task than is often the case. It has been a rewarding experience to work with the contributors to this volume. Also, I want to thank Davida, Debbie and Bill Weiss for their patience during the many hours I spent preparing the final version of this volume and for their assistance in preparation of the subject index. Finally, the most important of all acknowledgements is due to Roma L. Chapin who did a superlative job in preparing the final copy of this entire volume.

George B. Weiss

CONTENTS

SECTION   Page

Chapter

SECTION   Page

SECTION I

ANALYSIS AND ALTERATION OF CALCIUM ION

DISTRIBUTION AND MOVEMENTS

The chapters in this first section focus especially on how movement of Ca^{2+} occurs across the cell membrane, how this movement is facilitated or regulated, and how drug-induced alterations in Ca^{2+} movements can produce changes in cellular responsiveness. The primary concern, in each case, is the cellular basis of the role of Ca^{2+} in coupling excitation to contraction. Though the techniques employed are varied and the approaches appear quite dissimilar, the actual conclusions derived are not basically different.

In the first chapter, evidence is summarized for the entry of Ca^{2+} current through a specific Ca^{2+} channel and the manner in which inorganic (divalent and trivalent ions) and organic (verapamil and related compounds) Ca^{2+} antagonists alter Ca^{2+} binding and entry. By use of structural comparisons of Ca^{2+} antagonists and of Ca^{2+} ionophore actions as well, the possibility is raised that comparative data obtained with these agents might help to elucidate the molecular nature of the Ca^{2+} entry processes. In the second chapter, the sarcolemmal origin of that Ca^{2+} important in excitation-contraction coupling in heart cells is delineated. Altered permeabilities of cultured heart cell membranes are employed to examine mechanisms of Ca^{2+} entry as well as effects of stimulatory and inhibitory agents on superficial Ca^{2+} binding. The third chapter is concerned with the binding of Ca^{2+} at two types of sites and the quantitative relationships between these two sites and corresponding Ca^{2+} uptake and washout components. The fourth chapter discusses mechanisms by which Ca^{2+} is transported across cell membranes from depots and/or transport

sites. Both the third and fourth chapters consider drug actions
in terms of alterations induced in Ca^{2+} binding and uptake parameters.

All four of these initial chapters are concerned with the
quantitative aspects of Ca^{2+} distribution and movements in smooth
or cardiac muscle systems. The variety of techniques successfully
employed include electron microscopic, histochemical, isotopic
and electrophysiological ones. The level and precision of these
approaches are increasingly cellular in nature and provide varied
evidence of the primary involvement of Ca^{2+} as an essential modulator of actions of various drugs.

CHAPTER 1

CALCIUM, CALCIUM TRANSLOCATION, AND
SPECIFIC CALCIUM ANTAGONISTS

L. Rosenberger and D. J. Triggle

Department of Biochemical Pharmacology
State University of New York
Buffalo, New York 14214

INTRODUCTION

It is now almost one hundred years since Sidney Ringer (1882) described the importance of Ca^{2+} in the maintenance of frog heart contractility. Subsequent to this observation, it has been increasingly recognized that Ca^{2+} plays a critical and central role in a multitude of biological events at both the intra- and extracellular levels (Duncan, 1976; Kretsinger, 1976a; Table 1). However, Ca^{2+} distribution across the cell membrane is far from equilibrium, since if the resting membrane potential ($\sim-60mV$) were equal to the Ca^{2+} equilibrium potential, then the intracellular Ca^{2+} activity should be some 100-fold greater than the extracellular activity. This is quite clearly not so and although accurate measurements of free ionized intracellular Ca^{2+} concentrations have not been made in many systems the concensus of evidence firmly indicates that $[Ca^{2+}_{int}] < 10^{-7}M$ (Baker, 1972; 1976; Blaustein, 1974; Reuter, 1973). Such a low intracellular Ca^{2+} concentration accords with the binding constants of Ca^{2+} for those intracellular proteins whose activity is known to be modulated by Ca^{2+} (pK_D values $\sim$ 6-7; Kretsinger, 1976a,b) and indicates the "trigger" function of an increased intracellular Ca^{2+} concentration (Heilbrunn, 1956).

The very large driving force for Ca^{2+} entry indicates that there must exist specific mechanisms for the removal of intracellular Ca^{2+}. A schematic representation of the several processes that are involved in the regulation of intracellular Ca^{2+} is given in Figure 1. Subsequent to entry Ca^{2+} may be removed through complexation with cytoplasmic constituents (including the internal membrane surface), or by sequestration into the intracellular

TABLE I.   PARTIAL LISTING OF CALCIUM-DEPENDENT EVENTS

Excitation-contraction coupling   *Stimulus-secretion coupling*
Ciliary motility   *Blood clotting cascade*
Modulation of activities of intra-
  cellular enzymes (phosphorylase b
  kinase; adenylate and guanylate
  cyclases; phosphodiesterase acti-
  vator protein, etc.)
Lymphocyte transformation   *Egg cell activation*
Cell aggregation and adhesion   *Membrane stabilization and*
                                             fusion
Regulation of membrane excitability
  (electrical and chemical)   *Microtubule assembly*

---

structures, mitochondria (Lehninger, 1974; Carafoli and Crompton, 1976) and sarcoplasmic reticulum (MacLennan and Holland, 1975; Carafoli *et al.*, 1975). Although there can be no doubt as to the importance of Ca^{2+} uptake by the active transport processes mediated by mitochondria and sarcoplasmic reticulum the cell must, in order to maintain its total Ca^{2+} sensibly constant, ultimately transport Ca^{2+} to the external medium. Two major processes for such removal of intracellular Ca^{2+} have been described: in one process the extrusion of Ca^{2+} is directly coupled to the hydrolysis of ATP and in the second process the extrusion of Ca^{2+} is coupled to an influx of Na^+.

Active Ca^{2+} transport across the cell membrane mediated by a Mg^{2+}, Ca^{2+}-activated ATPase has been best described for the red blood cell (Schatzmann, 1975), but it likely operates in a number of other systems including L cells (Lamb and Lindsay, 1971), brain (Nakamura and Schwartz, 1971) and smooth muscle (Hurwitz *et al.*, 1973), and in general this transport system shows a considerable resemblance to that of sarcoplasmic reticulum. A second system for moving Ca^{2+} across cell membranes is Na^+ - Ca^{2+} coupled transport. The most detailed knowledge of this system derives from studies with squid axons (Baker, 1972; Blaustein and Russell, 1975; Baker and McNaughton, 1976), but the system is widely distributed (Blaustein, 1974) and appears to be of major importance in the regulation of intracellular Ca^{2+} levels. Ca^{2+} extrusion by this process depends upon the presence of external Na^+ and is generally described as insensitive to inhibitors of Na^+, K^+ - ATPase or metabolic poisons and only indirectly coupled to ATP-utilizing processes. The energy for the uphill transport of Ca^{2+} is presumed to be derived from the coupling of Ca^{2+} extrusion to the movement of Na^+ down its electrochemical gradient, the nature of

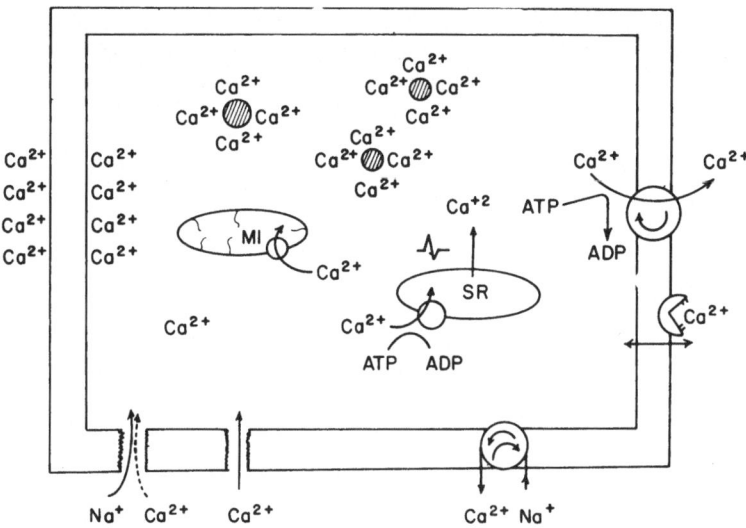

Fig. 1. A schematic representation of cellular calcium regulation. Intracellular calcium may be bound to intracellular proteins (⊘), to the internal surface of the cell membrane or sequestrated in mitochondria or sarcoplasmic reticulum. Calcium pumping across the plasma membrane is represented by a Ca^{2+} - ATPase and a Na^+ - Ca^{2+} exchange mechanism. Specific entry mechanisms for calcium include the "Na^+" and the "Ca^{2+}" channels. Additionally, ionophoric species may bypass specific calcium entry and exit routes.

the coupling determining the steepness of the Ca^{2+} gradient achieved. The most recent studies in squid axon (Baker and McNaughton, 1976) do suggest a role for ATP in maintaining Na^+-dependent Ca^{2+} efflux, but it is not established whether ATP hydrolysis occurs or whether ATP acts in allosteric fashion to control the affinities of Ca^{2+} and Na^+ binding sites. It is likely that the process is electrogenic with 3 Na^+ entering for each Ca^{2+} leaving, a stoichiometry that can generate the physiological Ca^{2+} gradient. Ca^{2+} entry can be observed if the Na^+ gradient is reversed, this process presumably representing operation of the carrier system in reverse.

THE Ca^{2+} ENTRY PROCESS

Given the existence of the several mechanisms that operate to maintain a low intracellular free Ca^{2+} concentration it is clear that there must also exist mechanisms that serve to increase [Ca^{2+}_{int}] and couple membrane excitation to intracellular Ca^{2+}-modulated events. This Ca^{2+} may be derived from intracellular stores or from extracellular sources (Figure 1). Although initial emphasis was placed by Hodgkin and Huxley (1952) on Na^+ and K^+ as the current carrying species during squid axon excitation, there is now substantial evidence for this, and many other tissues, that Ca^{2+} entry through "specific calcium channels" also contributes to the total membrane current (Baker, 1972; Reuter, 1973; Hagiwara, 1975; Triggle and Triggle, 1976). Thus, early work with crustacean muscles (Fatt and Katz, 1953; Fatt and Ginsborg, 1958; Hagiwara, 1975) showed that long lasting action potentials could be observed in the presence of tetraethylammonium (TEA - a K^+ channel antagonist), that neither Na^+ nor Mg^{2+} was essential to the maintenance of excitation, that Ca^{2+} removal abolished action potentials, that the amplitudes and durations of the action potentials increased with increased [Ca^{2+}_{ext}] and that Ca^{2+} could be replaced by Sr^{2+} or Ba^{2+}.

Although the inward current of the squid axon action potential contains only a very small Ca^{2+} component (0.001 % of the Na^+ entry), this preparation has facilitated the characterization of the Ca^{2+} current (Baker, 1972; Baker and Glitsch, 1975). The photoprotein aequorin emits light in the presence of ionized Ca^{2+} (Blinks et al., 1976) and its injection into squid axons has permitted the differentiation of two quite distinct components of Ca^{2+} entry. An early phase of Ca^{2+} entry associated with short depolarizing pulses parallels the rise in Na^+ permeability and is abolished by tetrodotoxin whereas the later phase of Ca^{2+} entry associated with longer depolarizing pulses is insensitive to tetrodotoxin or TEA (Figure 2). Apparently, the initial phase of Ca^{2+} entry uses the fast sodium channels which are approximately 100 times more permeable to Na^+ than to Ca^{2+}. The delayed Ca^{2+} entry is through channels apparently quite distinct from those used by Na^+ (TTX - sensitive) or K^+ (TEA - sensitive) and with an ion selectivity, $Ca^{2+}:Na^+:K^+$, 1:0.01:0.01, quite distinct from that of the sodium channel (Reuter and Scholz, 1977). The slow calcium channels do, however, have properties consistent with a Hodgkin-Huxley system since they show voltage- and time-dependent activation and inactivation; these properties are, however, markedly different from those of the early sodium channel since the calcium current is activated at a more positive membrane potential (and indeed can be seen when the Na^+ current has been inactivated by a depolarizing pulse), has a more positive equilibrium potential and is inactivated much less rapidly (Bassingthwaighte and Reuter, 1972; Reuter, 1973; Kohlhardt, 1975).

Further distinction between the fast sodium and slow calcium currents is provided by observations that these currents are associated with kinetically distinct gating currents associated with particle displacement in the opening and closing of ion channels (Armstrong, 1975; Goldman, 1976; Adams and Gage, 1976) and, of

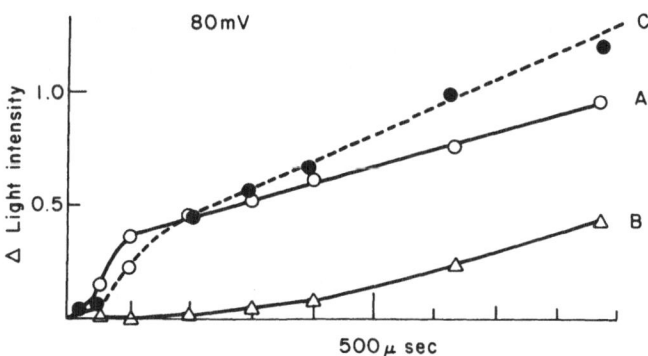

Fig. 2.   The two phases of calcium entry in squid axon (measured by aequorin light response) showing the relation between the voltage-clamp pulse (80 mV depolarization) duration (abscissa) and the increased light intensity per pulse. A, before TTX; B, in presence of TTX; C, after removal of TTX. (Reproduced with permission from Baker, Progr. Biophys. Mol. Biol., 24, 177. Copyright Pergamon Press).

particular importance, pharmacological differentiation of the Na^+, K^+ and Ca^{2+} channels is possible with selective antagonists. Tetrodotoxin and tetraethylammonium are well known for their actions on Na^+ and K^+ channels respectively (Hille, 1970) and the inorganic ions Mg^{2+}, Mn^{2+}, Ni^{2+}, Co^{2+}, La^{3+} and the organic agents verapamil (I), D-600 (II) and Nifedipine (BAY-1040; III) have gained prominence as Ca^{2+} channel antagonists (Fleckenstein, 1971, 1972; Reuter, 1973). There is an obvious analogy between this differentiation of ion channels and the differentiation of pharmacological receptors through specific antagonist action.

I. R = H
II. R = OMe

III

There is now considerable evidence that a calcium entry process similar to that seen in the squid axon occurs in a number of excitable tissues and that a calcium channel is utilized that is distinct from that carrying the early sodium current. The basis for the differentiation of such a process rests on the following properties:
     a.   Membrane currents and potential changes can be seen

in Na^+-free solution but are very rapidly abolished
in the absence of both Na^+ and Ca^{2+}. Potential
changes measured in Na^+-free solution are basically
identical to those seen in Na^+-containing media in
the presence of TTX or in preparations where the
Na^+ channel has been inactivated by prior depolarization.

b.   The calcium current is insensitive to TTX and TEA
     but is sensitive to antagonism by Mg^{2+}, Mn^{2+}, Co^{2+},
     La^{3+}, verapamil, D-600 and Nifedipine.

c. Sr^{2+} and Ba^{2+} can substitute for Ca^{2+}.

d.   The threshold, voltage- and time-dependent activa-
     tion and inactivation parameters and gating currents
     are quite distinct from those determined for the
     early sodium current.

As judged by the application of the criteria listed above
calcium channels mediating calcium translocation have been described in a wide variety of preparations, from protozoan to
mammalian (Table II), although it must be noted that in many instances complete ionic, electrophysiological and pharmacological
characterization is not available. Analysis of the calcium channel
activity has not yet reached the stage achieved for the sodium
channel where it has been possible to determine single channel
conductances and to measure channel density, the latter being of
the order of 50-500 TTX binding sites/μM^2 (Ritchie et $al.$, 1976).
However, calcium current density in cardiac muscle is at least a
hundred-fold less than the sodium current density; whether this
reflects a corresponding reduction in channel density and/or flux
rate through the channel is not known.

CALCIUM CHANNEL ANTAGONISTS

The di- and trivalent cations, Mn^{2+}, Ni^{2+}, Co^{2+}, La^{3+} and
the organic molecules verapamil, D-600 and Nifedipine are defined
as calcium channel antagonists and their actions serve as one
important component of the definition of calcium channels. It
must be emphasized, however, that neither the sites nor the mechanisms of action of these antagonists have been precisely defined.

It is plausible that the calcium channel organization is
basically similar to that suggested for the sodium channel by
Hille (1975). An important component of Hille's model is the
channel cation coordination site which constitutes a rate limiting selectivity filter. The energetics of cation interaction at

TABLE II. PARTIAL LISTING OF SLOW CALCIUM-CHANNEL-DEPENDENT EVENTS

System	*Reference*
Neurones	
Squid axon	*Baker (1972); Baker and Glitsch (1975)*
Squid giant synapse	*Katz and Miledi (1969)*
Aplysia	*Stinnakre and Tauc (1973)*
Crayfish X-organ	*Kuroda (1976)*
Helix	*Eckert and Lux (1976); Standen (1957)*
Muscle (skeletal)	
Barnacle	*Hagiwara (1975)*
Amphioxus	*Hagiwara and Kidokoro (1971)*
Frog (slow muscle)	*Kaumann and Uchitel (1976)*
Muscle (cardiac)	*Bassingthwaighte and Reuter (1972); Reuter (1973); Kohlhardt et al. (1972); Horackova and Vassort (1976); Reuter and Scholz (1977)*
Muscle (smooth)	
Guinea-pig taenia coli	*Tomita (1970); Reimer et al. (1974)*
Guinea-pig vas deferens	*Bennett (1967)*
Guinea-pig portal vein	*Golenhofen and Hermstein (1975)*
Rat portal vein	*Bilek et al. (1974)*
Rat uterus	*Reiner and Marshall (1975)*
Rabbit aorta and mesenteric artery	*Schümann et al. (1975)*
Tunicate egg cell	*Okamoto et al. (1976)*
Secretory Systems	*Douglas (1968, 1974)*
Squid giant synapse	*Katz and Miledi (1969)*
Pituitary gland	*Eto et al. (1974)*
Pancreatic isleto	*Malaisse et al. (1976)*
Adrenal gland	*Pinto and Trifaro (1976); Brandt et al. (1976)*
Protozoa	
Paramecium (ciliary) motility)	*Naitoh et al. (1972)*
Chlamydamonas (ciliary motility)	*Schmidt and Eckert (1976)*

this site determine whether a cation is a permeant or nonpermeant species. In the case of the sodium channel Na^+ binds the least well and is the most permeant. The geometry and ligand characteristics of this proposed site will determine the selectivity between monovalent and divalent cations (Diamond and Wright, 1969; Williams,

1970) and, in the case of the calcium channel, divalent cations with ionic radii similar to that of Ca^{2+} (Table III) may be expected to interact with this site and, to serve as substitutes for or antagonists of calcium permeation. There is a paucity of quantitative data for ion interactions at the calcium channel but it is clear that for antagonism, $M^{3+} > M^{2+}$ (Figure 3; Hagiwara, 1973; Baker and Glitsch, 1975), that amongst divalent cations the order of permeation is $Ba^{2+} > Sr^{2+} > Ca^{2+} \gg Mg^{2+}$, that Ni^{2+} and Co^{2+} serve as antagonists and that Mn^{2+} acts as both an antagonist and permeant species (Ochi, 1976). This suggests that ionic radius and hydration energy may be important factors in determining cation interaction and permeation in the calcium channel.

Although these inorganic cations do antagonize calcium channel function it is also clear that they exert other important effects on excitable membranes. Thus, Blaustein and Goldman (1968) observed that Co^{2+} and Ni^{+} reduce sodium current in lobster axon, and Mn^{2+}, Co^{2+} and Ni^{2+}, which abolish the calcium current in squid axon also reduce sodium current significantly while leaving the potassium current unaffected (Baker *et al.*, 1973). Similarly in cardiac tissue these cations are not without effect on the fast sodium current (Kohlhardt *et al.*, 1973; Katzung *et al.*, 1973) and Tsien (1974; Kass and Tsien, 1975) has also noted that concentrations of Mn^{2+} and La^{3+} which block the calcium current shift the voltage dependent activation of the Na current, the pacemaker potassium current and the slow outward current in the positive direction. Additionally, both Ba^{2+} and Ca^{2+} are known to modulate potassium conductance (Werman and Grundfest, 1961; Meech, 1972; Meech and Standen, 1975).

TABLE III. PHYSICAL PROPERTIES OF DIVALENT CATIONS

Cation	Ionic radius	Hydration energy	Coordination no.
	Å	$k J \, mol^{-1}$	
Ca^{2+}	0.99	- 1577	6,8
Sr^{2+}	1.13	- 1433	6,8
Ba^{2+}	1.35	- 1305	6,8
Mn^{2+}	0.80	- 1841	4,5,6
Cd^{2+}	0.97	- 1807	4,5,6
Co^{2+}	0.74	- 1996	4,5,6
Ni^{2+}	0.69	- 2105	4,5,6
Tm^{3+}	0.85	- 3600	7,8,9

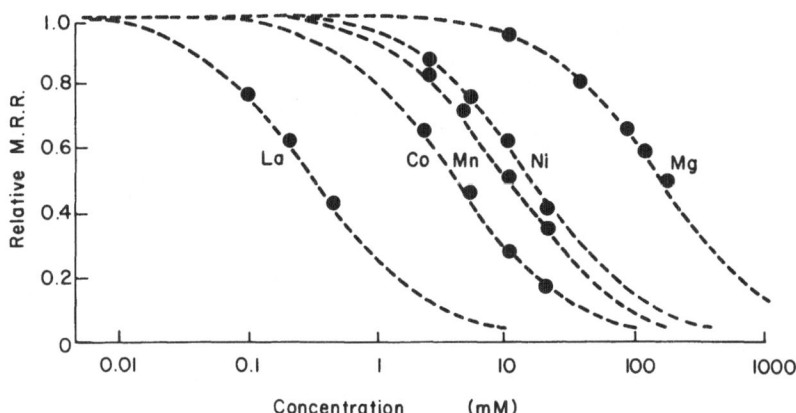

Fig. 3. Blocking effect of di- and trivalent cations on Ca-dependent action potential in barnacle muscle (the external solution contained 41 mM Ca²⁺). (Reproduced with permission from Hagiwara, Progr. Biophys., 4, 71 [1973].)

Many of these effects of di- and trivalent cations are likely related to a general adsorption to negatively charged membrane sites. Thus, it has long been known that an increase in [Ca^{2+}_{ext}] produces a positive shift of the threshold potential for spike generation (Frankenhaeuser and Hodgkin, 1957; Triggle, 1972). Such stabilization may arise from Ca^{2+} binding to or screening of surface negative charge (McLaughlin *et al.*, 1971; D'Arrigo, 1973) thus increasing the electric field within the membrane and so modifying voltage sensitive membrane events (Brown, 1975). These effects of Ca^{2+} are shared by other divalent and trivalent cations including Sr^{2+}, Ba^{2+}, Ni^{2+}, Co^{2+}, Mn^{2+}, La^{3+}, etc. in the sequence $M^{3+} > M^{2+}$ and it is clear that there exists a very general role for multivalent cation interaction at anionic sites in the regulation of membrane excitation. Finally, it is worth noting that the lanthanide series of cations are calcium channel antagonists probably by virtue of their rather general ability to substitute for Ca^{2+} at Ca^{2+} binding sites (Nieboer, 1975; Mikkelsen, 1976).

The organic calcium antagonists verapamil, D-600 and, to a lesser extent, Nifedipine have achieved prominence in recent years being classified, largely on the basis of electrophysiological evidence in cardiac preparations, as specific calcium channel antagonists (Fleckenstein, 1971, 1972, 1974, 1976; Fleckenstein *et al.*, 1972). In the concentration range 10^{-6}-10^{-8}M these agents produce a selective antagonism of the slow calcium current with minimal effect on the fast sodium current (Figure 4) and thus produce electromechanical decoupling of the heart in the activity sequence Nifedipine > D-600 > verapamil (Fleckenstein, 1972, 1976; Kohlhardt *et al.*, 1972, 1973a,b; Tritthart *et al.*, 1973). The

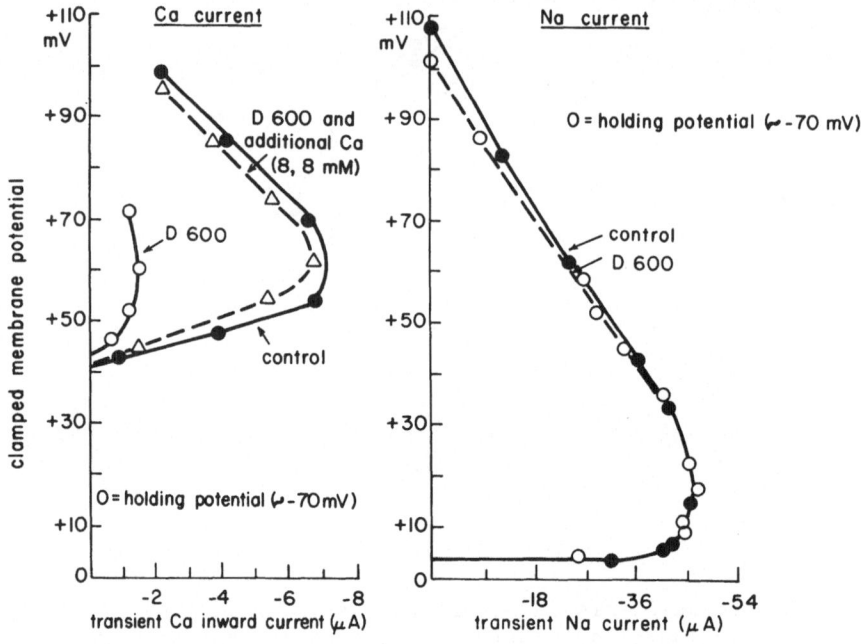

*Fig. 4. The influence of D-600 on the current-voltage relation-
ships of the transmembrane Ca and Na currents. D-600 (10^{-6}M) has
a negligible effect on the Na current but inhibits the Ca^{2+}
current, an effect which is overcome by increased [Ca^{2+}_{ext}].
(Reproduced with permission from Kohlhardt, Bauer, Krause and
Fleckenstein, Pflüg. Arch., 335, 309 [1972].)*

effects of these agents are overcome by increased [Ca^{2+}_{ext}] as
well as by Sr^{2+} and Ba^{2+} which are also permeant species and D-600
has been shown to be equally effective in suppressing the slow
current carried by either Ca^{2+} or Sr^{2+} (Kohlhardt *et al.*, 1973b).

    Because of the high activity and apparent selectivity of
action of these agents their activity in other calcium-utilizing
systems can be viewed as evidence that basically similar slow
calcium channels are operative in a variety of secretory and
mechanical processes (Tables IV-VI). It must be noted that for
many of these processes a complete characterization of the calcium
current is not available. However, the similar activities of
these antagonists in a variety of cardiac and smooth muscle and
secretory systems are certainly highly suggestive of a common
basis of action. In a few preparations widely different activities have been noted according to the stimulus employed and this
is probably indicative of different modes of calcium translocation.
Thus, in rabbit mesenteric artery, verapamil is some 1000 times

TABLE IV.   EFFECTS OF VERAPAMIL AND D-600 ON CALCIUM EVENTS IN CARDIAC TISSUE

Preparation (References)	Effect	Agent	ID_{50}, M (Approx.)
G.P. papillary (Fleckenstein et al., 1972)	Contraction	VP	5×10^{-7}
G.P. atria (Gorlitz et al., 1975)	Contraction	D-600	$< 10^{-7}$
Cat papillary (Tritthart et al., 1973)	Ca^{2+} current	D-600	2×10^{-6}
Cat ventricular trabeculae (Kohlhardt et al., 1972, 1973)	Ca^{2+} current	VP	$< 10^{-6}$
Cat ventricular trabeculae (Kohlhardt et al., 1973)	Sr^{2+} current	D-600	$< 10^{-6}$

more active against K^+ than against norepinephrine-induced contractions, suggesting that norepinephrine and K^+ employ principally intracellular and extracellular calcium sources, respectively (Schümann *et al.*, 1975; Table V). In contrast K^+ and muscarinic receptor-induced contractions of guinea-pig ileal longitudinal smooth muscle appear, as judged by antagonist activities, to employ identical calcium translocation mechanisms (Table V).

Where kinetic evidence is available verapamil, D-600 and Nifedipine appear to act noncompetitively against agonists and competitively against Ca^{2+} (Table VII). An exceptional situation appears to be indicated in cardiac tissue where the effects of these agents can be overcome by increasing [Ca^+_{ext}] and by catecholamines (Fleckenstein, 1971, 1972, 1976) so that a competitive relationship appears to exist also between β-agonists and the calcium antagonists (Gorlitz *et al.*, 1975; Endoh *et al.*, 1975). A likely explanation for this behaviour is that the action of catecholamines at the cardiac β-receptor is to increase the number of available calcium channels, perhaps by a c-AMP-dependent mechanism (Reuter, 1974, 1977).

Nifedipine, which shows no apparent structural similarity to verapamil or D-600, appears to behave in a fundamentally similar fashion. Nifedipine is a light-sensitive agent but the photochemical decomposition is unrelated to its pharmacological activity since the photochemical (IV) and the oxidation product (V) are at least one thousand times less active than Nifedipine itself.

TABLE V.   EFFECTS OF VERAPAMIL AND D-600 ON EXCITATION-CONTRACTION COUPLING IN SMOOTH MUSCLE

Preparation (References)	Activity	Antagonist	ID_{50}, M
G.P. taenia coli (Reimer et al., 1974)	spontaneous	VP	$\sim 3 \times 10^{-7}$
G.P. aorta (Golenhofen and Hermstein, 1975)	NE	VP	3×10^{-4}
G.P. portal vein (Golenhofen et al., 1973)	spontaneous	VP	$\sim 5 \times 10^{-7}$
G.P. portal vein (Golenhofen and Hermstein, 1975)	NE	VP	$\sim 10^{-6}$
G.P. portal vein (Golenhofen et al., 1973)	K^+	VP	$\sim 10^{-6}$
Rabbit aorta (Schümann et al., 1975)	NE	VP	1.2×10^{-4}
Rabbit aorta (Schümann et al., 1975)	Ca^{2+}/K^+	VP	2.7×10^{-8}
Rabbit mesenteric (Schümann et al., 1975)	NE	VP	4.5×10^{-5}
Rabbit mesenteric (Schümann et al., 1975)	Ca^{2+}/K^+	VP	5.4×10^{-8}
Rabbit ear artery (Golenhofen and Weston, 1976)	NE	D-600	$> 10^{-4}$
Rat uterus (Reiner and Marshall, 1975)	spontaneous	D-600	$\sim 10^{-7}$
Rat uterus (Reiner and Marshall, 1975)	electrical	D-600	$\sim 10^{-7}$
Rat aorta (Peiper et al., 1971)	NE	VP	$> 10^{-4}$
Rat aorta (Peiper et al., 1971)	K^+	VP	$\sim 10^{-6}$
G.P. ileum (long) (Rosenberger, Ticku and Triggle)	ACh	D-600	2.7×10^{-8}
G.P. ileum (long) (Rosenberger, Ticku and Triggle)	K^+	D-600	3.0×10^{-8}

TABLE VI. EFFECTS OF VERAPAMIL AND D-600 ON STIMULUS-SECRETION COUPLING

Preparation	Activity	Antagonist	ID_{50}, M
Pancreatic islets (Malaisse et al., 1976)	Insulin release, glucose stimulation	D-600	~ 2 x 10^{-6}
Pancreatic islets (Somers et al., 1976)	Ba^{2+} stimulation - insulin release	VP	~ 5 x 10^{-6}
Neurohypophysis (Dreifuss et al., 1975)	Oxytocin release	D-600	~ 10^{-5}
Pituitary (Eto et al., (1974)	ACTH, GH, TSH release: K^+ stimulation releasing factor	VP VP	~ 10^{-5} ineffective
Adrenal (Pinto and Trifaro, 1976)	Catecholamine release: ACh stimulation K^+ stimulation Na^+ reduction	D-600 D-600 D-600	~ 5 x 10^{-5} ~ 5 x 10^{-5} ineffective

TABLE VII. K_I *VALUES OF ORGANIC CALCIUM ANTAGONISTS IN SMOOTH*
MUSCLE PREPARATIONS

E-C COUPLING SMOOTH MUSCLE

Preparation (References)	Stimulus	Agent	K_I, M
G.P. taenia coli (Reimer et al., 1974)	Ca^{2+}/K^+	VP	1.4×10^{-8}
Rabbit pulmonary artery (Haeusler, 1972)	Ca^{2+}/K^+	VP	2.5×10^{-8}
Rat portal vein (Chona and Triggle)	Ca^{2+}/NE	D-600	2.5×10^{-8}
G.P. ileum (long.) (Rosenberger and Triggle)	Ca^{2+}/ACh	D-600	1.8×10^{-8}
G.P. ileum (long.) (Rosenberger and Triggle)	Ca^{2+}/ACh	Nifedipine	4.8×10^{-9}

Structure-activity studies are incomplete but the limited data
available (Table VIII) indicates that nonpolar substitution at
the 4-position of the 1,4-dihydropyridine ring increases activity
and that ortho substitution in 4-phenyl substituted compounds enhances activity whilst para-substitution is distinctly detrimental.
Quite possibly the active conformation of these agents requires
non-coplanarity of the phenyl and 1,4-dihydropyridine rings.

Little is known of the machanism(s) or the site(s) of action
of the organic calcium channel antagonists. Although they stand
in competitive relationship to Ca^{2+} it is perhaps unlikely that
they compete directly with the Ca^{2+} for the divalent cation coordination of the slow calcium channel. An allosteric mode of
action is therefore to be postulated. Voltage clamp studies in
cardiac tissue indicate that D-600, in addition to reducing the
membrane conductance to Ca^{2+} also reduces the rate of activation
of the Ca^{2+} conductance and impairs the recovery of calcium
channel activity from the inactivated state (Kohlhardt *et al.*,
1974, 1975; Nawrath *et al.*, 1977). The sites of these actions
are not known. Intracellular D-600 is ineffective in inhibiting
Ca^{2+} current in barnacle muscle (Rojas and Luxoro, 1974), but it

TABLE VIII. *STRUCTURE-ACTIVITY RELATIONSHIPS OF 1,4-DIHYDROPYRIDINES[a]*

Ar =	Phasic	ID_{50}, M[b] Tonic
C_6H_5	1.2×10^{-7}	2.8×10^{-8}
$2\text{-}O_2NC_6H_4$	2.0×10^{-8}	5.1×10^{-9}
$4\text{-}O_2NC_6H_4$	5.8×10^{-6}	3.2×10^{-6}
$2\text{-}FC_6H_4$	1.0×10^{-8}	3.7×10^{-9}
$4\text{-}FC_6H_4$	9.0×10^{-6}	7.0×10^{-6}
H	5.0×10^{-5}	7.0×10^{-5}
C_2H_5	1.6×10^{-5}	1.0×10^{-5}
$(CH_2)_5Me$	2.0×10^{-6}	1.0×10^{-7}
	1.0×10^{-4}	1.0×10^{-5}
$D\text{-}600$, MeBr	$\sim 10^{-4}$	$\sim 10^{-5}$

[a]*Rosenberger, Ticku and Triggle*

[b]*Concentration required to reduce by 50% the responses of guinea-pig ileal longitudinal smooth muscle to a supramaximal muscarinic stimulation.*

is of interest that the quaternary methobromide salt of D-600 and
the pyridinium analog of Nifedipine are quite ineffective in the
guinea-pig ileal preparation (Table VIII). A common site of
action of the inorganic and organic calcium channel antagonists
is also rendered unlikely by the finding that in TTX-treated 5-6
day embryonic chick hearts the remaining slow current is blocked
by verapamil but not by Mn^{2+} (Shigenobu et al., 1974).

There is no question but that verapamil, D-600 and Nifedipine
act as potent antagonists of the slow inward calcium current.
There is also evidence that these agents may have important effects
on other ionic processes. Verapamil and D-600, at the fairly
high concentrations used in the squid axon (2 x $10^{-4}M$), do reduce
the fast Na current and in cardiac fibers these agents also appear
to have some effect on both the Na^+ and K^+ currents (Cranefield
et al., 1974; Kass and Tsien, 1975). However, some part of the
effects of these agents on K^+ currents is likely due to the dependence of the latter upon Ca^{2+} entry (Bassingthwaighte et al., 1976).

Of particular interest to the questions of the sites and
mechanisms of action of D-600 are the observations that in cat
papillary muscles these agents produce frequency-dependent inhibition of contractions, being more effective at higher stimulation
frequences (Bayer et al., 1975a,b). Furthermore, the normal positive staircase seen with frequency jumps is drastically modified
by these agents so that an initial negative staircase is produced,
an effect which is seen only with the (-) isomers of verapamil
and D-600 and which is not seen with reduced Ca^{2+} or with Mn^{2+}
and La^{3+}. Detailed analysis of these findings suggests that both
verapamil and D-600 modify not only the slow inward Ca^{2+} current
but also a second calcium process namely a time- and voltage-
sensitive process that controls the restitution kinetics of calcium
availability (Kaufmann et al., 1974). The (+)-enantiomers of
verapamil and D-600 are significantly less effective as negative
inotropic agents and, additionally, do not appear to have any
effect on the kinetics of calcium availability. It is thus unlikely that the enantiomers of verapamil and D-600 modify cardiac
excitation-contraction coupling at a common site. Further differentiation of the actions of these enantiomers is revealed by their
actions on cardiac action potentials (Bayer et al., 1975c). In
papillary muscles the (+)-isomers are more effective in depressing
maximum velocity of depolarization, conductance velocity and increasing threshold stimulus whereas the (-)-isomers are more
effective in depressing plateau height. Possibly, the (-)-
enantiomers of verapamil and D-600 have selectivity as Ca^{2+} channel
antagonists whereas the (+)-enantiomers have selectivity as Na^+
channel antagonists. Not only is this a most unusual differentiation of enantiomeric action, but the concept of an agent where the
(+)- and (-)-isomers show selectivity for sodium and calcium

channels respectively is of possible importance to the understanding of the structural basis of the sites controlling Na^+ and Ca^{2+} permeation.

Whether Nifedipine, which is generally assumed to be a Ca^{2+} channel antagonist acting similarly to verapamil and D-600 but of higher activity, shares these other actions of verapamil and D-600 is not fully established. However, Nifedipine does exert a greater depressant effect on guinea pig atria with increasing stimulus frequency suggesting that it too modifies the kinetics of the Ca^{2+} restitution processes (Baumann, 1976). That compounds of such differing structure as verapamil and Nifedipine exert similar effects on both the Ca^{2+} permeation and restitution processes is perhaps suggestive that both processes are controlled through interaction at a common site.

IONOPHORE-INDUCED CALCIUM ENTRY

In recent years, considerable attention has been paid to ionophores, agents that act as carriers (or channel forming species) for ions across cell membranes (Simon *et al*., 1975; McLaughlin and Eisenberg, 1975; Pressman, 1976). Of particular interest to calcium transport are two agents X-537A (VI) and A23187 (VII), which exhibit divalent cation selectivity, A23187 being considerably more selective in this regard (Pfeiffer *et al*., 1974; Pfeiffer and Lardy, 1976; Degani and Friedman, 1974) and transporting Ca^{2+} by an electroneutral cation exchange process. A fairly extensive literature documents the ability of A23187 in the presence of

extracellular Ca^{2+} to mimic Ca^{2+}-dependent effects. A representative selection of A23187-initiated events is shown in Table IX,
and these findings are quite simply accomodated by the hypothesis
that this agent permits Ca^{2+} influx which bypasses the physiological Ca^{2+} entry route to produce the observed responses (Fig. 1).
In some situations, however, this view may be an oversimplifica-
tion and A23187 can initiate events by transporting divalent
cations other than calcium (Swamy *et al.*, 1975).

In a number of instances A23187 produces effects that are
apparently independent of extracellular Ca^{2+} (Table IX), thus
suggesting that it can enter the cell and release Ca^{2+} from intracellular sources. In at least two systems the effects of A23187
have been shown to depend upon the presence of *both* extracellular
Ca^{2+} and Na^+. In pancreatic acinar cells depolarization and
amylase release by A23187 is gradelly dependent on $[\ Ca^{2+}_{ext}\ ]$;
however, depolarization is also dependent upon the presence of
$[\ Na^+_{ext}\ ]$ (Poulsen and Williams, 1977). Similarly, A23187-induced
contractions of guinea-pig ileal longitudinal muscle are gradelly
dependent upon both $[\ Ca^{2+}_{ext}\ ]$ (Triggle *et al.*, 1975; Swamy *et al.*,
1975) and $[\ Na^+_{ext}\ ]$. Poulsen and Williams (1977) suggest that an
initial A23187-induced Ca^{2+} entry may trigger a subsequent depolarizing Na^+ influx. Alternatively, Na^+ transport by A23187 itself
(as an A_2HM complex, Table X) might provide the basis for direct
depolarization. Regardless of the precise details, the depolarizing Na^+ entry may activate the voltage-sensitive Ca^{2+} channel,
thus permitting calcium entry and response (Fig. 5). Supporting
evidence for this proposed mechanism of action is provided by the
antagonistic action of D-600 against A23187 responses that has
been observed in a few systems (Table XI), and where D-600 appears
to be equally active against ionophore and K^+-induced responses.

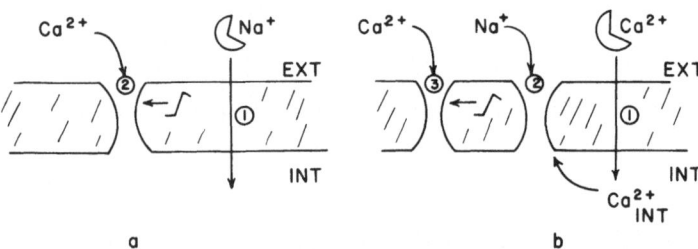

Fig. 5. *Possible mechanisms to explain the role of Na^+ in A23187-*
mediated responses. In a, Na^+ entry by the ionophore may cause
depolarization and subsequent activation of the Ca^{2+} channel. In
b, Ca^{2+} entry by the ionophore causes an increase in free intra-
cellular Ca^{2+}, which activates the Na^+ current and subsequently
the Ca^{2+} current.

TABLE IX.   A23187-INDUCED EVENTS

A. *Events Dependent upon Ca^{2+}_{ext}*

System	Reference
Stimulus-secretion coupling (adrenal medulla)	Cochrane et al., 1975
Smooth muscle contraction	Murray et al., 1975
Skeletal muscle contraction	Desmedt and Hainaut, 1976
Ca^{2+} release from sarcoplasmic reticulum	Scarpa et al., 1972
Lymphocyte activation	Greene et al., 1976
Increased K^+ permeability in erythrocytes	Reed, 1976
Platelet secretion and aggregation	Feinstein and Fraser, 1975
Inhibition of gluconeogenesis	Zahlten et al., 1973
Inhibition of cell agglutination	Hart et al., 1976
Neutrophil chemotaxis	Estendsen et al., 1976
Inhibition of microtubule assembly	Poste and Nicolson, 1976
H^+ - Ca^{2+} (Mg^{2+}) exchange in mitochondria	Reed and Lardy, 1972

B. *Events Independent of Ca^{2+}_{ext}*

System	Reference
Insulin release from pancreatic islets	Karl et al., 1975, Ashby and Spenk, 1975
Activation of unfertilized eggs (sea-urchin, bat-star, toad)	Chambers et al., 1974 Steinhardt et al., 1974
Platelet secretion and aggregation (partial)	Feinstein and Fraser, 1975
Protein synthesis inhibition (C_6 glioma cells)	Battenstein and Vellis, 1976
Frog egg contractility	Schroeder and Strickland, 1974
Skeletal muscle contraction (partial)	Desmedt and Hainaut, 1976
Smooth muscle contraction (partial)	Murray et al., 1975

TABLE X.   FORMATION CONSTANTS[a] FOR A23187-CATION COMPLEXES[b]

Divalent cation	K_f[c]	Monovalent cation	K_f[d]
Mg^{2+}	1.3×10^{-7}	Li^+	$4.9 \times 10^{-2}M^{-1}$
Ca^{2+}	3.7×10^{-7}	Na^+	$6.0 \times 10^{-4}M^{-1}$
Sr^{2+}	1.1×10^{-9}	K^+	$7.3 \times 10^{-5}M^{-1}$
Ba^{2+}	1.7×10^{-12}		

[a] *Determined by two phase (toluene/butanol - water) extraction technique.*

[b] *Pfeiffer and Lardy, 1976*

[c] *Refers to* $2\ AH_{org} + M^{2+}_{aq} \rightleftharpoons A_2M^{2+}_{org} + 2H^+_{aq}$,

$$K_f = [A_2M^{2+}]_{org}\ [H^+]^2_{aq}\ /\ [M^{2+}]_{aq}\ [AH]^2_{org}$$

[d] *Refers to* $2AH_{org} + M^+_{aq} \rightleftharpoons A_2HM_{org} + H^+_{aq}$

TABLE XI.   ANTAGONISM OF A23187   RESPONSES BY D-600

System[a]	Stimulant		D-600, M
Rat, bovine neurohypophysis	A23187		2.0×10^{-5} (marked inhib.)
- vasopressin release (Russel and Thorn, 1974; Thorn et al., 1975)	K^+/elec.		$< 10^{-5}$ ($\sim ID_{50}$)
G.P. ileal long. smooth muscle - contractions (Rosenberger and Triggle)	A23187	phasic	3.0×10^{-7} (ID_{50})
		tonic	1.2×10^{-8} (ID_{50})
	K^+	phasic	8.0×10^{-7} (ID_{50})
		tonic	3.0×10^{-8} (ID_{50})

[a] *Antagonism of A23187 contractions in G.P. taenia coli by D-600 has been reported by Mandrek and Golenhofen (1976).*

SUMMARY

There is strong evidence that calcium entry through an electro-physiologically and pharmacologically defined calcium channel is an important calcium entry route in many cells. A group of agents, including verapamil, D-600 and Nifedipine appear to act as quite selective inhibitors of ion translocation through this channel. However the mechanism(s) of action of these agents remain to be defined. Although these agents appear to be very useful as probes of calcium entry processes in cellular systems, their possible actions at other sites should not be ignored.

Acknowledgements

This work was supported in part by grants from the National Institutes of Health (HL 16003 and 50-G004).

REFERENCES

Adams, D. J., and Gage, P. W., 1976, Gating currents associated with sodium and calcium currents in an Aplysia neuron, *Science* 192: 783.

Armstrong, C. M., 1975, Ionic pores, gates and gating currents, *Quart. Rev. Biophys.* 7: 179.

Ashby, J. P., and Speake, R. N., 1975, Insulin and glucagon secretion from isolated islets of Langerhans, *Biochem. J.* 150: 89.

Baker, P. F., 1972, Transport and metabolism of calcium ions in nerve, *Progr. Biophys. Mol. Biol.* 24: 177.

Baker, P. F., and Glitsch, H. G., 1975, Voltage-dependent changes in the permeability of nerve membranes to calcium and other divalent cations, *Phil. Trans. R. Soc. London, Ser. B.* 270: 389.

Baker, P. F., and McNaughton, P. A., 1976, Kinetics and energetics of calcium efflux from intact squid giant axons, *J. Physiol. (London)* 259: 103.

Baker, P. F., Meves, H., and Ridgway, E. B., 1973, Effects of manganese and other agents on the calcium uptake that follows depolarization of squid axons, *J. Physiol. (London)* 231: 511.

Bassingthwaighte, J. B., Fry, C. H., and McGuigan, J. A. S., 1976, Relationship between internal calcium and outward current in mammalian ventricular muscle: a mechanism for the control of the action potential duration, *J. Physiol. (London)* 262: 15.

Bassingthwaighte, J. B., and Reuter, H., 1972, Calcium movements and excitation-contraction coupling in cardiac cells, *in* "Electrical Phenomena in the Heart", (W. C. De Mello, ed.), pp. 353-395, Academic Press, New York.

Baumann, K., 1976, On the action of Nifedipine under conditions of variable stimulation patterns and [Ca^{2+}]$_o$ in guinea-pig atrium,

Naunyn-Schmied. Arch. Pharmacol. 294: 161.

Bayer, R., Hennekes, R., Kaufmann, R., and Mannhold, R., 1975a, Inotropic and electrophysiological actions of verapamil and D-600 in mammalian myocardium. I. Pattern of inotropic effects of the racemic compounds, *Naunyn-Schmied. Arch. Pharmacol.* 290: 49.

Bayer, R., Kaufman, R., and Mannhold, R., 1975b, Inotropic and electrophysiological actions of verapamil and D-600 in mammalian myocardium. II. Pattern of inotropic effects of the optical isomers, *Naunyn-Schmied. Arch. Pharmacol.* 290:69.

Bayer, R., Kalusche, D., Kaufmann, R., and Mannhold, R., 1975c, Inotropic and electrophysiological actions of verapamil and D-600 in mammalian myocardium. III. Effects of the optical isomers on transmembrane action potentials, *Naunyn-Schmied. Arch. Pharmacol.* 290: 81.

Bennett, M. R., 1967, The effect of cations on the electrical properties of the smooth muscle cells of the guinea-pig vas deferens, *J. Physiol. (London)* 190: 465.

Bilek, I., Laven, R., Peiper, U., and Regnat, K., 1974, Effect of verapamil on the response to noradrenaline or to potassium depolarization in isolated vascular strips, *Microvasc. Res.* 7: 181.

Blaustein, M. P., 1974, The interrelationship between sodium and calcium fluxes across cell membranes, *Rev. Physiol. Biochem. Pharmacol.* 70: 33.

Blaustein, M. P., and Goldman, D. E., 1968, The action of certain polyvalent cations on the voltage clamped lobster axon, *J. gen. Physiol.* 51: 279.

Blaustein, M. P., and Russell, J. M., 1975, Sodium-calcium exchange and calcium-calcium exchange in internally dialysed squid axons, *J. Memb. Biol.* 22: 285.

Blinks, J. R., Prendergast, F. G., and Allen, D. G., 1976, Photo-proteins as biological indicators, *Pharmacol. Rev.* 28: 1.

Bottenstein, J. E., and Vellis, J. de., 1976, Divalent cation ionophore A23187. A potent protein synthesis inhibitor, *Biochem. Biophys. Res. Commun.* 73: 486.

Brandt, B. L., Hagiwara, S., Kidokoro, Y., and Miyazaki, S., 1976, Action potentials in the rat chromaffin cell and effects of acetylcholine, *J. Physiol. (London)* 263: 417.

Brown, R. H., 1975, Membrane surface charge: discrete and uniform modelling, *Progr. Biophys. Mol. Biol.* 28: 343.

Carafoli, E., Clementi, F., Drabikowski, W., and Margreth, A. (Editors), 1975, "Calcium Transport in Contraction and Secretion", North-Holland Publishing Company, Amsterdam.

Carafoli, E., and Crampton, M., 1976, Calcium ions and mitochondria, *in* "Calcium in Biological Systems" (C. J. Duncan, ed.), pp. 89-115, Symposium XXX of Society for Experimental Biology, Cambridge University Press, Cambridge.

Chambers, E. L., Pressmen, B. C., and Rose, B., 1974, The activation of sea-urchin eggs by the divalent cation ionophores A23187 and X-537A, *Biochem. Biophys. Res. Commun.* 60: 126.

Cochrane, D. E., and Douglas, W. W., 1974, Calcium-induced extrusion of secretory granules (exocytosis) in mast cells exposed to 48/80 or the ionophores A-23187 and X-537A, *Proc. Nat. Acad. Sci. U.S.A.* 71: 408.

Cochrane, D. E., Douglas, W. W., Mouri, T., and Nakazato, Y., 1975, Calcium and stimulus-secretion coupling in the adrenal medulla: contrasting stimulating effects of the ionophores X-537A and A23187 on catecholamine output, *J. Physiol. (London)* 252: 363.

Cranefield, P. F., Aronson, R. S., and Wit, A. L., 1974, Effect of verapamil on the normal action potential and on a calcium-dependent slow response of canine cardiac Purkinje fibres, *Circ. Res.* 34: 204.

D'Arrigo, J. S., 1973, Possible screening of surface charges on crayfish axons by polyvalent metal ions, *J. Physiol. (London)* 231: 117.

Desmedt, J. E., and Hainaut, K., 1976, The effect of A23187 ionophore on calcium movements and contraction processes in single barnacle muscle fibres, *J. Physiol. (London)* 257: 87.

Diamond, J. M., and Wright, E. M., 1969, Biological Membranes: the physical basis of ion and nonelectrolyte selectivity, *Annu. Rev. Physiol.* 31: 581.

Douglas, W. W., 1968, Stimulus-secretion coupling: the concept and clues from chromaffin cells, *Brit. J. Pharmacol.* 34: 451.

Douglas, W. W., 1974, Involvement of calcium in exocytosis and the exocytosis-vesiculation sequence, *Biochem. Soc. Symp.* 39: 1.

Dreifuss, J. J., Grau, J. D., and Nordmann, J. J., Calcium movements related to neurohypophysial hormone secretion, *in* "Calcium Transport in Contraction and Secretion" (E. Carafoli, F. Clementi, W. Drabikowski, eds.), pp. 271-279, North-Holland Publishing Company, Amsterdam.

Duncan, C. J. (Editor), 1976, "Calcium in Biological Systems", Symposium of The Society for Experimental Biology, XXX, Cambridge University Press, Cambridge.

Eckert, R., and Lux, H. D., 1976, A voltage-sensitive persistent calcium conductance in neuronal somata of Helix, *J. Physiol. (London)* 254: 129.

Endoh. M., Wagner, J., and Schümann, H. J., 1975, Influence of temperature on the positive inotropic effects mediated by α and β-adrenoreceptors in the isolated rabbit papillary muscle, *Naunyn-Schmied. Arch. Pharmacol.* 287: 61.

Estendsen, R. D., Reusch, M. E., Epstein, M. L. and Hill, H. R., 1976, Role of Ca^{2+} and Mg^{2+} in some human neutrophil functions as indicated by ionophore A23187, *Infection and Immunity* 13: 146.

Eto, S., Wood, J., Hutchins, M., and Fleischer, N., 1974, Pituitary $^{45}Ca^{++}$ uptake and release of ACTH, GH and TSH: effect of verapamil, *Amer. J. Physiol.* 226: 1315.

Fatt, P., and Katz, B., 1953, The electrical properties of crustacean muscle fibres, *J. Physiol. (London)* 120: 171.

Fatt, P., and Ginsborg, B. L., 1958, The ionic requirements for the production of action potentials in crustacean muscle fibres, *J. Physiol. (London)* 142: 516.

Feinstein, M. B., and Fraser, C., 1975, Human platelet secretion and aggregation induced by calcium ionophores, *J. gen. Physiol.* 66: 561.

Fleckenstein, A., 1971, Specific inhibitors and promoters of calcium action in the excitation-contraction coupling of heart muscle and their role in the prevention or production of myocardial lesions, *in* "Calcium and the Heart" (P. Harris and L. H. Opie, eds.), pp. 135-188, Academic Press, London and New York.

Fleckenstein, A., 1972, Physiologie und Pharmakologie der trans-membranären natrium-, kalium- und calcium-bewegunen, *Arz.-Forsch.* 22:2019.

Fleckenstein, A., 1974, Drug-induced changes in cardiac energy, *Adv. Cardiol.* 12: 183.

Fleckenstein, A., 1976, Adalat, A powerful Ca-antagonistic drug, *in* "New Therapy of Ischemic Heart Disease", (W. Lochner, ed.), pp. 56-65, Springer, Berlin.

Fleckenstein, A., Tritthart, H., Döring, H.-J., and Byon, K. Y., 1972, Bayer 1040-ein hochaktiver Ca^{++}-antagonisticher inhibitor der elektro-mechanischen koppelungsprozesse um warmblütermyokard, *Arz.-Forsch.* 22: 22.

Frankenhaeuser, B., and Hodgkin, A. L., 1957, The action of calcium on the electrical properties of squid axons, *J. Physiol. (London)* 137: 218.

Goldman, L., 1976, Kinetics of channel gating in excitable membranes, *Quart. Rev. Biophys.* 9: 491.

Golenhofen, K., Hermstein, N., and Lammel, E., 1973, Membrane potential and contraction of vascular smooth muscle (portal vein) during application of noradrenaline and high potassium and selective inhibitory effects of iproveratril (verapamil), *Microvasc. Res.* 5: 73.

Golenhofen, K., and Hermstein, N., 1975, Differentiation of calcium activation mechanisms in vascular smooth muscle by selective suppression with verapamil and D-600, *Blood Vessels* 12: 21.

Golenhofen, K., and Weston, A. H., 1976, Differentiation of calcium activation systems in vascular smooth muscle, *in* "Ionic Actions on Vascular Smooth Muscle", (E. Betz, ed.), pp. 21-25, Springer-Verlag, Berlin.

Gorlitz, B. D., Wagner, J., and Schümann, H., 1975, Functional antagonism between calcium-antagonists and noradrenaline in isolated guinea-pig atria, *Naunyn-Schmied. Arch. Pharmacol.* 238: 311.

Greene, W. C., Parker, C. M., and Parker, W. C., 1976, Calcium and lymphocyte activation, *Cell Immunol.* 25: 74.

Hagiwara, S., 1973, The calcium channel, *Adv. Biophysics* 4: 71.

Hagiwara, S., 1975, Ca-dependent action potential, *in* "Dynamic Properties of Lipid Membranes and Bilayers" (G. Eisenman, ed.), pp. 359-381, Dekker, New York.

Hagiwara, S., and Kidokoro, Y., 1971, Na and Ca components of action potential in Amphioxus muscle cells, *J. Physiol. (London)* 219: 217.

Heilbrunn, L. V., 1956, "The Dynamics of Living Protoplasm", Academic Press, New York.

Hille, B., 1970, Ionic channels in nerve membranes, *Progr. Biophys. Mol. Biol.* 21: 1.

Hart, C. A., Fisher, D., Hallinan, T., and Lucy, J. A., 1976, Effect of calcium ions and the bivalent cation ionophore A23187 on the agglutination and fusion of chicken erythrocytes by Sendai virus, *Biochem. J.* 158: 141.

Hodgkin, A. L., and Huxley, A. F., 1952, A quantitative description of membrane current and its application to conduction and excitation in nerve, *J. Physiol. (London)* 117: 500.

Horackova, M., and Vassort, G., 1976, Calcium conductance in relation to contractility in frog myocardium, *J. Physiol. (London)* 259: 597.

Hurwitz, L., Fitzpatrick, D. F., Debbas, G., and Landon, E. J., 1973, Localization of calcium pump activity in smooth muscle, *Science* 179: 384.

Karl, R. C., Zawalich, W. S., Ferrendelli, J. A., and Matschinsky, F. M., 1975, The role of Ca^{2+} and cyclic adenosine 3':5'-monophosphate in insulin release induced in vitro by the divalent cation ionophore A23187, *J. Biol. Chem.* 239: 4575.

Kass, R. S., and Tsien, R. W., 1975, Multiple effects of calcium antagonists on plateau currents in cardiac Purkinje fibers, *J. gen. Physiol.* 66: 169.

Katzung, B. G., Reuter, H., and Porzig, H., 1973, Lanthanum inhibits Ca inward current but not Na-Ca exchange in cardiac muscle, *Experientia* 29: 1073.

Katz, B., and Miledi, R., 1969, Tetrodotoxin - resistant electrical activity in presynaptic terminals, *J. Physiol. (London)* 203: 459.

Kaufmann, R., Bayer, R., Fürniss, T., Krause, H., and Tritthart, H., 1974, Calcium-movement controlling cardiac contractility II. Analog computation of cardiac excitation-contraction coupling on the basis of calcium kinetics in a multi-compartment model, *J. Mol. Cell. Cardiol.* 6: 543.

Kaumann, A. J., and Uchitel, O., 1976, Reversible inhibition of potassium contractions by optical isomers of verapamil and D-600 on slow muscle fibers of the frog, *Naunyn.-Schmied. Arch. Pharmacol.* 292: 21.

Kohlhardt, M., Bauer, B., Krause, H., and Fleckenstein, A., 1972, Differentiation of the transmembrane Na and Ca channels in mammalian cardiac fibres by the use of specific inhibitors, *Pflügers Arch.* 335: 309.

Kohlhardt, M., Bauer, B., Krause, H., and Fleckenstein, A., 1973a, Selective inhibition of the transmembrane Ca conductivity of mammalian myocardial fibres by Ni, Co and Mn ions, *Pflügers Arch.* 338: 115.

Kohlhardt, M., Herdey, A., and Kübler, M., 1973b, Interchangeabi-
    lity of Ca ions and Sr ions as charge carriers of the slow inward
    current in mammalian myocardial fibres, *Pflügers Arch.* 344: 149.
Kohlhardt, M., Krause, H., Kübler, M., and Herdey, A., 1975,
    Kinetics of inactivation and recovery of the slow inward current
    in the mammalian ventricular myocardium, *Pflügers Arch.* 355: 1.
Kohlhardt, M., Kübler, M., and Herdey, A., 1974, Characteristics
    of the recovery process of the Ca membrane channel in myocardial
    fibers, *Pflügers Arch.* 347: R2.
Kretsinger, R. H., 1976a, Calcium in biological systems, *Coord.
    Chem. Rev.* 18: 29.
Kretsinger, R. H., 1976b, Evolution and function of calcium-bind-
    ing proteins, *Int. Rev. Cytol.* 56: 323.
Kuroda, T., 1976, The effects of D-600 and verapamil on action
    potential in X-organ neuron of the crayfish, *Jpn. J. Physiol.*
    26: 189.
Lamb, J. F., and Lindsay, R., 1971, Effect of Na, metabolic inhi-
    bitors and ATP on Ca movements in L cells, *J. Physiol. (London)*
    218: 691.
Lehninger, A. L., 1974, Ca^{2+} transport by mitochondria and its
    possible role in the cardiac contraction-relaxation cycle, *Circ.
    Res. Suppl.* III, 83.
MacLennan, D. H., and Holland, P. C., 1975, Calcium transport in
    sarcoplasmic reticulum, *Annu. Rev. Biophys. Bioeng.* 4: 377.
Malaisse, W. J., Devis, G., Pipeleers, D. G., and Somers, G.,
    1976, Calcium antagonists and islet function. IV. Effect of
    D-600, *Diabetologia* 12: 77.
Mandrek, K., and Golenhofen, K., 1976, Activation of gastrointes-
    tinal smooth muscle induced by the calcium ionophore A23187, *in*
    "Smooth Muscle Pharmacology and Physiology" (M. Worcel and G.
    Vassort, eds.), pp. 343-352, Inserm, Paris.
McLaughlin, S., and Eisenberg, M., 1975, Antibiotics and membrane
    biology, *Annu. Rev. Biophys. Bioeng.* 4: 335.
McLaughlin, S. G. A., Szabo, G., and Eisenman, G., 1971, Divalent
    ions and the surface potential of charged phospholipid membranes,
    J. gen. Physiol. 58: 667.
Meech, R. W., 1972, Intracellular calcium injection causes in-
    creased potassium conductance in Aplysia nerve cells, *Comp.
    Biochem. Physiol.* 42A: 493.
Meech, R. W., and Standen, N. B., 1975, Potassium activation in
    Helix aspersa neurones under voltage clamp: a component mediated
    by calcium influx, *J. Physiol. (London)* 249: 211.
Mikkelsen, R. B., 1976, Lanthanides as calcium probes in biomem-
    branes, *in* "Biological Membranes", Vol. 3 (D. Chapman and D. F.
    H. Wallach, eds.), pp. 153-190, Academic Press, New York.
Murray, J. W., Reed, P. W., and Fay, F. S., 1975, Contraction of
    isolated smooth muscle cells by ionophore A23187, *Proc. Nat.
    Acad. Sci. U.S.A.* 72: 4459.

Naitoh, Y., Eckert, R., and Friedman, K., 1972, A regenerative calcium response in Paramecium, *J. Exp. Biol.* 56: 667.

Nakamura, Y., and Schwartz, A., 1971, Adenosine triphosphate-dependent calcium-binding vesicles: magnesium, calcium, adenosine triphosphatase and sodium-potassium adenosine triphosphatase distributions in dog brain, *Arch. Biochem. Biophys.* 144: 16.

Nawrath, H., Ten Eick, R. E., McDonald, T. F., and Trautwein, W., 1977, On the mechanism underlying the action of D-600 on slow inward current and tension in mammalian myocardium, *Circ. Res.* 40: 408.

Nieboer, E., 1975, The lanthanide ions as structural probes in biological and model systems, *Structure and Bonding* 22: 1.

Ochi, R., 1976, Manganese-dependent propagated action potentials and their depression by electrical stimulation in guinea-pig myocardium perfused by sodium-free media, *J. Physiol. (London)* 263: 139.

Okamota, A., Takahashi, K., and Yoshii, M., Two components of the calcium current in the egg cell membrane of the tunicate, *J. Physiol. (London)* 225: 527.

Peiper, U., Griebel, L., and Wende, W., 1971, Activation of vascular smooth muscle of rat aorta by noradrenaline and depolarization: two different mechanisms, *Pflügers Arch.* 330: 74.

Pfeiffer, D. R., and Lardy, H. A., 1976, Ionophore A23187: the effect of H^+ concentration on complex formation with divalent and monovalent cations and the demonstration of K^+ transport in mitochondria mediated by A23187, *Biochemistry* 15: 935.

Pfeiffer, D. R., Reed, P. W., and Lardy, H. A., 1974, Ultraviolet and fluorescent spectral properties of the divalent cation ionophore A23187 and its metal ion complexes, *Biochemistry* 13: 4007.

Pinto, J. E. B., and Trifaro, J. M., 1976, The different effects of D-600 (methoxy verapamil) on the release of catecholamines induced by acetylcholine, high potassium or sodium deprivation, *Brit. J. Pharmacol.* 57: 127.

Poste, G., and Nicolson, G. L., 1976, Calcium ionophores A23187 and X-537A affect cell agglutination by lectins and capping of lymphocyte surface immunoglobulins, *Biochim. Biophys. Acta.* 426: 148.

Poulsen, J. H., and Williams, J. A., 1977, Effects of the calcium ionophore A23187 on pancreatic acinar cell membrane potential and amylase release, *J. Physiol. (London)* 264: 323.

Pressman, B. C., 1976, Biological applications of ionophores, *Annu. Rev. Biochem.* 45: 501.

Reed, P. W., 1976, Effects of the divalent cation ionophore A23187 on potassium permeability of rat erythrocytes, *J. Biol. Chem.* 251: 3489.

Reed, P. W., and Lardy, H. A., 1972, A23187: a divalent cation ionophore, *J. Biol. Chem.* 247: 6970.

Reimer, J., Dörfler, F., Mayer, C.-J., and Ulbrecht, G., 1974, Calcium-antagonistic effects on the spontaneous activity of guinea-pig taenia coli, *Pflügers Arch.* 351: 241.

Reiner, O., and Marshall, J. M., 1975, Action of D-600 on spontaneous and electrically stimulated activity of the parturient rat uterus, *Naunyn-Schmied. Arch. Pharmacol.* 290: 21.

Reuter, H., 1973, Divalent cations as charge carriers in excitable membranes, *Progr. Biophys. Mol. Biol.* 26: 1.

Reuter, H., 1974, Localization of beta-adrenergic receptors and effects of noradrenaline and cyclic nucleotides on action potentials, ionic currents and tension in mammalian cardiac muscle, *J. Physiol. (London)* 264: 17.

Reuter, H., 1977, The regulation of the calcium conductance of cardiac muscle by adrenaline, *J. Physiol. (London)* 264: 49.

Reuter, H., and Scholz, H., 1977, A study of the ion selectivity and the kinetic properties of the calcium dependent slow inward current in mammalian cardiac muscle, *J. Physiol. (London)* 264: 17.

Ringer, S., 1883, A further contribution regarding the influence of the different constituents of the blood on the contraction of the heart, *J. Physiol. (London)* 4: 29.

Ritchie, J. M., Rogart, R. B., and Strichartz, G. R., 1976, A new method for labelling saxitoxin and its binding to non-myelinated fibres of the rabbit vagus, lobster walking leg, and garfish olfactory nerves, *J. Physiol. (London)* 261: 477.

Rojas, E., and Luxoro, M., 1974, Coupling between ionic conductance changes and contractions in barnacle muscle fibres under membrane potential control, *in* "Actualities Neurophysiologiques", (A. M. Monnier, ed.), pp. 159-169, Masson, Paris.

Russell, J. T., and Thorn, N. A., 1974, Calcium and stimulus-secretion coupling in the neurohypophysis, *Acta Endocrin.* 76: 471.

Scarpa, A., Baldassare, J., and Inesi, G., 1972, The effect of calcium ionophores on fragmented sarcoplasmic reticulum, *J. gen. Physiol.* 60: 735.

Schatzmann, H. J., 1975, Active calcium transport and Ca^{2+}-activated ATPase in human red cells, *Current Topics in Membranes and Transport* 6: 125.

Schmidt, J. A., and Eckert, R., 1976, Calcium couples flagellar reversal to photostimulation in Chlamydomonas reinhardti, *Nature* 262: 713.

Schroeder, T. E., and Strickland, D. L., 1974, Ionophore A23187, calcium and contractility in frog eggs, *Exp. Cell. Res.* 83: 139.

Schumann, H. J., Görlitz, B. D., and Wagner, J., 1975, Influence of papaverine, D-600 and Nifedipine on the effects of noradrenaline and calcium on the isolated aorta and mesenteric artery of the rabbit, *Naunyn-Schmied. Arch. Pharmacol.* 289: 409.

Shigenobu, K., Schneider, J. A., and Sperelakis, N., 1974, Verapamil blockade of slow Na^+ and Ca^{++} responses in myocardiac cells, *J. Pharmacol. Exp. Ther.* 190: 280.

Simon, W., Morf, W. E., and Meier, P. Ch., 1975, Specificity for alkali and alkaline earth cations of synthetic and natural organic complexing agents in membranes, *Structure and Bonding* 16: 113.

Somers, G., Devis, G., Van Obberghen, E., and Malaisse, W. J., 1976, Calcium antagonists and islet function. VI. Effect of barium, *Pflügers Arch.* 365: 21.

Standen, N. B., 1975, Calcium and sodium ions as charge carriers in the action potential of an identified snail neurone, *J. Physiol. (London)* 249: 241.

Steinhardt, R. A., Epel, D., and Carrol, E. J., 1974, Is calcium ionophore a universal activator for unfertilized eggs, *Nature* 252: 41.

Stinnakre, J., and Tauc, L., 1973, Calcium influx in active Aplysia neurones detected by injected aequorin, *Nature* 242: 113.

Swamy, V. C., Ticku, M. K., Triggle, C. R., and Triggle, D. J., 1975, The action of the ionophores, X-537A and A23187, on smooth muscle, *Can. J. Physiol. Pharmacol.* 53: 1108.

Thorn, N. A., Russell, J. T., and Robinson, I. C. A. F., 1975, Factors affecting intracellular concentration of free calcium ions in neurosecretory nerve endings, *in* "Calcium Transport in Contraction and Secretion", (E. Carafoli, F. Clementi, W. Drabikowski, and A. Margreth, eds.), pp. 261-269, North-Holland Publishing Company, Amsterdam.

Tomita, T., 1970, Electrical properties of mammalian smooth muscle, *in* "Smooth Muscle", (E. Bülbring, A. F. Brading, A. W. Jones, and T. Tomita, eds.), Williams and Wilkins, Baltimore, Md.

Triggle, D. J., 1972, Effect of calcium on excitable membranes and neurotransmitter action, *Progr. Surface and Memb. Sci.* 5: 267.

Triggle, D. J., and Triggle, C. R., 1976, "Chemical Pharmacology of the Synapse", Chapter IV, Academic Press, London and New York.

Triggle, C. R., Grant, W. F., and Triggle, D. J., 1975, Intestinal smooth muscle contraction and the effects of cadmium and A23187, *J. Pharmacol. Exp. Ther.* 194: 182.

Tritthart, H., Volkmann, R., Weiss, R., and Fleckenstein, A., 1973, Calcium-mediated action potentials in mammalian myocardium, *Naunyn-Schmied. Arch. Pharmacol.* 280: 239.

Tsien, R. W., 1974, Mode of action of chronotropic agents in cardiac Purkinje fibers, *J. gen. Physiol.* 64: 320.

Werman, R., and Grundfest, H., 1961, Graded and all-or-none electrogenesis in arthropod muscle II. The effects of alkali-earth and onium ions on lobster muscle fibers, *J. gen. Physiol.* 44: 997.

Williams, R. J. P., 1970, The biochemistry of sodium, potassium, magnesium and calcium, *Quart. Revs. Chem. Soc.* 24: 331.

Zahlten, R. N., Stratman, F. W., and Lardy, H. A. 1973, Regulation of glucose synthesis in hormone-sensitive isolated rat hepatocytes, *Proc. Nat. Acad. Sci. U.S.A.* 70: 3213.

CHAPTER 2

SURFACE CALCIUM IN THE HEART: ITS FUNCTION AND ROLE IN DRUG ACTION

Joy S. Frank

Department of Physiology and Cardiovascular Research
Laboratory, UCLA Center for the Health Sciences
Los Angeles, California 90024

INTRODUCTION

It is well documented that activation of the myofilaments in striated muscle is controlled by an increase in calcium (Ca^{2+}) delivery to troponin sites on the myofilaments (Solaro *et al.*, 1974; Ebashi, 1963). Calcium ions enter the cytoplasm from surface membrane sites and intracellular storage sites in response to membrane depolarization. In skeletal muscle the Ca^{2+} involved in the E-C coupling process is released and sequestered entirely intracellularly (Armstrong *et al.*, 1972; Winegrad, 1970). Cellular Ca^{2+} exchanges in skeletal muscle at a slow rate and reacts slowly to alterations of the external Ca^{2+} concentration (Rich and Langer, 1975; Lüllmann *et al.*, 1974). When a skeletal muscle is perfused with a Ca^{2+}-free medium the decline of tension has a $T_{\frac{1}{2}}$ of 23 min (Fig. 1). The large lateral sacs of the sarcoplasmic reticulum serve in skeletal muscle as storage and release sites for activator Ca^{2+} (Endo and Nakajima, 1973; Winegrad, 1968).

Cardiac muscle on the other hand has some distinctive morphological and functional features that are quite different from skeletal muscle and point to a different mechanism involved in E-C coupling (Shine *et al.*, 1971; Fawcett and McNutt, 1969). The sarcoplasmic reticulum of heart muscle is a simple tubular system with very small cisternae situated just under the surface membrane and adjacent to the transverse tubular membrane. There are no large lateral sacs as in skeletal muscle. If the heart is perfused with a Ca^{2+}-free medium force development falls immediately with a $T_{\frac{1}{2}}$ of a min or less (Fig. 1) (Rich and Langer, 1975). This striking illustration of the myocardium's dependence on a source of interstitial Ca^{2+} is in marked contrast to skeletal muscle.

33

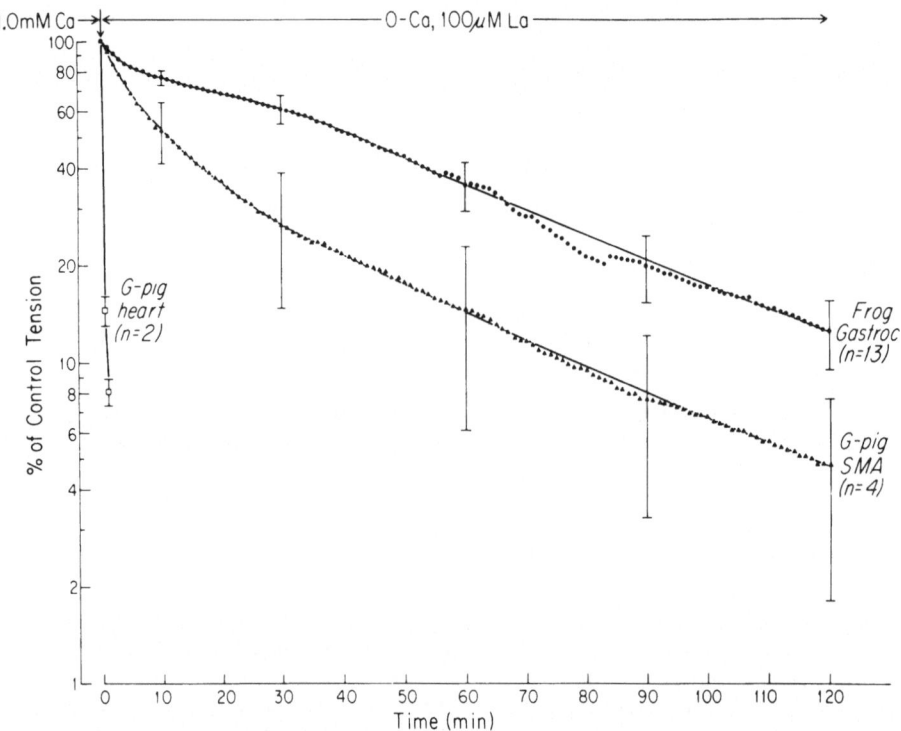

Figure 1. Rate of tension decline of intra-arterially perfused guinea pig interventricular septa and semimembranosus accessorius (SMA) muscles and frog gastrocnemius (FG) muscles during calcium-free perfusion. 100 μM La^{3+} added to zero Ca^{2+} solutions to maintain resting membrane potential and excitability. Each point is the mean of n observations, normalized as % of control, with one standard error of the mean (S.E.M.) shown in brackets. Reproduced with permission from T. Rich and G. A. Langer (1975).

However, the source of contractile dependent Ca^{2+} in the heart is still a matter of debate (Langer *et al.*, 1976a; Fabiato and Fabiato, 1977). The controversy centers about whether all the Ca^{2+} required for full activation, approximately 90 μmoles Ca^{2+}/kg wet wt, comes from superficial sites on the cell or whether intracellular deposits play a role in Ca^{2+} release. Many studies have consistently indicated that in the myocardium, contractile dependent Ca^{2+} originates from sites on and around the sarcolemma (Shine *et al.*, 1971; Langer and Frank, 1972). The specific location and nature of these Ca^{2+} binding sites are unknown although recent studies have pointed to the negatively charged glycoproteins at the surface of the sarcolemma as important in E-C coupling

(Langer *et al.*, 1976b). The external portion of the sarcolemma, a region of the cell whose function has been overlooked, is now the focus of studies attempting to locate the Ca^{2+} involved in E-C coupling in the heart.

Many of these studies on the cell surface have been done on myoblasts grown in culture. Since cultured cells are grown as a monolayer there is direct access to the surface without inter-position of capillary membrane and interstitium. The first portion of this chapter will consider the ultrastructure of the sarcolemma in both adult and cultured cells and integrate the structural findings with what is known about the function of the cell surface. The final portion of the chapter will explore the possibility that cardioactive drugs alter contractile performance through their ability to effect the accumulation and exchange of Ca^{2+} by the cell membrane.

ULTRASTRUCTURE OF THE MYOCARDIAL SARCOLEMMA

The cell membranes of a wide variety of mammalian cells appear to be more complex than previously realized and our morphological definition of the membrane as only the trilaminar (7.5-9 nm) "unit" membrane is too limited and should be expanded to include the carbohydrate layers which form the outermost boundary of the cell. The term sarcolemma as used here includes 1) the lipid bilayer or "unit" membrane 2) the glycoprotein cell coat located on the imme-diate outer surface of the lipid bilayer and an integral part of the membrane 3) the external lamina or carbohydrate coating just superficial to the cell coat. While it has been known that all cell membranes have carbohydrate layers which are negatively charged, this important component of the membrane has not been well studied in cardiac cells. Research on cell membrane pro-gresses most rapidly when a high yield of pure plasma membranes is available for study. Unfortunately, the complexity of the cardiac sarcolemma has prevented easy isolation.

When routine electron microscopy techniques are used on intact cells the sarcolemmal surface is seen as a uniformly thick ($\sim$ 50 nm) mat or feltwork of fine filaments. In most preparations of adult tissue the surface appears layered with a less dense inner zone ($\sim$ 20 nm) referred to as the surface coat, and a slightly denser outer zone of approximately 30 nm referred to here as the external lamina (Fig. 2). Whether this layering is representative of a true structural and chemical difference is not known. Parsons and Subjeck (1972), in a study of cell coats, point out that the glycoprotein chains of the surface coat probably extend out from the lipoprotein layer about 20-30 nm but that, under conditions of tissue preservation, the filaments may collapse and form the

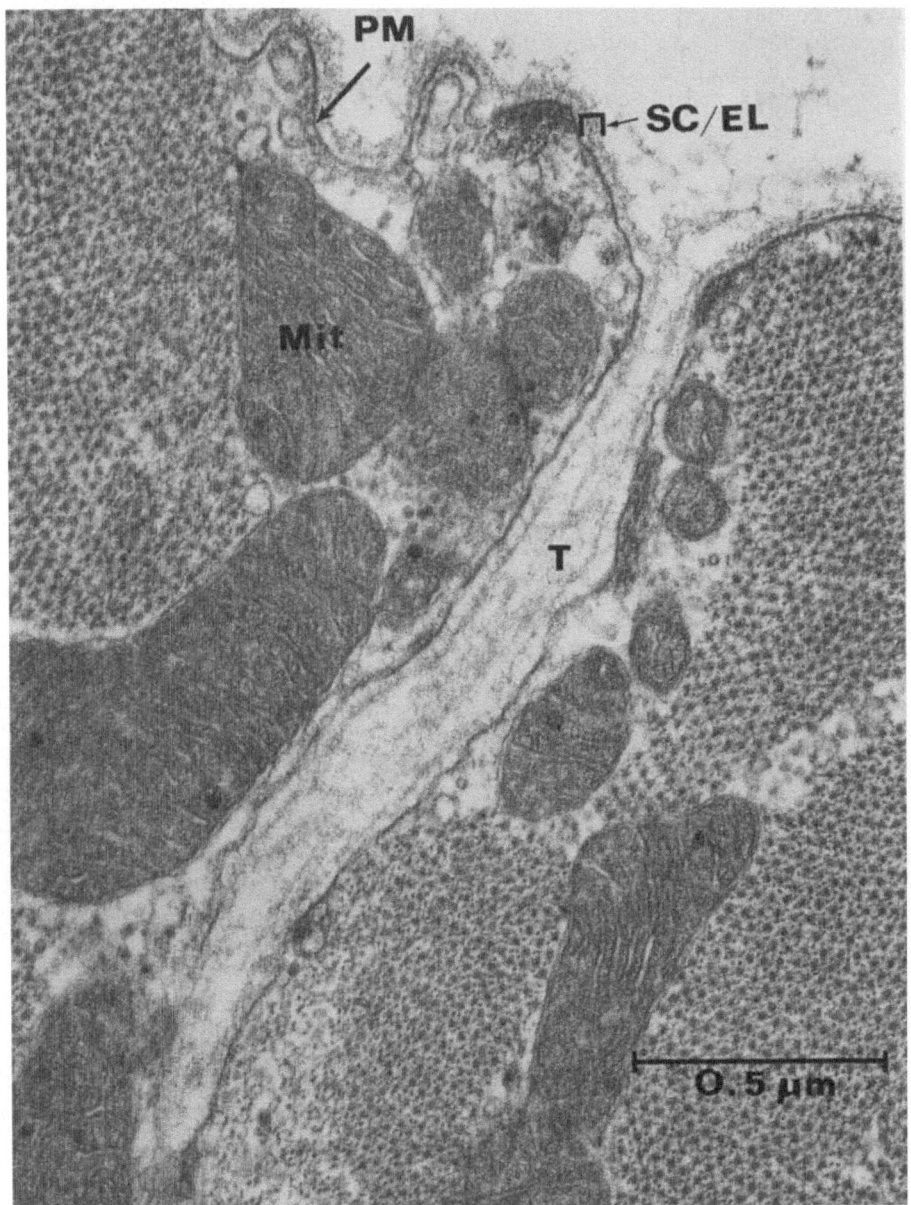

Figure 2. Electron micrograph of cross-section of rabbit myo-cardial cell, showing the plasmalemmal unit membrane (PM) and the associated surface coat (SC) and external lamina (EL). The cell membrane invaginates to form transverse tubule (T). Mit, mitochondria.

mat-like network seen in the electron microscope. The cell surface
of rat myoblasts grown in culture is more amorphous without the
varying densities visible in routine staining in the adult heart.
The dimensions of the surface layer (including the surface coat
and external lamina) ranges between 50-80 nm but, because of the
shape of the cells, oblique cuts through the membrane are extremely
common and make accurate measurements difficult.

     To get further definition of the morphology of the cellular
surface special stains are needed. Since the cell surface carbohydrates (glycoproteins and glycolipids) are rich in acidic residues,
the cell surface is negatively charged (Winzler, 1970). The stains
used to render the surface of the cell more visible are basically
polycationic colloids (like ruthenium red, alcian blue, colloidal
iron, lanthanum and cationic ferritin) which bind to the negatively
charged surface rendering it more dense and thus more visible in
the electron microscope. All of these stains have been used in
identifying the cell coat, outlining its distribution and in some
cases indicating its chemistry. For example, ruthenium red and
alcian blue react with polysaccharides while colloidal iron appears
to be specific for sialic acid residues (Martinez-Palomo, 1970).
All of the polycationic stains have been used in both adult heart
and myoblast cells and, as expected, the sarcolemma and its invaginations (transverse tubular membrane) react strongly indicating
the presence of negatively charged moieties (Howse *et al.*, 1970;
Gros and Challice, 1975; Frank *et al.*, 1977). Lanthanum and
ruthenium red react with the "unit" trilaminar membrane as well as
the surface coat and external lamina (Fig. 3). The particles of
cationic ferritin are confined to areas (surface coat/external
lamina) superficial to the bilayer. Whether this distribution is
indicative of a true affinity difference is unknown. There is a
probable explanation in the particle size of these colloids.
Cationic ferritin has a very uniform particle size of approximately
3 nm while both ruthenium red and lanthanum tend to form aggregates
of varying size.

     Colloidal iron stain has been used in sheep and crayfish
hearts as well as in adult rabbit hearts and rat tissue culture
cells (Howse *et al.*, 1970; Frank *et al.*, 1977). In all cases,
colloidal iron stains the cell surface but with a unique two layered pattern. Colloidal iron particles are found uniformly on the
surface coat, and a second layer of stain is found on the outermost
region of the external lamina, leaving an area of approximately 30
nm between the layer free of stain. This unique staining pattern
indicates that sialic acid molecules with their negatively charged
carboxy groups are present next to the lipid bilayer and on the
external lamina at the interstitial interface (Fig. 4).

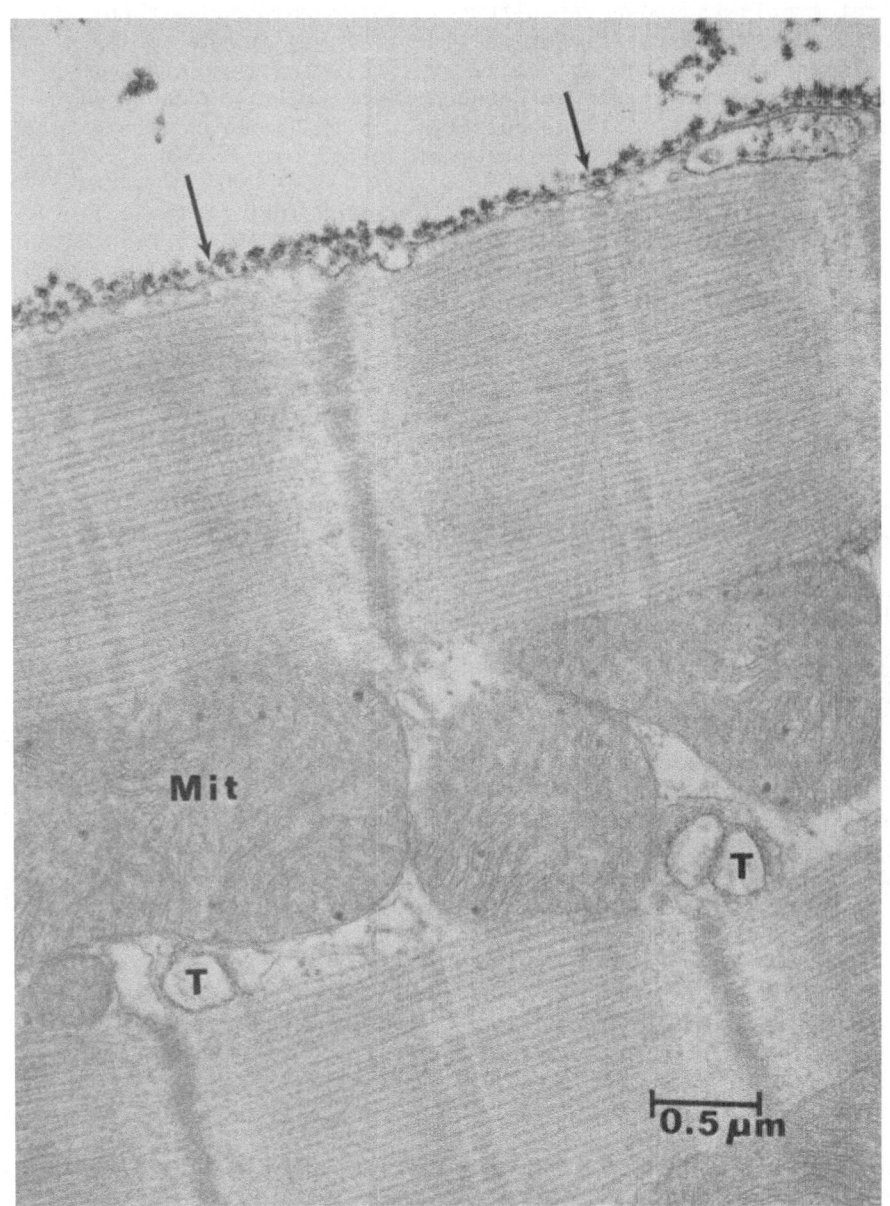

Figure 3.   Myocardial cells from rabbit perfused with 0.5 mM LaCl₃. Note intense La staining on the entire membrane complex (arrows) and as well on the transverse tubular membrane.   T, transverse tubule; Mit, mitochondria.

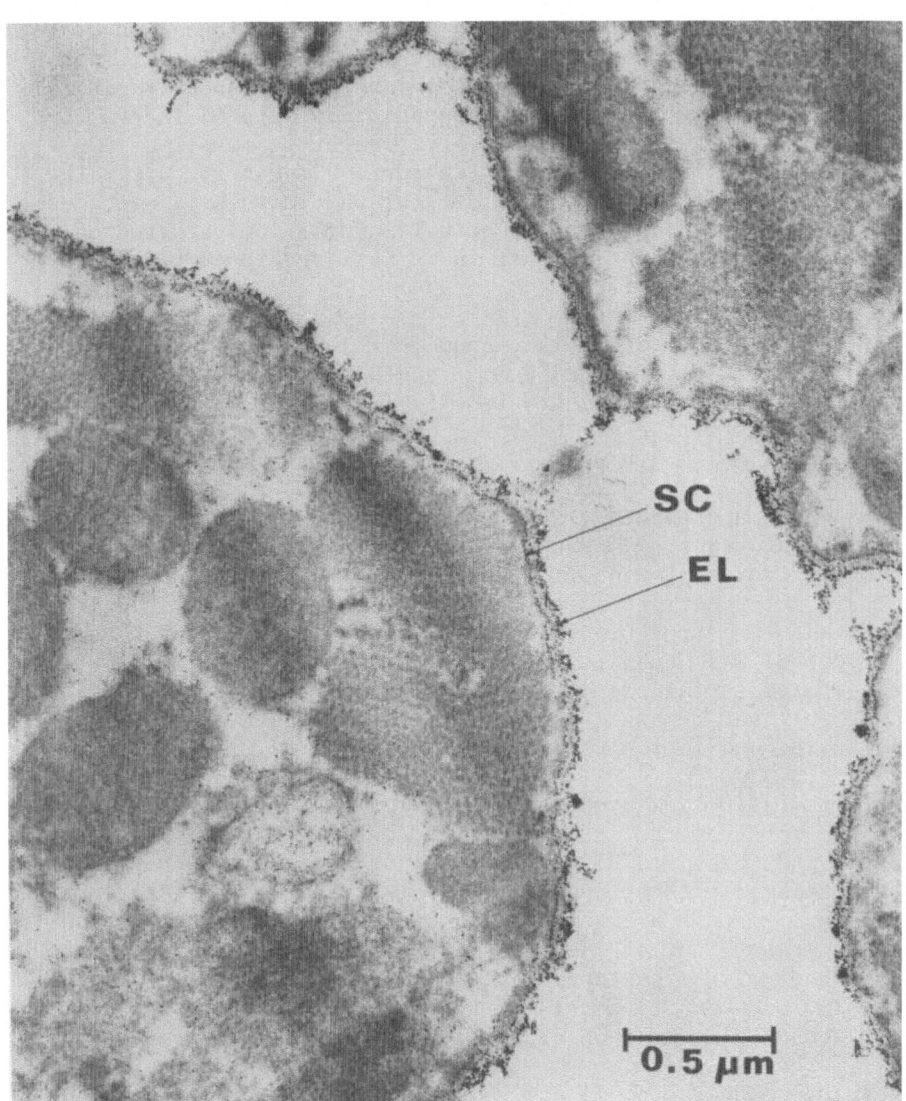

Figure 4. Electron micrograph of two rabbit myocardial cells stained with colloidal iron hydroxide (CIH). Note double layered pattern of the stain. CIH stains the outermost region of the external lamina (EL) and stains the surface coat (SC) just super-ficial to lipid bilayer leaving an area of approximately 30 nm free of stain.

HISTOCHEMICAL STUDIES: LANTHANUM

The histochemistry of the myocardial cell surface has identified the presence of sialic acid and other acidic carbohydrates.
But just how this important part of the cell membrane functions
in regulating ionic binding is a complex issue. As early as 1963
Bennett first suggested that the surface coatings of the sarcolemma or "glycocalyx" as he called it, might be involved in
selective ion permeability and transport. It was not until the
early 1970's that the histochemistry of the sarcolemma was coupled
to functional studies and some actual information gathered on
Bennett's early suggestion. It is in this regard that lanthanum
has been a unique tool.

The trivalent cation lanthanum (La^{3+}) is one of a series of
cations (others - Ca^{2+}, Zn^{2+}, Mn^{2+} and Mg^{2+}) which will uncouple
excitation from contraction. La^{3+} is one of the most potent in
the series, as little as 40 μmoles will reduce force development
to zero within 2-3 min while leaving the action potential intact.

Sanborn and Langer (1970), in studies on the perfused rabbit
septum, found that La^{3+} displaced ^{45}Ca from its binding sites
and uncoupled excitation from contraction. They indicated that
La^{3+} did not penetrate across the cell membrane. La^{3+} had been
localized ultrastructurally in the perfused rabbit septum and,
as expected, was bound to the sarcolemmal membrane complex. In
the perfused septal preparation La^{3+} was never found in the interior
of the cell but remained confined to the surfaces of myocardial,
endothelial and fibroblastic cells (Frank *et al.*, 1977).

With the use of myocardial cells grown in culture it is
possible to study the effects of La^{3+} on cellular Ca^{2+} exchange
(Langer and Frank, 1972). The technique depends on the growth
of a monolayer of beating cells on the surface of polystyrene
discs that contain a scintillation material. This permits continuous measurement of ^{45}Ca activity of the cells during uptake
and washout of the isotope. The addition of 0.5 mM La^{3+} to the
perfusion medium during the course of ^{45}Ca uptake produces an
immediate displacement of 515 μmoles/kg wet weight from these
cells. The Ca^{2+} displaced by La^{3+} is all within the rapidly exchangeable compartment ($\lambda = 0.77$ min^{-1}). Exposure of the cells
to La^{3+} 9 to 10 minutes after the ^{45}Ca washout has begun and after
the rapidly exchangeable component is washed out produces no ^{45}Ca
displacement but slows subsequent efflux (Fig. 5 & 6). La^{3+} was
localized ultrastructurally to the cell surface of the myoblasts.
The localization of La^{3+} to sites on the sarcolemmal membrane has
been a consistent finding in all studies in adult, neonatal and
cultured heart cells. Indeed, only when the cell membrane has been
compromised and its permeability altered has La^{3+} been found

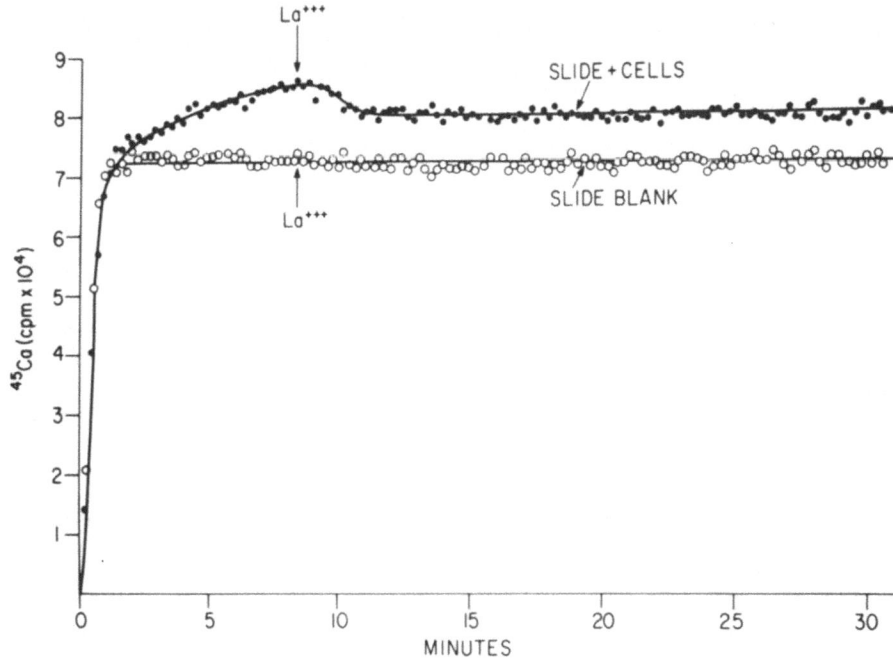

Figure 5. ^{45}*Ca uptake as affected by the addition of 0.5 mM LaCl₃*
to the perfusate at 8.5 min. LaCl₃ remained in the solution for
the 30 min course of the uptake. Reproduced with permission from
G. A. Langer and J. S. Frank (1972).

intracellularly. In conditions which alter the permeability of the
membrane (i.e. enzymatic digestion, extended Ca^{2+}-free perfusion)
La^{3+} is found intracellularly bound mainly to mitochondrial membranes (see below).

It is instructive to compare the effect of La^{3+} on skeletal
muscle, keeping in mind that skeletal muscle will develop tension
for a considerable period of time without an extracellular source
of Ca^{2+}. The effect of La^{3+} on twitch tension of perfused guinea
pig semimembranosus muscle is strikingly different from that found
in the perfused myocardium (Rich and Langer, 1975). Over a 10
min perfusion period, 50 μM La^{3+} fails to reduce twitch tension
by more than 20% in this skeletal muscle - indicating a fundamental
difference in E-C coupling process of skeletal and cardiac tissue.

The data from cardiac muscles show that 1) La^{3+} is capable
of displacing some 10-20% of the total exchangeable Ca^{2+} in addition to eliminating further Ca^{2+} exchange across the membrane and

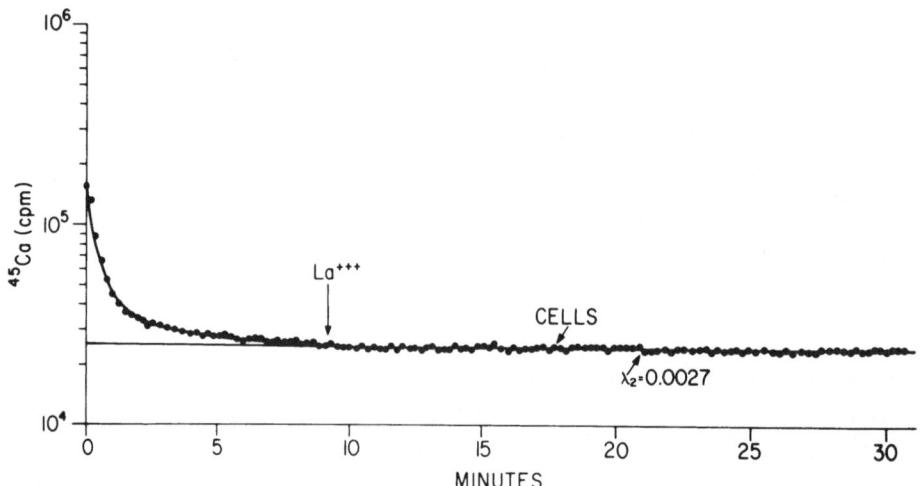

Figure 6.   The effect of 0.5 mM LaCl$_3$ introduced at the 9th min of ^{45}Ca washout.   Note that there is no evidence of ^{45}Ca displacement but only a slowing of the subsequent washout.   Reproduced with permission from G. A. Langer and J. S. Frank (1972).

2) this La^{3+} is bound to a set of sites on the surface of the sarcolemma. Clearly, this data indicates that there exists within the confines of the sarcolemma a significant amount of Ca^{2+} which is essential for maintenance of contraction.

Lanthanum's ability to bind to the surface of cells and displace Ca^{2+} from its binding sites is not limited to cardiac muscle. In the giant muscle fibers of a barnacle there are a fixed number of sites within the membrane that normally bind the Ca^{2+} that acts as a carrier of current during the Ca^{2+} spike. Henkart and Hagiwara (1976) found that La^{3+} can bind to these membrane sites and behaves as a competitive inhibitor of the Ca^{2+} spike. Weiss and Goodman (1969), in studies on the ileal longitudinal smooth muscle, indicated that La^{3+} displaced Ca^{2+} from surface sites, and while bound to these sites prevented an inward release of Ca^{2+} from less accessible membrane sites.

Which molecules on the cell surface bind the Ca^{2+} essential in E-C coupling is still unknown. The histochemical disposition of La^{3+} within the sarcolemma complex covers many moieties such as glycoproteins, glycolipids as well as phospholipids within the bilayer. It is known from studies in other tissues that protein, phospholipid and neuraminic acid components of the plasma membrane are all capable of binding Ca^{2+}, and that the selective attack by proteolytic enzymes, phospholipase C and neuraminidase decrease Ca^{2+} binding.

In isolated membranes from tissue other than muscle Ca^{2+} binding could be directly attributed to sialic acid although studies differ as to the magnitude of the binding. Long and Mouat (1971), working with red blood cell membranes, found that 65% of the total Ca^{2+} bound was attributed to sialic acid moieties. Schlatz and Marinetti (1971) found in rat liver membranes that sialic acid accounted for about 30% of the Ca^{2+} binding with acidic phospholipids accounting for the remainder.

In one of the few studies on isolated cardiac membranes, Williamson *et al.* (1975) showed that membranes isolated from guinea pig hearts bound appreciable amounts of Ca^{2+} in the absence of ATP or oxalate but that Ca^{2+} binding to the sarcolemma could be increased up to 3-fold by addition of ATP. They found both high and low affinity binding sites and they suggested that the low affinity Ca^{2+} binding may represent specific sites for Ca^{2+} entry on the surface of the sarcolemma. The apparent association constant for Ca^{2+} binding to the low affinity sites was similar to the overall association constant for Ca^{2+} required to increase myocardial contractility in intact hearts. In a more recent study on Ca-binding sites on isolated rat heart membranes, Limas (1977) also identified high and low affinity sites for Ca^{2+}. Interestingly, ruthenium red, the general stain for surface polysaccharides decreased Ca^{2+} binding in a nonspecific manner, that is, it affected both high and low affinity sites, while La^{3+} was effective only on low-affinity sites.

CALCIUM BINDING SITES AT THE CELL SURFACE AND THE ROLE OF SIALIC ACID

It is possible to speculate that sialic acid residues on the surface membrane of heart cells bind Ca^{2+} as a first step in the Ca^{2+} influx mechanism. Certainly the histochemistry data show an abundance of sialic acid in the glycoprotein layers of the membrane and studies on other tissues have shown that cell surface sialic acid binds Ca^{2+}. Sialic acid can be removed from the cell surface with a very specific neuraminidase preparation and the loss of this component of the surface coat/external lamina can be evaluated in terms of structure and function of the membrane.

All the studies discussed below were performed in cultured heart cells where there is direct access to the cell surface and the attachment of the cells to the isotopic detector (scintillator plastic) permitted continuous counting of ^{45}Ca uptake and elimination from the cell layer (Langer *et al.*, 1976b). Figure 7 shows the pattern of ^{45}Ca uptake and washout from two cultures of myoblasts that had been treated identically, except that the "neuraminidase" curve represents data from cells exposed to the enzyme

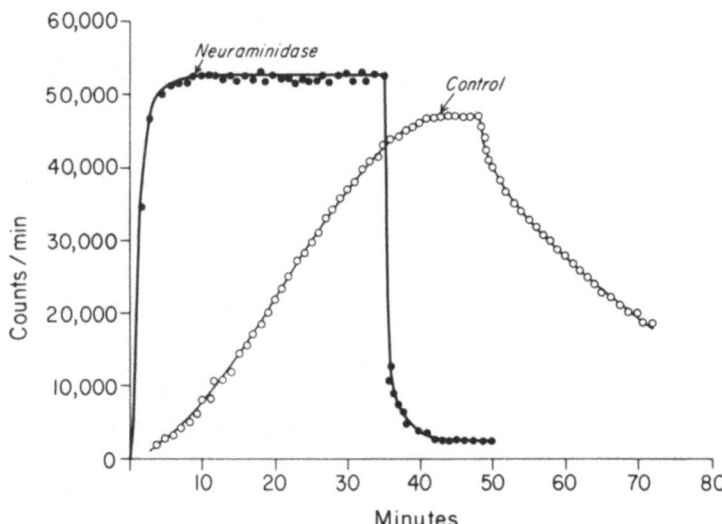

Figure 7. ^{45}Ca-uptake and washout in control and neuraminidase
treated cultured heart cells. The neuraminidase curve is data
from cells treated with 0.25 unit/ml neuraminidase for 13 min
prior to exposure to 45Ca. The ^{45}Ca washout was begun after
asymptote labeling had been achieved. Reproduced with permission
from Langer et al. (1976b).

at a concentration of 0.25 units/ml for 13 minutes prior to exposure to ^{45}Ca labeled perfusate. The pattern of ^{45}Ca uptake and
washout as shown for the control is typical for cultured heart
cells. Asymptotic ^{45}Ca activity is reached after 40-50 min of
labeling. In a series of 24 control experiments the exchangeable
Ca^{2+} at asymptotic labeling was 16.2 $\pm$ 1.4 (S.E.) mmole/kg
(dry wt). The removal of sialic acid from the cells with neuraminidase (some 49.3 x 10^{-9} moles/mg sialic acid released or 61%
total cellular sialic acid) had a marked effect on Ca^{2+} exchange.
As figure 7 shows in neuraminidase treated cells asymptotic values
were reached within 8-10 min or 4-5 times more rapidly than control.
In 18 cultures so treated the exchangeable Ca^{2+} at asymptote was
18.5 $\pm$ 1.4 mmoles Ca^{2+}/Kg, a content not significantly different
from control. The major effect is the marked increase in rate of
Ca^{2+} exchange across the cell - 96% of ^{45}Ca was eliminated within
8 min. The effect of sialic acid removal on Ca^{2+} exchangeability
is in marked contrast to its effect on K^+ exchange across the cell.
In control and neuraminidase treated cultures the K^+ exchangeability was evaluated by a comparison of the pattern of ^{42}K washout.
In two preparations the rate constants were not found to be significantly different. The control rate constant was 0.059 $\pm$ 0.004

min^{-1} and neuraminidase treated 0.061 ± 0.008 min^{-1}. Therefore sialic acid removal did not disrupt cellular permeability in a nonspecific manner but had a dramatic effect on the rate at which Ca^{2+} crossed the membrane. Since we know that La^{3+} does not penetrate the sarcolemma complex under normal conditions the reaction of La^{3+} in neuraminidase treated cells was investigated. In control cells, 0.5 mM $LaCl_3$ was introduced after the cells reached asymptote (50 min). This produced a displacement of 11.5% (2.3 mmoles/kg) of labeled Ca^{2+} within 10 min. In neuraminidase treated cells on the other hand, 0.5 mM $LaCl_3$ produced a displacement of 83% (15.6 ± 1.27 mmoles) of labeled Ca^{2+}, indicating that in conditions where sialic acid is removed from the cell surface La^{3+} now displaces Ca^{2+} from additional sites presumably from within the cell. Indeed the ultrastructure of neuraminidase-treated cells exposed to La^{3+} shows only sparse La^{3+} deposits on the cell surface while considerable amounts of La^{3+} were found within the cell (Fig. 8). The kinetic data from sialic acid stripped cells is summarized in Table I. Cell surface sialic appears then to have a critical role in the control of Ca^{2+} flux across the cell and to inhibit the entry of cations such as La^{3+}. Sialic acid is always the terminal group on the saccharide side chains of the glycoproteins (Cook, 1968). It is this terminal location and the fact that it is negatively charged at physiological pH which makes it an excellent candidate for Ca^{2+}-binding.

In an interesting study by Ishiyama et al., (1975), the effect of sialic acid removal on Ca^{2+} binding and on contractility in guinea pig taenia coli was investigated. After the removal of sialic acid from these cells they found a 50% inhibition of the KCl and the histamine induced contractions. The Scatchard plot for Ca^{2+} binding on the taenia coli muscle cell membrane indicates the presence of at least two types of binding sites with a high and low affinity constant for Ca^{2+}. Treatment of this smooth muscle with neuraminidase completely removed the low affinity Ca^{2+} binding sites. These authors speculate, as well, that the carboxyl groups of sialic acid are the primary sites of Ca^{2+} influx.

While there is no direct evidence of Ca^{2+} binding to sialic acid moieties in the heart the findings in cultured heart cells have shown that removal of sialic acid essentially destroys the ability of the cell to regulate its Ca^{2+} exchange and in addition permits entry into the cell a competitive cation such as La^{3+}. In addition La^{3+} binding to the cell surface is markedly decreased. Our earlier speculations that Ca^{2+} binding to sialic acid residues in the surface coat/external lamina complex play a crucial role in the regulation of transmembrane Ca^{2+} flux in the heart seem not unreasonable.

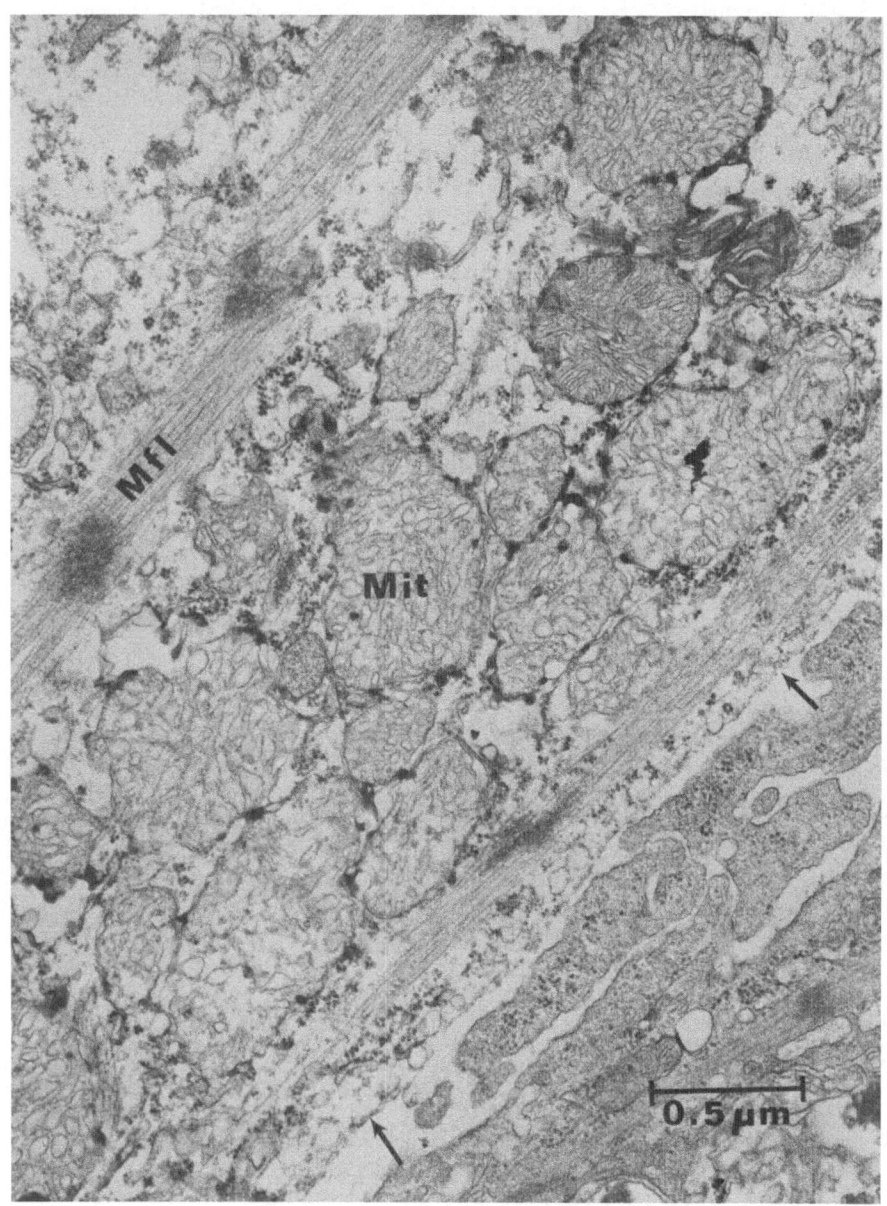

Figure 8. Electron microscope of rat myoblast grown in tissue culture. Cells were exposed to 0.25 units/ml neuraminidase for 13 min, then incubated in 0.5 mM LaCl₃ for 5 min and finally fixed for electron microscopy. Note with the removal of sialic acid La³⁺ is found in the cell around the mitochondria, while the cell surface appears free of stain (arrows). Mfl, myofilaments; Mit, mitochondria.

TABLE I

KINETIC DATA FROM CULTURED MYOBLASTS

	Time to Asymptote Labeling of ^{45}Ca	Exchangeable Ca^{2+} Calculated at Asymptote	Amount of Ca^{2+} Displaced By 0.5 mM $LaCl_3$	K^+ Exchange Constants
Control Cultures	40-50 min	16.2 ± 1.4 (S.E.) mmoles Ca²⁺/kg dry cells n = 24 wet wt:dry wt = 5.85	1.84 ± 0.13 (S.E.) mmoles Ca²⁺/kg dry cells or 11.4% labeled Ca²⁺ n = 10	0.059 ± 0.004 min⁻¹ n = 4
Neuraminidase treated cultures (0.25 units/mL) for 15 min prior to ^{45}Ca labeling	8-10 min	18.2 ± 1.4 (S.E.) mmoles Ca²⁺/kg dry cells n = 18 P > 0.25	15.6 ± 1.27 (S.E.) mmoles Ca²⁺/kg dry cells or 83% labeled Ca²⁺ n = 11 P < 0.001	0.061 ± 0.008 min⁻¹ n = 4

EFFECTS OF CALCIUM REMOVAL

The presence of Ca^{2+} within the cell membrane complex is essential for its structural and functional integrity. Perfusion of isolated hearts with Ca^{2+}-free medium has been shown to produce cessation of contractility, disturbance of electrical activity and definite ultrastructural changes in the cell membrane (Zimmerman and Husmann, 1966; Paradise and Visscher, 1975; Yates and Dhalla, 1975). In an ultrastructural study Muir (1967) first noted that the "basement membrane" was separated from the surface of rat myocardial cells that had been perfused with a "Ca^{2+}-free" medium. Tomlinson *et al*. (1976) described similar changes. When the rabbit interventricular septum is perfused with a medium containing less than 5 µM Ca^{2+}, processed for electron microscopy and then stained with colloidal iron, it is evident that the external lamina separates from the surface coat (Figure 9). The external lamina remains anchored to the cell at the transverse tubule. It appears that a Ca^{2+} dependent connection between the external lamina and surface coat is broken and subsequently the two layers are separated by a fluid filled space.

From the numerous studies on the effects of "zero" Ca^{2+} perfusion in heart it is obvious that, functionally, the sarcolemmal permeability is compromised after more than 10 minutes without Ca^{2+}. Paradise and Visscher (1975) in the rabbit and Yates and Dhalla (1975) in the rat found that, after exposure to "zero" Ca^{2+}, a marked contracture was produced upon the reintroduction of Ca^{2+}. An increase in the Ca^{2+} content of the rat hearts was also observed. Zimmerman *et al*. (1966) were the first to demonstrate an efflux of myoglobin, lactic dehydrogenase and creatine phosphokinase from the rat myocardium after restoration of Ca^{2+} to the perfusion medium following a Ca^{2+}-free perfusion. They termed this sequence of events the "Ca paradox".

In a recent study on Ca^{2+}-free perfusion in the interventricular septum of the rabbit, Crevey *et al*. (in press) were able to demonstrate an increased influx in ^{45}Ca after previous exposure to "zero" Ca^{2+} medium. In addition, they noted a large increase in the K^+ permeability which did not require the reintroduction of Ca^{2+} into the medium for its initiation, but the K^+ loss occurred throughout the "zero" Ca^{2+} perfusion. In cultured myoblasts as well, the increased K^+ permeability of these cells occurs almost immediately upon exposure to "zero" Ca^{2+} solutions. In the interventricular septum of the rabbit La^{3+} was localized within the cell after 20 min exposure to "zero" Ca^{2+} medium (Frank *et al*., 1977). It appears that Ca^{2+} depletion has increased the membrane's permeability in a very non-specific way with an increase in its permeability to ions such as K^+, Ca^{2+} and La^{3+}, as well as to larger molecules such as intracellular enzymes. This response to

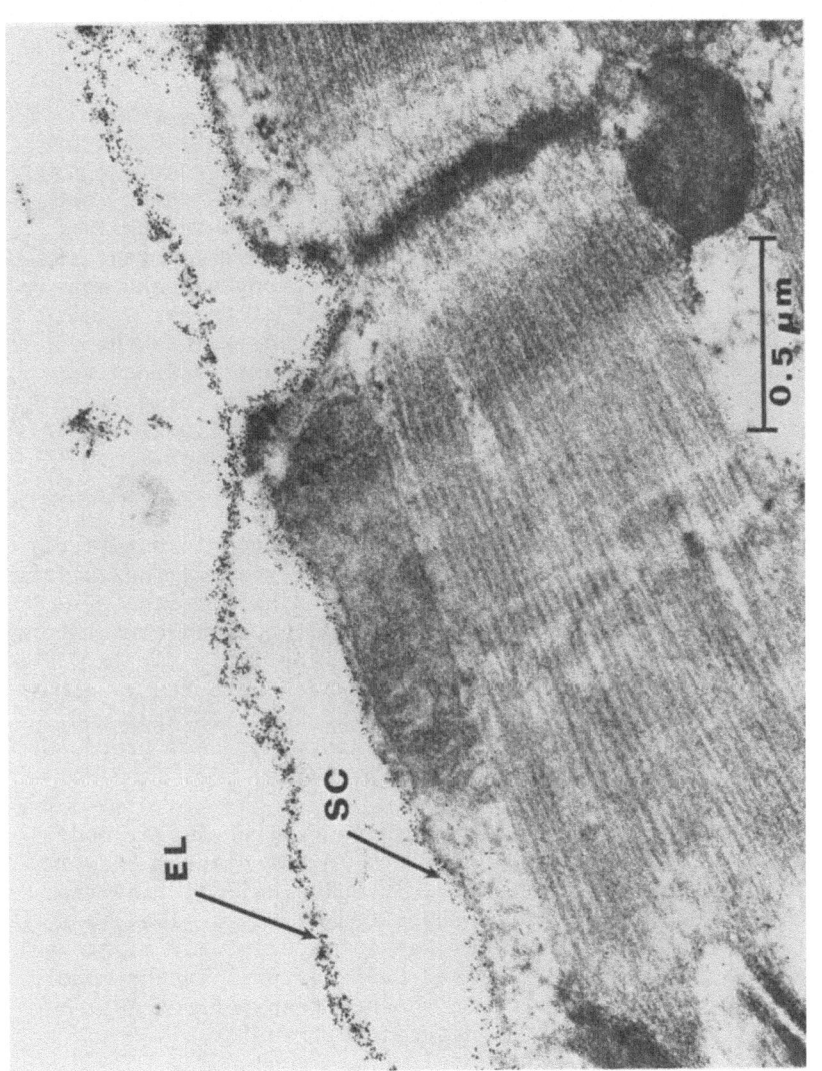

Figure 9. Portion of an adult rabbit myocardial cell. The heart was perfused with "zero" Ca solution for 20 min, then perfusion fixed and stained with colloidal iron hydroxide (CIH). CIH stains the surface coat (SC) and external lamina (EL) but note the wide separation between the two, forming what appears to be a fluid filled bleb.

removal of Ca^{2+} from the membrane can be contrasted with the more specific removal of sialic acid residues where only the Ca^{2+} and La^{3+} permeability was increased. The Ca^{2+} depletion experiments suggest an effect on the lipid bilayer as well as more superficial parts of the membrane. Whether the ultrastructural changes that occur in heart cells stripped of Ca^{2+} are related to the functional changes that occur in the membrane is not known. Until more is known about the structure of the sarcolemma the ways in which Ca^{2+} influences the permeability will remain obscure.

As demonstrated in myoblasts grown in culture, the removal of negative charges from the cell surface markedly effects Ca^{2+} permeability across the membrane. One of the important controlling factors in the regulation of the rate with which Ca^{2+} enters the myocardial cell appears to be the binding of Ca^{2+} to the cell surface. Just how Ca^{2+} moves across the sarcolemmal membrane is still unknown. There is evidence for both electrogenic and non-electrogenic (carrier-mediated) movement of Ca^{2+}. Langer *et al.* (1976a) has suggested a working model for Ca^{2+} entry into the cell which incorporates these two mechanisms and is instructive because it is based on current understanding of cardiac membrane function and structure. A diagram of the model is illustrated in Figure 10 and for a more detailed explanation see Langer *et al.* (1976a).

The model takes into account that Ca^{2+} is bound to negatively charged sites (possibly sialic acid) in the external lamina/surface coat. These sites are obviously in rapid equilibrium with Ca^{2+} in the interstitium. Calcium may move across the sarcolemma through pores formed by protein subunits embedded in the lipid matrix. The protein subunits are the integral proteins which have their carbohydrate moieties exposed to the extracellular space (Singer and Nicolson, 1972). This subunit "channel" theory has been proposed as a possible route for cation transport.

The other Ca^{2+} transport system outlined in the Langer model for the myocardium is designated "carrier" in the diagram and is based on data derived from experiments in which Na^+-Ca^{2+} interaction was evaluated. It has been suggested by Repke (1964) and by Langer (1965) that an increase of Na^+ intracellularly might be one of the first signals for increased Ca^{2+} influx. In the model the movement of a carrier results in the net transport of Na^+ outward and Ca^{2+} inward without a net charge transfer.

Both pore and carrier are accessible to influences from the interstitium through the surface coat/external lamina - this is an essential feature of this model and is in keeping with experimental evidence in the heart. The cation uncouplers of excitation and contraction (La^{3+}, Cd^{2+}, Zn^{2+} and Mn^{2+}) would displace Ca^{2+}

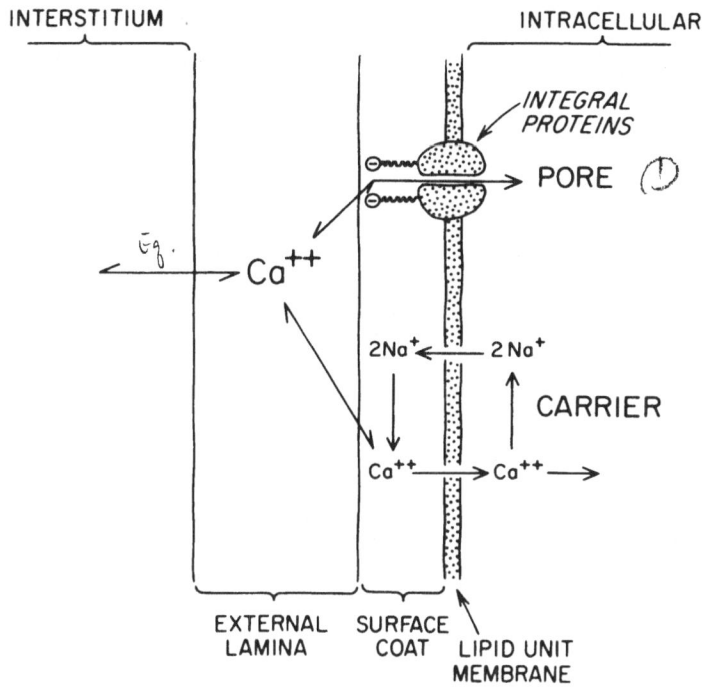

Figure 10. A model for calcium movement. Ca^{2+} is bound to nega-
tively charged sites in the external lamina that are in equilibrium
with Ca^{2+} in the interstitium. Ca^{2+} is proposed to move across
the membrane via two routes: 1) through pores formed by the integral
proteins embedded in the lipid membrane. Movement through this
system would be electrogenic. 2) With a carrier (probably coupled
to outward Na movement) such that movement via this system is
electroneutral. Reproduced with permission from Langer et al.
(1976a)

from the external lamina/surface coat while competing for Ca^{2+}
binding sites at both the pore and carrier.

DRUG-INDUCED CHANGES IN SUPERFICIAL CALCIUM SITES

The importance of superficial stores of Ca^{2+} in the regulation of contractile force in the heart raises the possibility that
some cardioactive drugs may act either by altering the amount of
Ca^{2+} available for influx from the cell surface or may interfere
with the movement of Ca^{2+} across the membrane. Certainly, very
small changes in Ca^{2+} delivery to the cell produces large effects

on contractility, i.e. an increase of only 13 μmoles of Ca^{2+}/kg
wet wt per beat will augment tension from 50 to 90% of maximum
(Solaro et $al.$, 1974).

Two powerful cardioactive drugs, digitalis glycoside and
verapamil, have been shown to affect Ca^{2+} influx in the myocardium.
The basic mechanism in which digitalis exerts its enhancement of
contractility is still not resolved. However, the increase in
Ca^{2+} influx that occurs across the membrane with its application
is well established. Langer (1972) has postulated that digitalis
inhibits the Na^+ pump activity causing a small net accumulation
of $[Na]_i$. This increase in intracellular Na^+ acts to stimulate
an increase in Ca^{2+} influx via the Na^+-Ca^{2+} exchange system proposed in Figure 10.

Verapamil has cardiac depressant activity. It inhibits cardiac
contractility and abbreviates the plateau phase of the action potential (Fleckenstein, 1971). It does not appear to displace Ca^{2+}
from its surface binding sites as do other uncouplers (La^{3+}, Cd^{2+},
Mn^{2+}) but inhibits a component of Ca^{2+} influx (Langer et $al.$,
1975). When 100 μM verapamil was added to cultured myoblasts after
the cells were labeled with ^{45}Ca for 60 min, there was no abrupt
loss of ^{45}Ca (as with the cationic uncouplers) but rather a steady
gradual decline of Ca^{2+}. It appears that the drug prevents surface
Ca^{2+} binding sites from being replenished. In isolated cardiac
membranes from guinea pigs, Williamson et $al.$ (1975) showed that
1 μg/ml of verapamil specifically inhibited the low affinity Ca^{2+}
binding and had little effect on the high affinity Ca binding. In
isolated rat sarcolemmal membranes La^{3+} was also found to inhibit
only the low-affinity Ca^{2+} binding sites.

The evidence, while indirect, suggests that cardioactive
drugs such as digitalis and verapamil have their known effects on
myocardial contractility by induction of perturbations in the
superficially bound Ca^{2+}. Nayler et $al.$ (1976), in a series of
studies set out to investigate this possibility for glycoside and
verapamil using La^{3+} as a probe. In dog trabecular muscle, she
found that doses of ouabain which would increase the peak tension
developed during contraction also increased the amount of Ca^{2+}
displacable by La^{3+}. Conversely, concentrations of verapamil which
would reduce peak tension developed in rabbit papillary muscles
reduced the amount of Ca^{2+} which La^{3+} could displace, i.e. 1.0
μg/ml of verapamil reduced peak tension considerably and reduced
the amount of Ca^{2+} displaced by La^{3+} by 29%.

SUMMARY

While the basic principles of excitation-contraction coupling are well defined, there are many questions that remain to be
answered before this sequence can be accurately described and
understood at a molecular level. A critical consideration of the
existing data from heart and skeletal muscle shows important differences in E-C coupling in these two muscles. The dependence on
a superficial store of contractile dependent Ca^{2+} in the heart is
striking. The key to understanding of the molecular basis of
E-C coupling and drug action in the heart lies in unraveling the
chemistry of the sarcolemmal membrane. Only limited information
is available at present concerning the interactions between and
the organization of the lipids and proteins of membranes. Much
of this information has come from other tissues where preparations
of isolated membranes are more readily available.

One approach to this problem is to perturb intact membranes
in different well-defined ways and by the use of a variety of
techniques determine the effects of the perturbation on the
function and structure of the cell. The myocardial tissue culture
preparation is well suited to this type of experimentation. The
studies where sialic acid was removed from cultured cells and the
effects on ionic permeability and cell membrane structure analyzed
shows the usefulness of this type of approach. Neuraminidase
treated myoblasts have altered permeabilities to Ca^{2+} and La^{3+}
which were manifest by kinetic and ultrastructural analysis and
focus attention on the role of glycoproteins in the regulation of
Ca^{2+} movement into myocardial cell.

More experimentation along this line is needed. In isolated
systems phospholipids are known to bind Ca^{2+} (Seimiya and Ohki,
1973). Lenard and Singer (1966) have shown that in the intact
membrane the polar groups of phospholipids are in contact with
the bulk aqueous phase and thus accessible to interstitial influences. The importance of the role of phospholipid interaction
with Ca^{2+} in the myocardial membrane warrants investigation.

Acknowledgements

This work was supported by Grant HL 11351-10 from the
National Institutes of Health.

REFERENCES

Armstrong, C. M., Bezanilla, F. M., and Horowicz, P., 1972, Twitches in the presence of ethylene glycol bis (β-aminoethyl-ether) - N, N'-tetraacetic acid, *Biochem. Biophys. Acta* 267: 605.

Bennett, H. S., 1963, Morphological aspects of extracellular poly-saccharides, *J. Histochem. Cytochem.* 11: 14.

Cook, G. M., 1968, Glycoproteins in membranes, *Biol. Rev.* 43: 363.

Crevey, B. J., Langer, G. A. and Frank, J. S., 1977, Structural and functional role of Ca ion in the rabbit sarcolemma, *In Press*.

Ebashi, E., 1963, Third component participating in the superpre-cipitation of "natural" actomyosin, *Nature* 200: 1010.

Endo, M., and Nakajima, I., 1973, Release of calcium induced by "depolarization" of the sarcoplasmic reticulum membrane, *Nature* (New Biol.) 246: 216.

Fabiato, A., and Fabiato, F., 1977, Calcium release from the sarcoplasmic reticulum, *Circ. Res.* 40: 191.

Fawcett, D. W., and McNutt, N. S., 1969, Ultrastructure of the cat myocardium: I. Ventricular papillary muscle, *J. Cell. Biol.* 42: 1.

Fleckenstein, A., 1971, Specific inhibition and promoters of calcium action in the excitation-contraction coupling of heart muscle and their role in the prevention or production of myo-cardial lesions, *in* "Calcium in the Heart" (P. Harris and L. H. Opie, eds.), pp. 135-188, Academic Press, New York.

Frank, J. S., Langer, G. A., Nudd, L. M., and Seraydarian, K., 1977, The myocardial cell surface: Its histochemistry and the effect of sialic acid and calcium removal in its structure and cellular ionic exchange, *Circ. Res.* 41: November 1977.

Gros, D., and Challice, C. E., 1975, The coating of mouse myo-cardial cells. A cytochemical electron microscopical study, *J. Histochem. Cytochem.* 23: 727.

Henkart, M., and Hagiwara, S., 1976, Localization of calcium bind-ing sites associated with the calcium spike in barnacle muscle, *J. Memb. Biol.* 27: 1.

Howse, H. D., Ferrans, V. J., and Hibbs, R. G., 1970, A compara-tive histochemical and electron microscopic study of the surface coatings of cardiac muscle cells, *J. Mol. Cell. Cardiol.* 1: 157.

Ishiyama, Y., Yabu, H. and Miyazaki, E., 1975, Changes in contract-ility and calcium binding of guinea pig *Taenia Coli* by treatment with enzymes which hydrolyze sialic acid, *Jpn. J. Physiol.* 25: 719.

Langer, G. A., 1965, Calcium exchange in dog ventricular muscle: relation to frequency of contraction and maintenance of contractility, *Circ. Res.* 17: 78.

Langer, G. A., 1972, Effects of digitalis in myocardial ionic exchange, *Circulation* 46: 180.

Langer, G. A., and Frank, J. S., 1972, Lanthanum in heart cell
    culture: Effect on calcium exchange correlated with its locali-
    zation, *J. Cell Biol.* 54: 441.
Langer, G. A., Frank, J. S., and Brady, A. J., 1976a, The myo-
    cardium, *in* "International Review of Physiology, Cardiovascular
    Physiology II" (A. C. Guyton and A. W. Cowley, eds.), 9: 191,
    University Park Press, Baltimore.
Langer, G. A., Frank, J. S., Nudd, L. M. and Seraydarian, K., 1976b,
    Sialic acid: Effect of removal on calcium exchangeability of
    cultured heart cells, *Science* 193: 1013.
Lenard, J., and Singer, S. J., 1966, Protein conformation in cell
    membrane preparation as studied by optical rotatory dispersion
    and circular dichroism, *Proc. Nat. Acad. Sci. U.S.A.* 56: 1828.
Limas, C. J., 1977, Calcium-binding sites in rat myocardial sar-
    colemma, *Arch. Biochem. Biophys.* 179: 302.
Long, C., and Mouat, B., 1971, The binding of calcium ions by
    human erythrocytes, *Biochem. J.* 121: 15.
Lullman, H., Preuner, J. and Sunano, S., 1974, One interaction
    of acetycholine, caffeine and altered Ca-concentrations upon
    excitation-contraction coupling in chronically denervated
    skeletal muscle, *Pflügers Arch.* 353: 279.
Martinez-Palomo, A., 1970, The surface coats of animal cells, *Int.
    Rev. Cytol.* 29: 29.
Muir, A. R., 1967, The effects of divalent cations on the ultra-
    structure of the perfused rat heart, *J. Anat.* 101: 239.
Nayler, W. G., Dunnett, J., and Sullivan, A., 1976, Drug-induced
    changes in the superficially located stores of calcium in
    heart sarcolemma, *in* "Recent Advances in Studies on Cardiac
    Structure and Metabolism" "The Sarcolemma" (P. E. Roy and N. S.
    Dhalla, eds.) 9: 53-70, University Park Press, Baltimore.
Paradise, N. F., and Visscher, M. B., 1975, K^+ and Mg^{++} net flux
    is in relation to zero $[Ca^{++}]$ perfusion and subsequent cardiac
    contracture, *Proc. Soc. Exp. Biol. and Med.* 149: 40.
Parsons, D. F., and Subjeck, J. R., 1972, The morphology of the
    polysaccharide coat of mammalian cells, *Biochim. Biophys. Acta*
    265: 85.
Repke, K., 1964, Über den biochemischer Wirkungsmodus von Digitalis,
    Klin. Wochenschr. 41: 157.
Rich, T. L., and Langer, G. A., 1975, A comparison of excitation-
    contraction coupling in heart and skeletal muscle: An examination
    of "Calcium-Induced Calcium-Release", *J. Mol. Cell. Cardiol.*
    7: 747.
Sanborn, W. G., and Langer, G. A., 1970, Specific uncoupling of
    excitation and contraction in mammalian cardiac tissue by
    lanthanum, *J. gen. Physiol.* 56: 191.
Seimiya, T., and Ohki, S., 1973, Ionic structure of phospholipid
    membrane and binding of calcium ions, *Biochim. Biophys. Acta*
    298: 546.
Shine, K. I., Serena, S. D. and Langer, G. A., 1971, Kinetic

localization of contractile calcium in rabbit myocardium, *Amer. J. Physiol.* 221: 1408.

Shlatz, L., and Marinetti, G. V., 1972, Calcium binding to the rat liver plasma membrane, *Biochim. Biophys. Acta* 290: 70.

Singer, S. J., and Nicolson, G. L., 1972, The fluid mosaic model of the structure of cell membranes, *Science* 175: 720.

Solaro, R. J., Wise, R. M., Shiner, J. S., and Briggs, F. N., 1974, Calcium requirements for cardiac myofibrillar activation, *Circ. Res.* 34: 525.

Tomlinson, C. W., Yates, J. C., and Dhalla, N. S., 1974, Relationship among changes in intracellular Ca stores, ultrastructure and contractility of myocardium, *in* "Recent Advances in Studies on Cardiac Structure and Metabolism" "The Sarcolemma" (N. S. Dhalla, ed.) 4:33, University Park Press, Baltimore.

Weiss, G. B., and Goodman, F. R., 1969, Effects of lanthanum on contraction, calcium distribution and Ca^{45} movements in intestinal smooth muscle, *J. Pharmacol. Exp. Ther.* 169: 46.

Williamson, J. R., Woodrow, M. L., and Scarpa, A., 1975, Calcium binding to cardiac sarcolemma *in* "Recent Advances in Studies in Cardiac Structure and Metabolism" "Basic Functions of Cations in Myocardial Activity" (A. Fleckenstein and N. S. Dhalla, eds) 5: 61, University Park Press, Baltimore.

Winegrad, S., 1968, Intracellular calcium movements of frog skeletal muscle during recovery from tetanus, *J. gen. Physiol.* 51: 65.

Winegrad, S., 1970, The intracellular site of calcium activation of contraction in frog skeletal muscle, *J. gen. Physiol.* 55: 77.

Winzler, R. J., 1970, Carbohydrates in cell surfaces, *Int. Rev. Cytol.* 29: 77.

Yates, J. C., and Dhalla, N. S., 1975, Structural and functional changes associated with failure and recovery of hearts after perfusion with Ca^{++}-free medium, *J. Mol. Cell. Cardiol.* 7: 91.

Zimmerman, A. N. E., and Husmann, W. C., 1966, Paradoxical influence of calcium ions in the permeability of the cell membranes of the isolated rat heart, *Nature* 211: 646.

CHAPTER 3

QUANTITATIVE MEASUREMENT OF BINDING SITES AND WASHOUT

COMPONENTS FOR CALCIUM ION IN VASCULAR SMOOTH MUSCLE

George B. Weiss

Department of Pharmacology
University of Texas Health Science Center
Dallas, Texas 75235

INTRODUCTION

In a recent review article (Weiss, 1977a), a general hypothesis was developed concerning the central importance of Ca^{2+} to
any comprehensive understanding of responsiveness of muscle systems
to pharmacological agents. Briefly, this view was that both the
qualitative and the quantitative nature of the muscle response
to a given agent is directly determined by the amounts of intracellular Ca^{2+} available and this, in turn, is a direct consequence
of differing Ca^{2+}-binding properties of the specific cytoarchitec-
ture present in each particular type of muscle. This is not to
say that other phases of the sequence beginning with the drug-
receptor interaction are not also essential. However, determination of the nature of the final response obtained is not a function
of receptor activation but, rather, a result of alterations in
membrane binding and permeability characteristics and, ultimately,
a direct function of the intracellular Ca^{2+} level. Though this
relationship exists in all types of muscle, elaboration of corre-
lations between muscle tension and Ca^{2+} distribution and movements
has not progressed as rapidly in smooth muscle as in striated
muscle. The sequence of events leading from membrane excitation
to muscle contraction in striated muscle has been convincingly
documented (see Sandow, 1965; Bianchi, 1968) and related to clearly
defined morphological structures. However, in smooth muscle
anatomical structures resembling those observed in striated muscle
are not as readily identified and, partly as a consequence of
this, specific cellular sources and sites for Ca^{2+} cannot be delineated in a parallel fashion.

One of the more useful ways of evaluating Ca^{2+} uptake, distribution and loss is by analysis of ^{45}Ca desaturation measurements
and the derivative rate coefficient plots. These approaches were
initially developed by Shanes and Bianchi (1959) to delineate ^{45}Ca
movements in frog sartorius muscle. The basic techniques have
been described elsewhere (Bianchi, 1965, 1968; Weiss, 1966). Desaturation curves indicate the amount of ^{45}Ca remaining in the
tissue after differing time intervals during the washout as a
percentage of the initial ^{45}Ca content; they are useful for analysis of relative and absolute sizes and half-times ($T_{\frac{1}{2}}$; reciprocals
of rate constants) of various washout components. Rate coefficient
curves show that fraction of the average amount of ^{45}Ca present in
the tissue during a specified time interval which leaves the tissue
during that period; they provide a sensitive estimation of changes
in the transient or maintained rate of loss of ^{45}Ca under various
conditions.

Desaturation curves for ^{45}Ca have been obtained in a number
of vascular smooth muscle preparations (for example, see Weiss,
1977a). Generally, the curves resolve into one slow component
and one or more rapid components. As noted previously (Weiss,
1977a), the critical question concerning ^{45}Ca washout components
is whether the values obtained have true physical meaning in terms
of delineation of ^{45}Ca loss from specific tissue compartments or
sites. In other words, do ^{45}Ca washout components correspond in
some fashion to tissue Ca^{2+} compartments? This type of question
cannot be answered simply by performing varied washout experiments
of the same general type. This is partly because of the presence
of additional factors such as binding of ^{45}Ca to cell fiber, exchange of ^{45}Ca with nonradioactive Ca^{2+}, and reuptake and rebinding
of a portion of the ^{45}Ca efflux component per unit time. Even
though each of these events can be quantitated to some extent,
the basic kinetic type of approach inherent in all of these experiments cannot define the cellular locations of different ^{45}Ca
washout components. Furthermore, the question of exchange of
^{45}Ca between different cellular Ca^{2+} components during the washout
superimposes an unknown set of variations which both prevent analysis of emergent ^{45}Ca in terms of conventional series or parallel
compartments and impede estimation of specific component magnitudes.

To obtain additional information about the magnitude of ^{45}Ca
tissue compartments, it was necessary to develop an alternative
approach which could measure binding of Ca^{2+} at tissue sites and
affinity of Ca^{2+} for these sites without permitting the type of
^{45}Ca-^{40}Ca exchange occurring during a conventional washout. The
next section of this chapter will outline an approach developed
to analyze Ca^{2+} uptake and binding by use of Scatchard plots and
will examine the effects of Sr^{2+} and Lu^{3+} on these parameters.

The subsequent section of this chapter will compare the effects of Sr^{2+} and Lu^{3+} on Ca^{2+} binding with the actions of these same two ions on ^{45}Ca desaturation components and rate coefficients under analogous conditions favoring either high or low affinity binding of Ca^{2+}.

DELINEATION OF TWO DIFFERENT BINDING SITES FOR CALCIUM IONS

When considering the question of how to quantitatively describe the binding of Ca^{2+}, a problem arises concerning the ability to distinguish between alterations in affinity of differing binding sites for Ca^{2+} and changes in the actual number of binding sites. A method designed to distinguish between these two possibilities has been developed and utilizes ^{45}Ca tissue/medium (T/M) ratios (expressed as ml/g tissue wet weight) obtained over a wide range of extracellular Ca^{2+} concentrations (from trace to 15 mM). Total Ca^{2+} uptake values (expressed as µmol/g tissue) can be calculated by adjusting the T/M ratios to exclude the contents of the extracellular space (measured with sucrose-^{14}C during each series of experiments) and to account for the differing specific activities of the ^{45}Ca incubation solutions. By utilizing the simplifying assumptions that (a) essentially all of the Ca^{2+} taken up by the cells exists in bound form (as bound Ca^{2+}) and (b) the extracellular Ca^{2+} concentration is equivalent to the free Ca^{2+} level, the ratio of bound Ca^{2+}/free Ca^{2+} vs. the bound Ca^{2+} can be plotted. This type of plot was originally devised by Scatchard (1949) to describe the binding of small molecules to macromolecules. Termed a "Scatchard plot", it has been used to estimate the relative affinity of sites and number of binding sites for such biological parameters as the binding of Tb^{3+} to ribosomes and RNA (Barela et al., 1976) and the effects of neuraminidase and phospholipase C on binding of Ca^{2+} in the guinea pig taenia coli membrane (Ishiyama et al., 1975). Similar approaches in this laboratory yield values for rabbit aortic smooth muscle (Weiss, 1977b) of the type illustrated in Figure 1. This plot, a summary derived from ^{45}Ca uptake values in muscles after 30 min and 60 min of incubation with ^{45}Ca in solutions of varying specific activities of Ca^{2+}, indicates that the Ca^{2+} taken up is bound at two different sites. One of these is a high affinity site which is clearly present at lower Ca^{2+} concentrations and the other is a low affinity site which is delineated at higher Ca^{2+} concentrations. An estimation of the relative number of binding sites (n) present per unit tissue (expressed as µmol Ca^{2+} bound per gram tissue) can be obtained from the x-axis intercept. The estimated number of binding sites as well as the calculation of the apparent dissociation constant, K_D (K_D = n/y intercept) are also included in Figure 1. From these values and the Scatchard plot, it is clear that the affinities for Ca^{2+} and the apparent number of

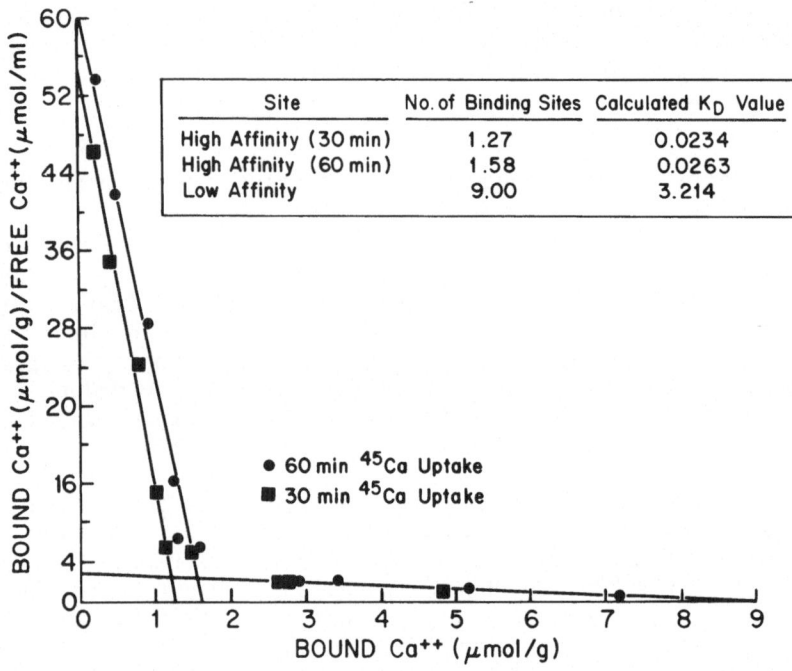

Figure 1. Scatchard plot of ^{45}Ca uptake after 30 min (■) or 60 min (●) incubation in solutions containing different extracellular Ca^{2+} concentrations into rabbit aortic smooth muscle (From Weiss, 1977b).

low affinity binding sites for Ca^{2+} are similar after both 30 min and 60 min of exposure to ^{45}Ca. In contrast to this, the apparent number of high affinity binding sites is less after 30 min than after 60 min of ^{45}Ca incubation. This demonstrates that binding of Ca^{2+} at high affinity sites is not completely equilibrated after 30 min exposure to ^{45}Ca. This may indicate that high affinity Ca^{2+} sites are less accessible to extracellular ^{45}Ca than are low affinity Ca^{2+} sites.

Of more general importance is the conclusion that all of the ^{45}Ca taken up may well be present at two specific types of membrane binding sites. If this is the case, then it becomes feasible to delineate actions of agents which inhibit Ca^{2+} uptake and/or binding in a more precise manner in terms of effects on either affinity of Ca^{2+} for sites or number of available sites for either high or low affinity sites. Two ions which appeared to be excellent initial candidates for evaluation in terms of effects on either of these two parameters were the divalent alkaline earth ion, Sr^{2+}, and the trivalent rare earth ion, Lu^{3+}. Strontium ion appears to substitute for Ca^{2+} in some but not all Ca^{2+}-dependent actions in vascular smooth muscle (see Weiss, 1977a), whereas the actions of Lu^{3+} resemble inhibitory actions of low (0.05-0.10 mM) concentrations of La^{3+} on smooth muscle tension and ^{45}Ca fluxes (Weiss and Goodman, 1975).

The effects of Sr^{2+} on vascular smooth muscle are consistent with the view that Sr^{2+} can replace Ca^{2+} at binding sites in vascular smooth muscle (Hudgins and Weiss, 1969a) but is not as readily released from these sites by stimulatory agents as is Ca^{2+} (Daniel, 1965). In accord with this, Sr^{2+} can act directly as does Ca^{2+} on contractile protein to initiate contraction (Bohr, 1964) and does support a high K^+-induced response (which depends on the extracellular divalent ion response) to a greater degree than the responses of stimulatory agents which are more resistant to Ca^{2+} depletion (Hudgins and Weiss, 1969b; Hudgins, 1969). The effects of Lu^{3+} on vascular smooth muscle, in contrast to those of Sr^{2+}, are entirely inhibitory in terms of actions of Ca^{2+}. In initial studies (Weiss and Goodman, 1975) it was observed that the inhibitory effect of Lu^{3+} on superficial binding of Ca^{2+} appeared to be somewhat greater than that on ^{45}Ca uptake. However, these effects on differing ^{45}Ca desaturation curve components could not be clearly dissociated.

In order to obtain Scatchard-type plots of the effects of Sr^{2+} and Lu^{3+} on ^{45}Ca distribution in rabbit aortic smooth muscle, it was first necessary to obtain paired ^{45}Ca T/M ratios for control muscles and for those exposed to Sr^{2+} and to Lu^{3+} over an appropriate range of extracellular Ca^{2+} concentrations. The results obtained are summarized in Table I. All ^{45}Ca incubation intervals were 60 min, a duration sufficient for equilibration of ^{45}Ca (Hudgins and Weiss, 1969a; Weiss and Goodman, 1975); the concentration of radioactive Ca^{2+} was approximately 0.001 mM. Examination of the magnitude of decrease in ^{45}Ca T/M ratios obtained with Sr^{2+} and Lu^{3+} indicates that the effects of these two ions were similar at the three lower extracellular Ca^{2+} concentrations but that the effect of Lu^{3+} was more pronounced than that of Sr^{2+} at higher extracellular Ca^{2+} concentrations. At the two highest extracellular Ca^{2+} levels, 1.5 mM Sr^{2+} did not have a significant inhibitory effect.

This divergence in effects of Sr^{2+} and Lu^{3+} is maintained when total Ca^{2+} uptakes are calculated from the values in Table I. The Ca^{2+} uptake values for control muscles and for paired Lu^{3+}-treated and Sr^{2+}-treated muscles are summarized in Table II. The percentage decrease in Ca^{2+} uptake in Lu^{3+} or Sr^{2+} is substantial (52-80%) for all pairs except those in Sr^{2+} at the three higher

TABLE I: EFFECT OF 1.5 mM Sr^{2+} AND Lu^{3+} ON ^{45}Ca TISSUE/MEDIUM (T/M)
           RATIOS IN PAIRED RABBIT AORTIC SMOOTH MUSCLES

A. Lu^{3+}:

Extracellular Ca^{2+}	^{45}Ca T/M Ratios in Control Tissues	^{45}Ca T/M Ratios in Lu^{3+}-Treated Tissues	Difference in T/M Ratios[a]
mM	ml/g ± S.E.		ml/g ± S.E.
0.011	17.966 ± 1.564	4.786 ± 0.221	13.181 ± 1.435
0.031	13.514 ± 1.181	4.371 ± 0.099	9.143 ± 1.087
0.101	8.520 ± 0.847	3.020 ± 0.074	5.500 ± 0.795
1.501	2.340 ± 0.092	1.196 ± 0.110	1.144 ± 0.038
5.001	1.439 ± 0.026	0.817 ± 0.025	0.622 ± 0.034
15.001	0.990 ± 0.025	0.656 ± 0.018	0.334 ± 0.019

B. Sr^{2+}:

Extracellular Ca^{2+}	^{45}Ca T/M Ratios in Control Tissues	^{45}Ca T/M Ratios in Sr^{2+}-Treated Tissues	Difference in T/M Ratios
mM	ml/g ± S.E.		ml/g ± S.E.
0.011	17.966 ± 1.564	3.837 ± 0.101	14.130 ± 1.479
0.031	13.514 ± 1.181	3.176 ± 0.075	10.338 ± 1.177
0.101	8.520 ± 0.847	2.962 ± 0.013	5.558 ± 0.845
1.501	2.340 ± 0.092	1.796 ± 0.122	0.567 ± 0.066
5.001	1.439 ± 0.026	1.382 ± 0.027	0.057 ± 0.037[*]
15.001	0.990 ± 0.025	0.958 ± 0.018	0.032 ± 0.023[*]

[a]$P<0.005$ for all paired differences except [*]($p>0.05$); N=4 except for
5.001 mM values (N=7) and 15.001 mM values (N=10).

extracellular Ca^{2+} concentrations. Inclusion of these data in
Scatchard-type plots is illustrated in Figure 2. The number of
binding sites and calculated K_D values for both high and low
affinity sites are also shown within Figure 2. For high affinity
sites, both Sr^{2+} and Lu^{3+} decrease the number of binding sites
and increase the calculated K_D value. The major difference is
that Lu^{3+} decreases the number of low affinity binding sites whereas

TABLE II: EFFECT OF 1.5 mM Sr^{2+} AND Lu^{3+} on Ca^{2+} UPTAKE IN PAIRED RABBIT AORTIC SMOOTH MUSCLES

A. Lu^{3+}:

Extracellular Ca^{2+}	Ca^{2+} Uptake in Control Tissues	Ca^{2+} Uptake in Lu^{3+}-Treated Tissues	Decrease in Ca^{2+} Uptake
mM	μmol/g ± S.E.		%
0.011	0.194 ± 0.017	0.049 ± 0.002	74.7
0.031	0.408 ± 0.037	0.125 ± 0.003	69.4
0.101	0.825 ± 0.086	0.270 ± 0.007	67.3
1.501	2.987 ± 0.138	1.270 ± 0.165	57.5
5.001	5.451 ± 0.130	2.335 ± 0.125	57.2
15.001	9.601 ± 0.375	4.590 ± 0.270	52.2

B. Sr^{2+}:

Extracellular Ca^{2+}	Ca^{2+} Uptake in Control Tissues	Ca^{2+} Uptake in Sr^{2+}-Treated Tissues	Decrease in Ca^{2+} Uptake
mM	μmol/g ± S.E.		%
0.011	0.194 ± 0.017	0.038 ± 0.001	80.4
0.031	0.408 ± 0.037	0.088 ± 0.002	78.4
0.101	0.825 ± 0.086	0.264 ± 0.001	68.0
1.501	2.987 ± 0.138	2.136 ± 0.183	28.4
5.001	5.451 ± 0.130	5.161 ± 0.135	5.3
15.001	9.601 ± 0.375	9.121 ± 0.270	5.0

Sr^{2+} does not. Thus, Lu^{3+} affects both high and low affinity Ca^{2+}-binding sites whereas Sr^{2+} appears to affect only high affinity binding sites.

RELATIONSHIPS BETWEEN CALCIUM DESATURATION COMPONENTS AND CALCIUM BINDING SITES

Whether the effects of Lu^{3+} and Sr^{2+} on Ca^{2+}-binding sites are due to direct or indirect actions of the two ions cannot be

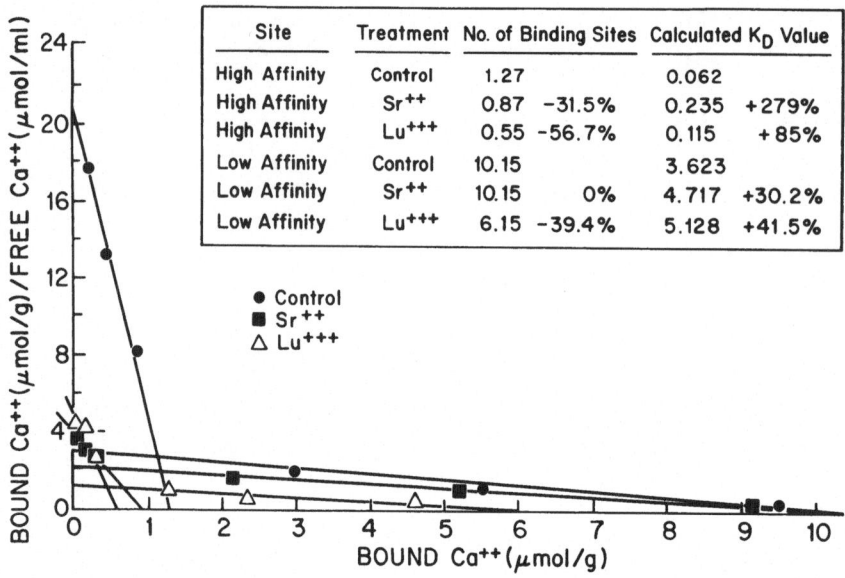

Site	Treatment	No. of Binding Sites		Calculated K_D Value	
High Affinity	Control	1.27		0.062	
High Affinity	Sr++	0.87	−31.5%	0.235	+279%
High Affinity	Lu+++	0.55	−56.7%	0.115	+85%
Low Affinity	Control	10.15		3.623	
Low Affinity	Sr++	10.15	0%	4.717	+30.2%
Low Affinity	Lu+++	6.15	−39.4%	5.128	+41.5%

● Control
■ Sr++
△ Lu+++

Figure 2. Scatchard plot of ^{45}Ca uptake from solutions containing different extracellular Ca^{2+} concentrations (●) as well as either 1.5 mM Sr^{2+} (■) or 1.5 mM Lu^{3+} (△).

determined from Scatchard plots. However, analogous experiments measuring effects of Sr^{2+} and Lu^{3+} on ^{45}Ca fluxes under conditions where either high or low Ca^{2+} affinity site binding is optimized could yield additional information regarding the nature of Sr^{2+}-Ca^{2+} and Lu^{3+}-Ca^{2+} exchange at each of these sites. Desaturation curves showing the effects of 1.5 mM Sr^{2+} or 1.5 mM Lu^{3+} on ^{45}Ca uptake in 0.031 mM or 5.001 mM Ca^{2+} solutions followed by washout in 0-Ca solutions (to minimize ^{45}Ca-^{40}Ca exchange) are summarized in Figure 3. Inspection of the desaturation curves indicates that Lu^{3+} does not change the curve greatly but Sr^{2+} decreases the relative size (percentage) of the slow washout component (and, conversely, increases the relative size of the fast washout component). Specific changes induced in one or another component can be ascertained by analysis of the components illustrated in Figure 3. These components and the corresponding calculated total Ca^{2+} uptakes and component Ca^{2+} uptakes are included in Table III. Though Table III is somewhat complex, the relevant information can be determined readily. First, in 0.031 mM Ca^{2+} (under conditions maximizing high affinity Ca^{2+} binding), both Sr^{2+} and Lu^{3+} markedly decrease the ^{45}Ca T/M ratios, the ^{45}Ca slow components and the corresponding ^{45}Ca uptakes. Both ions also inhibit

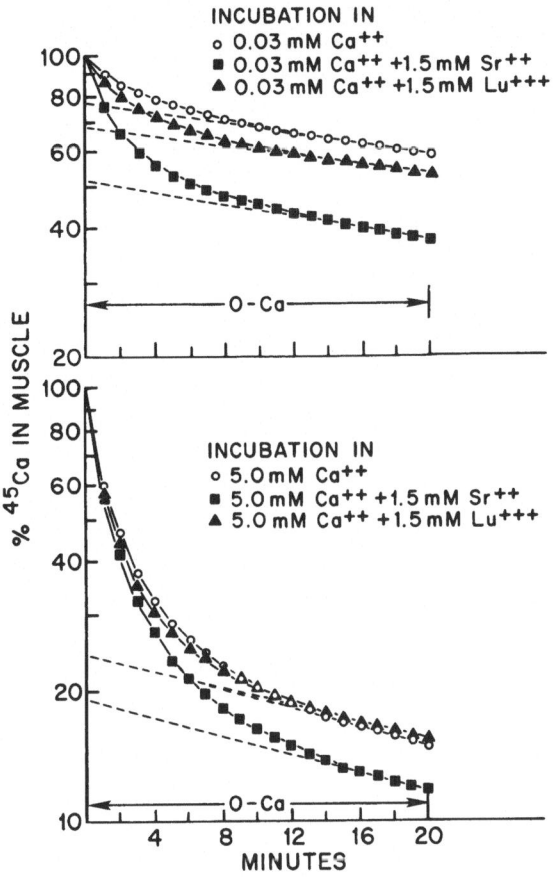

Figure 3. Effects of Sr^{2+} or Lu^{3+} on 60 min ^{45}Ca uptake in rabbit aortic smooth muscle prior to washout in O-Ca solution. Each desaturation curve is the average of values obtained with 8 (control) or 3 (Sr^{2+} and Lu^{3+}) muscles. Dashed lines indicate extrapolation of the slow washout component to the beginning of the washout.

the adjusted ^{45}Ca fast component, but the effect of Lu^{3+} (about 3/4 inhibited) is greater than that of Sr^{2+} (about 1/2 inhibited). Second, in 5.001 mM Ca^{2+} (under conditions maximizing low affinity Ca^{2+}-binding), both Sr^{2+} and Lu^{3+} have some inhibitory effect on the ^{45}Ca slow component T/M ratio (and corresponding Ca^{2+} uptake) but this is already low due to ^{40}Ca-^{45}Ca competition. However, the total ^{45}Ca T/M ratio, the ^{45}Ca fast component and the corresponding Ca^{2+} uptakes are decreased by Lu^{3+} but not by Sr^{2+}. In

TABLE III: ANALYSIS OF EFFECTS ON ^{45}Ca DESATURATION COMPONENTS^a OF INCUBATION IN 0.031 mM OR 5.001 mM Ca^{2+} ± 1.5 mM Sr^{2+} OR Lu^{3+}

	Incubation in 0.031 mM Ca^{2+}			Incubation in 5.001 mM Ca^{2+}		
	Control	1.5 mM Sr^{2+}	1.5 mM Lu^{3+}	Control	1.5 mM Sr^{2+}	1.5 mM Lu^{3+}
^{45}Ca T/M Ratio, ml/g	14.679	3.545	3.457	6.281	6.136	3.371
^{45}Ca Slow Component, ml/g	11.450	1.822	2.351	1.526	1.178	0.809
^{45}Ca Fast Component, ml/g	3.229	1.702	1.106	4.755	4.958	2.561
Adjusted ^{45}Ca Fast Component, ml/g^b	2.879	1.352	0.756	3.005	3.208	0.812
Ca^{2+} Uptake, μmol/g	0.455	0.110	0.107	1.256	1.226	0.673
Slow Component Ca^{2+} Uptake, μmol/g	0.355	0.057	0.073	0.305	0.235	0.161
Fast Component Ca^{2+} Uptake, μmol/g	0.100	0.053	0.034	0.951	0.991	0.512
Adjusted Fast Component Ca^{2+} Uptake, μmol/g^b	0.089	0.042	0.023	0.601	0.641	0.162

^{a}Data obtained from desaturation curves summarized in Figure 3.

^{b}Values corrected for an extracellular space of 0.350 ml/g or Ca^{2+} uptakes of either 0.011 μmol/ml (0.031 mM x 0.350 ml/g) or 1.750 μmol/ml (5.001 mM x 0.350 ml/g).

this high extracellular Ca^{2+} concentration, approximately 2/3 of the Ca^{2+} uptake (excluding extracellular space Ca^{2+}) is present as part of the fast washout component.

Thus, the one difference between the effects of Lu^{3+} and those of Sr^{2+} on ^{45}Ca uptake appears to be a lack of effect (or diminished effect) of Sr^{2+} on the fast washout component. Additional information concerning whether this effect corresponds in some manner to the diminished effect of Sr^{2+} on low affinity Ca^{2+}-binding sites (illustrated in Figure 2) can be obtained by performing a different type of ^{45}Ca desaturation experiment. In this approach, muscles are incubated for 60 min with ^{45}Ca in solutions containing either 0.03 mM or 5.0 mM added Ca^{2+}. Then all muscles are washed out in 0-Ca solution for the first 20 min of a 30-min washout. For the final 10 min of the washout either 1.5 mM Sr^{2+} or 1.5 mM Lu^{3+} are added to the 0-Ca washout solution. The desaturation curves obtained are summarized in Figure 4. In both the upper portion of Figure 4 (0.03 mM Ca^{2+}) and the lower portion (5.0 mM Ca^{2+}), addition of 1.5 mM Lu^{3+} resulted in a small maintained increase in ^{45}Ca efflux, whereas addition of 1.5 mM Sr^{2+} initiated a much larger and at least partially transient increase in ^{45}Ca efflux. Previously (see Weiss, 1977a), a transient increase in ^{45}Ca loss was interpreted as indicating either a temporary increase in membrane permeability to Ca^{2+} or displacement (and depletion) of ^{45}Ca from Ca^{2+} sites comprising a relatively limited portion of the total ^{45}Ca content of the tissue. Conversely, a maintained increase in ^{45}Ca efflux might represent a sustained Ca^{2+} permeability increase, an increased rate of ^{45}Ca loss from sites comprising the major portion of tissue ^{45}Ca, or a decreased rate of ^{45}Ca reuptake or backflux.

The pattern of ^{45}Ca loss observed after addition of either Lu^{3+} or Sr^{2+} to the washout solution can be more precisely diagrammed by a rate coefficient plot of the same data as in Figure 4. This is shown in Figure 5 and, even more than in the preceding figure, the maintained nature of the Lu^{3+}-induced effect on ^{45}Ca efflux is illustrated and the much larger but transient nature of the Sr^{2+}-induced effect is also shown. The effect of Sr^{2+} on ^{45}Ca loss is much greater in muscles previously incubated in 0.03 mM Ca^{2+} solution (i.e., under conditions optimizing high affinity Ca^{2+} binding) rather than in 5.0 mM Ca^{2+} solution (i.e., under conditions optimizing low affinity Ca^{2+} binding).

Further support for the idea that high affinity Ca^{2+} binding might correlate with slow component ^{45}Ca, whereas low affinity binding might be more closely associated with fast component ^{45}Ca is provided by an additional experiment in which ^{45}Ca desaturation components are measured after 60 min ^{45}Ca incubation under conditions favoring differing Ca^{2+} binding affinities. The Ca^{2+}

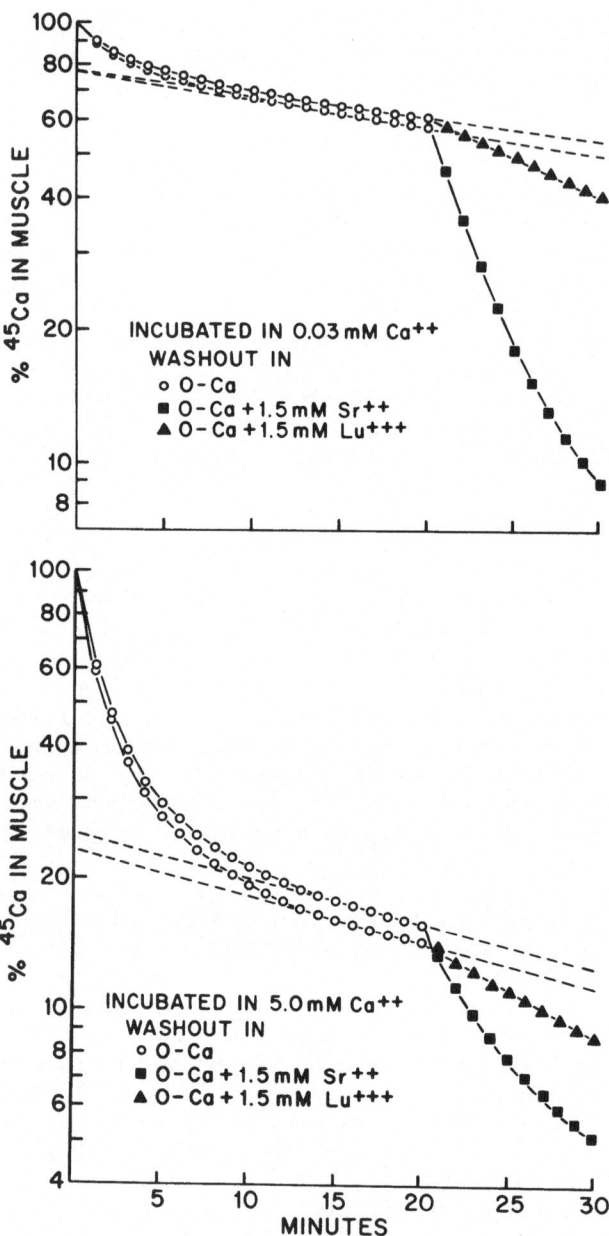

Figure 4.   Effects of addition of Sr^{2+} or Lu^{3+} on ^{45}Ca efflux from rabbit aortic smooth muscle.   Each desaturation curve is the average of values obtained with 4 (at 0.03 mM Ca^{2+}) or 5 (at 5.0 mM Ca^{2+}) muscles.   Muscles were incubated for 60 min with ^{45}Ca plus either 0.03 mM or 5.0 mM added Ca^{2+}.   Dashed lines represent extrapolation of the slow components of the initial portion of the washout.

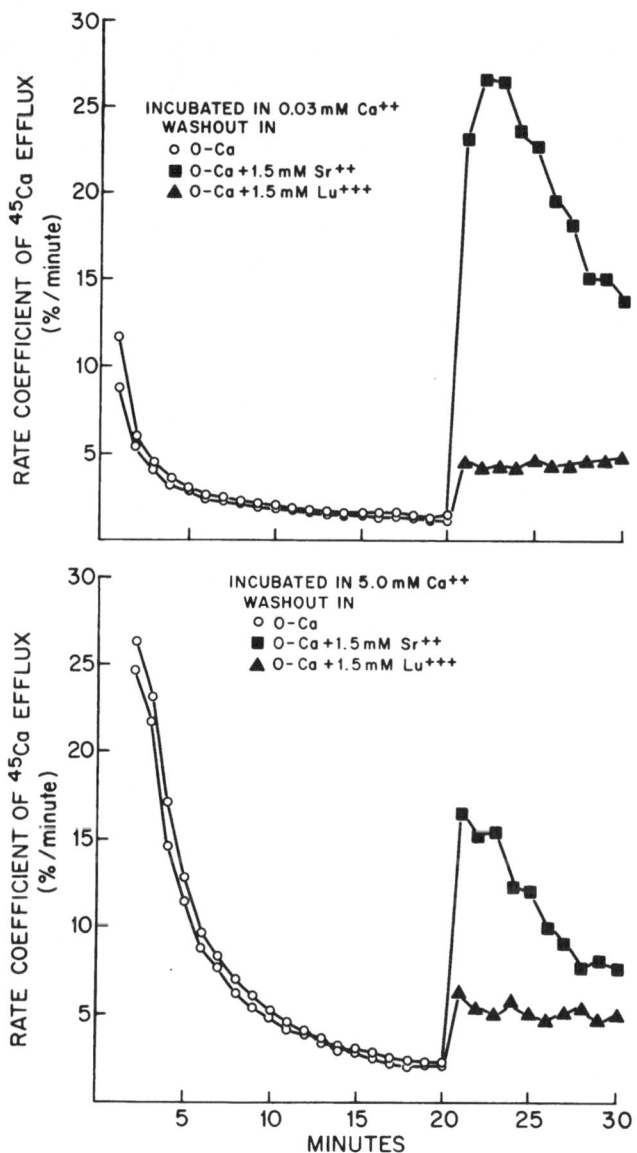

Figure 5. Effects of addition of Sr^{2+} or Lu^{3+} on ^{45}Ca efflux from rabbit aortic smooth muscle. Rate coefficient data employed in this figure were obtained from the same muscle sets as in figure 4.

incubation concentrations were selected to yield comparisons based upon the high and low affinity concentration ranges observed in the Scatchard plot (e.g., Figure 1). For example, the Ca^{2+} uptake in both washout components after incubation with ^{45}Ca at 0.021 mM extracellular Ca^{2+} concentration (approximately mid-way in the high affinity range) and at 0.201 mM extracellular Ca^{2+} concentration (approximately at the point where high and low affinity lines bisect) is compared to ascertain which ^{45}Ca component might be increasing more under high affinity ^{45}Ca-binding conditions. Similarly, Ca^{2+} uptake after incubation with ^{45}Ca at 0.201 mM extracellular Ca^{2+} concentration is also compared with 1.501 mM extracellular Ca^{2+} concentration (well within the low affinity range). All of these comparisons are included in Table IV. Clearly, the ^{45}Ca slow component uptake is greater than the ^{45}Ca fast component uptake under high affinity Ca^{2+}-binding conditions (0.021 mM Ca^{2+}) and less under low affinity conditions (1.501 mM Ca^{2+}). More pertinent to the intended comparison is the incremental gain in Ca^{2+} uptake over the two concentration ranges. Between Ca^{2+} incubation values of 0.201 mM Ca^{2+} and 0.021 mM Ca^{2+}, the Ca^{2+} uptake increased by 0.279 μmol/g in the adjusted fast component and by 0.663 μmol/g in the slow component. Conversely, between Ca^{2+} incubation values of 0.201 mM Ca^{2+} and 1.501 mM Ca^{2+}, the Ca^{2+} uptake increased by 1.544 μmol/g in the adjusted fast component and by 0.495 μmol/g in the slow component. Thus, increased Ca^{2+} uptake was greater into the slow component fraction in the high affinity Ca^{2+}-binding range and it was greater into the fast component fraction in the low affinity Ca^{2+}-binding range.

SUMMARY

From the experimental results obtained with rabbit aortic smooth muscle and presented in the preceding section, it appears that the slow washout component of the ^{45}Ca desaturation curve includes the major fraction of high affinity Ca^{2+} and the fast ^{45}Ca washout component includes the major portion of low affinity Ca^{2+}. This approximate correspondence between differing Ca^{2+} binding sites and ^{45}Ca desaturation components indicates that component analysis may well have some physical meaning in terms of Ca^{2+} accumulation, binding and loss at specific membrane and/or cellular sites.

By considering the effects of Sr^{2+} and Lu^{3+} on both desaturation curves and Scatchard plot components, we are able to delineate more precise mechanisms of action for these ions. Strontium ion clearly has a specific action on high affinity Ca^{2+}-binding sites and appears to act by displacing Ca^{2+} or competing with Ca^{2+} at these sites. It may also compete to some extent with Ca^{2+} for low

TABLE IV: COMPARISON OF Ca^{2+} DESATURATION COMPONENTS AFTER ^{45}CA INCUBATION UNDER CONDITIONS OF HIGH (0.021 mM), LOW (1.501 mM) AND INTERMEDIATE Ca^{2+} BINDING AFFINITIES[a]

	Incubation Solution Ca^{2+} Concentrations (mM)		
	0.021	0.201	1.501
^{45}Ca T/M Ratio, ml/g	23.133	7.381	2.619
^{45}Ca Slow Component, ml/g (%)	19.709(85.2)	5.359(72.6)	1.048(40.0)
^{45}Ca Fast Component, ml/g (%)	3.424(14.8)	2.022(27.4)	1.571(60.0)
Ca^{2+} Uptake, μmol/g	0.486	1.484	3.931
Fast Component Ca^{2+} Uptake, μmol/g	0.072	0.407	2.359
Adjusted Fast Component Ca^{2+} Uptake, μmol/g[b]	0.065	0.344	1.888
Slow Component Ca^{2+} Uptake, μmol/g	0.414	1.077	1.572
Adjusted Fast Component/ Slow Component	0.157	0.319	1.201

[a] All muscles were incubated with ^{45}Ca plus specified concentrations of nonradioactive Ca^{2+} for 60 min and then washed out in 0-Ca solution; N=4.

[b] Adjusted for extracellular space values of 0.314 ml/g x extracellular Ca^{2+} concentration.

affinity sites but the affinity of Ca^{2+} for these sites is such that, over the appropriate concentration range, Sr^{2+} is not effective. This lack of effect of Sr^{2+} on low affinity sites might provide an alternative explanation of why the K^+-induced contraction is not inhibited by Sr^{2+} to the same degree as is the norepinephrine-induced response (see Weiss, 1977b). Potassium ion may utilize low affinity Ca^{2+}, whereas the action of norepinephrine depends on the presence of high affinity Ca^{2+}. Thus, the high affinity Ca^{2+} corresponds to what has previously (Hinke, 1965; Hudgins and Weiss, 1968; Hiraoka et al., 1968) been termed depletion-resistant Ca^{2+} and the low affinity Ca^{2+} corresponds to more readily depleted Ca^{2+}.

The actions of Lu^{3+} on Scatchard plots of Ca^{2+} uptake are more pronounced than those of Sr^{2+} and indicate that Lu^{3+} inhibits both high and low affinity Ca^{2+}-binding. However, desaturation and rate coefficient plots show that Lu^{3+} does not displace high affinity Ca^{2+} and may act simply by blocking uptake of Ca^{2+} to these sites. The action of Lu^{3+} on low affinity Ca^{2+} is not as clear because this ^{45}Ca component may desaturate and/or exchange very rapidly, but Lu^{3+} may well act in a similar manner at these sites. Previous studies of the effects of Lu^{3+} on ^{45}Ca loss also do not show the presence of any large transient effects (Weiss and Goodman, 1975).

More important than the specific effects of Sr^{2+} and Lu^{3+} are the implications of these findings for drug action on vascular smooth muscle. In all types of muscle, only a very small portion of the Ca^{2+} is actually free in the intracellular compartment (see Bianchi, 1968). Thus, in rabbit aortic smooth muscle, virtually all of the Ca^{2+} is present at either high or low affinity sites - presumably in or on the cell membrane. Drugs which act to increase contractile tone would therefore act by releasing Ca^{2+} (or preventing rebinding of Ca^{2+}) at one or the other (or both) of these sites, whereas inhibitory agents would act by preventing release of Ca^{2+} (or increasing rebinding of Ca^{2+}) at one or the other (or both) of these sites. Thus, these approaches facilitate a more precise definition of the ways in which stimulatory and inhibitory agents act to alter binding and utilization of Ca^{2+} and, in this manner, to regulate vascular smooth muscle contractility.

The mechanisms by which drugs alter Ca^{2+}-related parameters in vascular smooth muscle should, by use of both desaturation curves and Scatchard plots, be characterized in terms of specific effects on affinity of Ca^{2+} for a particular type of binding site and the number of available Ca^{2+} binding sites of each type. This approach is analogous to that employed in recent years for description of drug-receptor interactions. These initial actions of drug molecules are delineated in terms of affinities for receptor sites and of intrinsic activities as measures of relative abilities to elicit responses. The usefulness of these concepts in characterization of drug-receptor interactions is particularly important when considering agents which elicit intermediate effects (e.g., effects of weak or partial agonists). Thus, these concepts have facilitated viewing of the results of actions of various drugs on a particular receptor as yielding a spectrum of possible effects rather than as "all-or-none" stimulatory or inhibitory effects. In a similar manner, the drug-receptor interaction might be viewed as initiating a series of responses (termed excitation-contraction coupling) which include modifications of affinity of Ca^{2+} for binding sites and changes in the number of available Ca^{2+} sites. These Ca^{2+}-related effects might well be as important determinants of the degree of eventual muscle contractile or relaxant response as is the initial drug-receptor interaction. Increased efforts to qualitatively and quantitatively delineate the alterations in Ca^{2+} affinity and binding sites elicited with various stimulatory and inhibitory drugs represent an important direction for future research in this field and these efforts should be extended to include characterization of drug-Ca^{2+} interactions in other types of smooth muscle.

Acknowledgements

Experimental work from this laboratory was supported by National Institutes of Health Grant HL 14775.

REFERENCES

Barela, T. D., Burchett, S., and Kizer, D. E., 1976, Terbium as a molecular probe of magnesium binding to ribosomes and ribosomal RNA, *Proc. 12th Rare Earth Conf.* 1: 223.

Bianchi, C. P., 1965, The effect of EDTA and SCN on radiocalcium movement in frog rectus abdominis muscle during contractures induced by calcium removal, *J. Pharmacol. Exp. Ther.* 147: 360.

Bianchi, C. P., 1968, "Cell Calcium," Butterworths, London.

Bohr, D. F., 1964, Contraction of vascular smooth muscle, *Can. Med. Assoc. J.* 90: 174.

Daniel, E. E., 1965, Attempted synthesis of data regarding divalent ions in muscle function, *in* "Muscle" (W. M. Paul, E. E. Daniel, C. M. Kay, and G. Monckton, eds.), pp. 295-313, Pergamon Press, New York.

Hinke, J. A. M., 1965, Calcium requirements for noradrenaline and high potassium ion concentration in arterial smooth muscle, *in* "Muscle" (W. M. Paul, E. E. Daniel, C. M. Kay, and G. Monckton, eds.), pp. 269-284, Pergamon Press, New York.

Hiraoka, M., Yamagishi, S., and Sano, T., 1968, Role of calcium ions in the contraction of vascular smooth muscle, *Amer. J. Physiol.* 214: 1084.

Hudgins, P. M., 1969, Some drug effects on calcium movements in aortic strips, *J. Pharmacol. Exp. Ther.* 170: 303.

Hudgins, P. M., and Weiss, G. B., 1968, Differential effects of calcium removal upon vascular smooth muscle contraction induced by norepinephrine, histamine and potassium, *J. Pharmacol. Exp. Ther.* 159: 91.

Hudgins, P. M., and Weiss, G. B., 1969a, Characteristics of ^{45}Ca binding in vascular smooth muscle, *Amer. J. Physiol.* 217: 1310.

Hudgins, P. M., and Weiss, G. B., 1969b, Effects of Ba, Sr and stimulatory agents on Ca movements and contraction in vascular smooth muscle, *Fed. Proc.* 28: 541.

Ishiyama, Y., Yabu, H., and Miyazaki, E., 1975, Changes in contractility and calcium binding of guinea pig taenia coli by treatment with enzymes which hydrolyze sialic acid, *Jpn. J. Physiol.* 25: 719.

Sandow, A., 1965, Excitation-contraction coupling in skeletal muscle, *Pharmacol. Rev.* 17: 265.

Scatchard, G., 1949, The attractions of proteins for small molecules and ions, *Ann. N.Y. Acad. Sci.* 51: 660.

Shanes, A. M., and Bianchi, C. P., 1959, The distribution and kinetics of release of radiocalcium in tendon and skeletal muscle, *J. gen. Physiol.* 42: 1123.

Weiss, G. B., 1966, The effects of potassium on nicotine-induced contracture and Ca^{45} movements in frog sartorius muscle, *J. Pharmacol. Exp. Ther.* 154: 595.

Weiss, G. B., 1977a, Calcium and contractility in vascular smooth muscle, *in* "Adv. Gen. Cell. Pharmacol." (T. Narahashi and C. P. Bianchi, eds.) Vol. 2, pp. 71-154, Plenum Press, New York.

Weiss, G. B., 1977b, Approaches to delineation of differing calcium binding sites in smooth muscle, *in* "Excitation-Contraction Coupling in Smooth Muscle" (R. Casteels, T. Godfraind, and J. C. Ruegg, eds.) pp. 253-260, Elsevier/North Holland Biomedical Press, Amsterdam.

Weiss, G. B., and Goodman, F. R., 1975, Interactions between several rare earth ions and calcium ion in vascular smooth muscle, *J. Pharmacol. Exp. Ther.* 195: 557.

CHAPTER 4

CALCIUM IN SMOOTH MUSCLE FUNCTION

Leon Hurwitz and Linda J. McGuffee

Department of Pharmacology
School of Medicine
University of New Mexico
Albuquerque, New Mexico 87131

INTRODUCTION

In smooth muscle (Prosser, 1974; Hurwitz and Suria, 1971; Somlyo and Somlyo, 1968), as in other types of muscle (Fuchs, 1974; Langer, 1968; Sandow, 1965), calcium is considered to be the agent that activates the contractile apparatus. Consequently, the cellular structures and reactions which act to regulate the concentration of Ca^{2+} available to the contractile proteins play a vital role in the contraction-relaxation cycle in smooth muscle cells. In the discussion which follows, major emphasis will be placed on those aspects of smooth muscle function which control the movements of Ca^{2+} in the cell. The first part of this chapter will be devoted to a brief overview of the excitation-contraction coupling mechanism which is assumed to operate during a drug or neurohormone-induced contractile response. The remainder of the chapter will deal more specifically with some of the characteristics of the transport system that facilitates the entry of Ca^{2+} into the cytoplasmic matrix and with the interaction between this system and other cellular processes associated with contraction in the smooth muscle cell.

CALCIUM MOVEMENTS DURING DRUG-INDUCED MECHANICAL ACTIVITY

A smooth muscle contraction induced by an excitatory agent, such as acetylcholine or norepinephrine, is considered to be the end result of a series of cellular reactions and processes. The initial reaction in the series consists, in most cases, of a rapid reversible interaction between the excitatory agent and

specific tissue receptors located in the plasma membrane of the
smooth muscle cell (Hurwitz and Suria, 1971; Triggle, 1971; Waud,
1968).   Based on current evidence (Hurwitz, 1975; Hurwitz and
Suria, 1971; Hurwitz and Joiner, 1970; Hurwitz and Joiner, 1969),
it is not unreasonable to view the interaction between the excitatory drug and the specific tissue receptors as providing the
stimulus which activates some sort of membrane transport or membrane releasing system or both.   The activated transport (or
releasing) system promotes the flow of Ca^{2+} from intra- and/or
extracellular storage depots into the cytoplasmic matrix.   As a
result the concentration of free Ca^{2+} in the vicinity of the
contractile proteins is increased.   These ions can then bind
reversibly to specific sites on the contractile proteins and,
thereby, initiate a mechanical response.

When the excitatory drug is withdrawn from the vicinity of
the smooth muscle, the flow of Ca^{2+} into the cytoplasm is substantially reduced and the contracted cells begin to relax.   Relaxation is thought to be initiated by the removal of free Ca^{2+}
from the cytoplasm (Prosser, 1974).   A gradual reduction in the
level of these divalent ions is accompanied by a gradual dissociation of Ca^{2+} from contractile elements and by a gradual diminution
in the capacity of the contractile elements to maintain tension.
Removal of the free cytoplasmic Ca^{2+} is presumably accomplished
by a metabolically dependent calcium pump located in the plasma
membrane and/or the membranes of intracellular organelles (Batra,
1973; Hurwitz *et al.*, 1973; Andersson, 1972; Andersson and
Nilsson, 1972; Fitzpatrick *et al.*, 1972; Carsten, 1969).   The pump
transports the divalent ions from the cytoplasm to sites where
these ions are sequestered or to the external medium (Batra, 1973;
Hurwitz *et al.*, 1973; Andersson, 1972; Fitzpatrick *et al.*, 1972;
Carsten, 1969).

From the above considerations it is reasonable to infer that
both the rate of inward flow or release of Ca^{2+} (from extra- or
intracellular calcium stores) initiated by the agonist, and the
simultaneous rate of removal of free cytoplasmic Ca^{2+} by the
energy linked calcium pump play an important role in determining
the final concentration of Ca^{2+} in the cytoplasmic matrix.   Since
these ions enter into a reversible interaction with specific
contractile proteins of the muscle cell, their concentration in
the cytoplasmic matrix will determine the extent to which they
complex the contractile proteins and elicit the mechanical response.
One may assume, therefore, that the concentration of the free Ca^{2+}
in the cytoplasmic matrix and, more indirectly, the rate at which
the calcium transport system delivers Ca^{2+} to the cytoplasmic
matrix serve as important determinants of the magnitude of the
mechanical response.

Different types of smooth muscle differ widely in their mechanical responses to an excitatory agent. Some smooth muscles respond to an agonist by undergoing rapid increases in tension (or rapid decreases in length) which come to a sharp peak and then within a short period of time return to their initial or very close to their initial levels of tension. Depending on the type of smooth muscle under consideration, the agonist may elicit either one or a train of these responses. At the other extreme, a smooth muscle such as the rat trachea responds to an agonist by undergoing a slow steady increase in tension until some particular level is reached. This level of tension is then reasonably well maintained until the agonist is withdrawn from the bathing medium. Others such as the longitudinal muscle of guinea pig ileum exhibit various degrees of both types of responses. These intricate patterns of response presumably reflect the complex dynamics that characterize the rate of movement of Ca^{2+} into the cytoplasmic matrix from several different calcium depots in the smooth muscle cell. They may also reflect complex dynamics that operate in the removal of free Ca^{2+} from the cytoplasm to various reservoirs by ATP-dependent calcium pumps. In those instances in which a well maintained submaximal contraction is established by some given concentration of agonist, the level of Ca^{2+} attained in the cytoplasmic matrix may be thought of as having reached a steady state level. That is to say, the rate of movement of Ca^{2+} into the cytoplasmic matrix is equal to its rate of removal from the cytoplasmic matrix.

SOURCES AND SINKS OF ACTIVATOR CALCIUM

A factor which is considered to have an important influence on the mechanical response in smooth muscle is the location(s) of the depot(s) from which an agonist mobilizes Ca^{2+} for contraction. Based on evidence from physiological studies (Hurwitz and Suria, 1971; Hudgins and Weiss, 1968; Hinke, 1965) in which various types of smooth muscle were examined, it would appear that at least two different mobilizable depots of Ca^{2+} exist in smooth muscle. One is a pool of Ca^{2+} that is present in the extracellular fluid or that is loosely bound to superficial sites in the muscle cell; the other is a tightly bound pool of Ca^{2+} that is presumed to be sequestered in some intracellular location (or locations) in the muscle fiber.

The finding that intracellular as well as extracellular or superficial sites may store the ions that are mobilized to activate the contractile machinery does not imply that both these sites play equally important physiological roles in all types of smooth muscles. In some smooth muscles, such as that found in the main pulmonary artery of the rabbit (Devine *et al.*, 1972) or

the rabbit aorta (Devine *et al.*, 1972; Hudgins and Weiss, 1968),
a firmly bound intracellular pool of Ca^{2+} appears to support
mechanical activity to a significant degree; in others, such as
that found in the taenia coli of the guinea pig (McGuffee and
Bagby, 1976), it is much less supportive; and in still others,
such as the longitudinal muscle of the guinea pig ileum (Hurwitz
and Joiner, 1970), a firmly bound pool of Ca^{2+} plays a negligible
role in mechanical activity.

While it may be reasonable to assume that the plasma membrane
is the site of at least part of the loosely bound pool, the locations of firmly held or sequestered Ca^{2+} is less obvious (Hurwitz
and Suria, 1971). With regard to the latter question, extensive
efforts have been made to find intracellular concentrations of
Ca^{2+} using both physiological and morphological techniques. The
application of physiological techniques has uncovered energy
dependent calcium concentrating systems in mitochondrial (Batra,
1973; Fitzpatrick *et al.*, 1972) and microsomal (Hurwitz *et al.*,
1973; Carsten, 1969) preparations from smooth muscle. These
findings suggest a possible role for mitochondria, sarcoplasmic
reticulum (SR) and/or plasma membrane as Ca^{2+} sequestering
structures which induce relaxation of smooth muscle *in vivo*.
They also introduce the possibility that these structures may
function as sites from which activator Ca^{2+} can be mobilized for
contraction. It should be emphasized, however, that Ca^{2+} uptake
by isolated subcellular fractions offers only suggestive evidence
that the organelles included in these fractions serve as sinks
for or sources of activator Ca^{2+} *in vivo*.

If areas of Ca^{2+} concentration in smooth muscle could be
viewed directly, this would serve to delineate sites where activator Ca^{2+} may possibly be stored. The simplest way to localize
intracellular areas of Ca^{2+} concentration would be to view the
Ca^{2+} pools with the electron microscope. Unfortunately, within
the physiological range of Ca^{2+} concentrations found in smooth
muscle, Ca^{2+} is not very electron opaque and cannot, therefore,
be seen in the electron microscope. However, a variety of
electron microscopic techniques have been employed in an attempt
to make the sites of Ca^{2+} sequestration visible. These methods
include precipitation of Ca^{2+} as electron opaque calcium salts
(Debbas *et al.*, 1975; Popescu and Diculescu, 1975; Jonas and
Zelck, 1974; Heumann, 1969), substitution of a more electron
opaque cation for Ca^{2+} (Somlyo *et al.*, 1974; Somlyo and Somlyo,
1971; Peachey, 1964), electron probe x-ray analysis (Somlyo *et al.*,
1974) and ^{45}Ca autoradiography (McGuffee and Bagby, 1976). While
these techniques do not disclose the physiological role of the
Ca^{2+} found in association with a given site, they do indicate
which cellular structures have the capacity to accumulate Ca^{2+}.
These studies have implicated the structures of the smooth muscle

cell illustrated in Figure 1. They include SR, mitochondria and
plasma membrane as possible sequestration sites for Ca^{2+}. However,
the pattern of distribution of Ca^{2+} among these sites was found
to vary considerably depending on the technique used (McGuffee
and Bagby, 1976; Debbas *et al.*, 1975; Popescu and Diculescu, 1975;
Jonas and Zelck, 1974; Somlyo *et al.*, 1974; Somlyo and Somlyo, 1971;
Heumann, 1969; Peachey, 1964). At least part of this variability
in distribution may be related to the fact that all of these
findings were made in tissues which have been dehydrated, fixed
and embedded using conventional electron microscopic techniques.
It is well established that diffusible substances may possibly be
translocated or removed from tissue during these procedures
(Appleton, 1974; Christensen, 1969; Stumpf and Roth, 1969;
Stirling and Kinter, 1967). For this reason the distribution of
electron opacities or developed ^{45}Ca grains observed in the studies
discussed above may not reflect the *in vivo* distribution of Ca^{2+}.
Freeze drying of tissue sections has been used successfully in
an effort to minimize the movement of diffusible substances in
tissues such as hamster intestine (Stirling and Kinter, 1967)
and rat liver and pancreas (Christensen, 1971). The feasibility
of using this technique to study the intracellular distribution
of Ca^{2+} in smooth muscle is currently under examination in
several laboratories.

MODES OF CALCIUM MOBILIZATION

Not only are there multiple stores of Ca^{2+} in smooth muscle
cells, but the capacity of different agonists to mobilize Ca^{2+}
from these stores varies. In addition, the mechanism by which
agonists mobilize Ca^{2+} from different stores appears to vary.
Results of studies, using vascular and nonvascular types of
smooth muscle, have suggested that membrane depolarization, be
it drug-induced or not, is associated with the mobilization predominantly of extracellular or loosely bound Ca^{2+} (Hiraoka *et al.*,
1968; Hudgins and Weiss, 1968; Jhamandas and Nash, 1967; Van
Breemen and Daniel, 1966, Daniel, 1965, Hinke, 1965; Hinke *et al.*,
1964). However, a change in membrane potential is not a prerequi-
site for the development of tension in all smooth muscles (Falk
and Landa, 1960). Norepinephrine, for example, can induce a
contraction without depolarization in the pulmonary artery of the
rabbit (Su *et al.*, 1964). This would suggest that the norepinephrine is capable of mobilizing Ca^{2+}, presumably from an intracellular site, in a manner that is independent of membrane depolarization. A voltage-independent mechanism may also operate to mobilize
calcium from extracellular pools. To complicate the matter even
further, the Ca^{2+} pools utilized for contraction may vary from
species to species. For example, the rat aorta relies to a greater
extent on extracellular Ca^{2+} than does the rabbit aorta (Krishna-

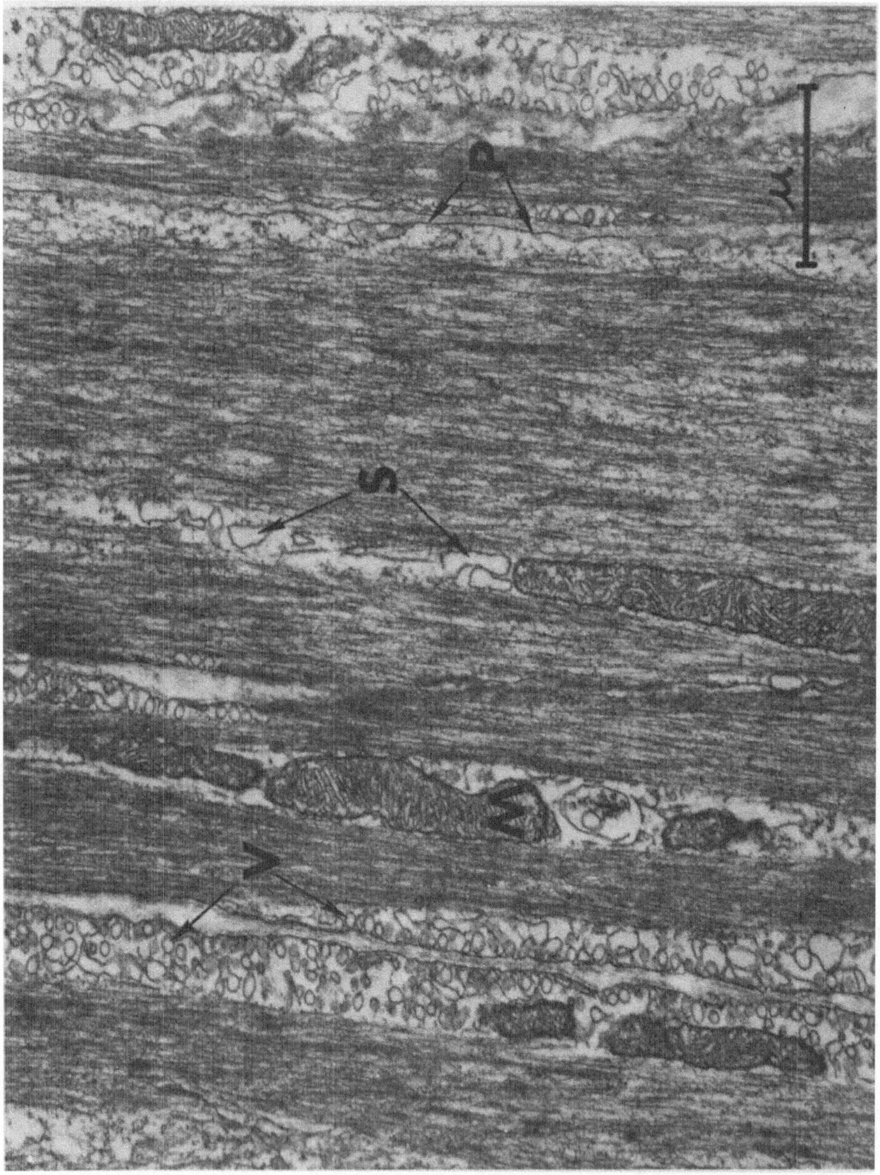

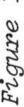

Figure 1

Figure 1. A longitudinal section through the longitudinal muscle of the guinea pig ileum as viewed through the electron microscope. Sarcoplasmic reticulum (S) and mitochondrian (M) are found within the cells. Surface vesicles (V) which are invaginations of the plasma membrane occur in clusters along the plasma membrane (P). The tissue was fixed in osmium tetroxide vapor, dehydrated in acetones and embedded in Araldite. After sectioning, the tissue was stained with uranyl acetate and post stained with Reynold's lead citrate.

murty and Grollman, 1976). Thus, it is extremely difficult to generalize about the manner in which an agonist mobilizes Ca^{2+} or about the source from which it mobilizes these ions in various types of smooth muscle cells.

SOME CHARACTERISTICS OF THE CALCIUM TRANSPORT SYSTEM

Whether or not membrane depolarization is an intermediate step in the action of an agonist, the end result is the activation of a calcium transport or releasing system which promotes the entry of Ca^{2+} into the cytoplasmic matrix of the smooth muscle cell. In view of the indispensible role played by this transport system a knowledge of its basic characteristics and of its interrelationship with the agonist-receptor complex is essential to a thorough understanding of smooth muscle function. Although the basic characteristics of the calcium transport system (or systems) in smooth muscle has not, as yet, been clearly elucidated, some of its properties may be inferred from experimental data that is currently available. These data lead to the suggestion that the calcium transport (or releasing) system in a smooth muscle consists of a finite number of specialized regions that are present within various membranes of the cell (Hurwitz *et al.*, 1972). One series of experiments which demonstrates this concept involves an interaction between Cd^{2+} and Mn^{2+} in the isolated longitudinal muscle from the guinea pig ileum. Triggle *et al.* (1975) have shown that the longitudinal muscle immersed in a calcium-free medium will take up Cd^{2+} ions in the presence of the ionophore, A23187. The uptake of cadmium ion into the muscle cell is accompanied by a smooth, slowly developing, increase in muscle tension. Whether this increase in tension is induced by the displacement of intracellularly bound Ca^{2+} by the Cd^{2+} or by a direct interaction between Cd^{2+} and the contractile proteins could not be determined from these data.

Uptake of Cd^{2+} into the longitudinal muscle can also be achieved without the use of an ionophore (Imai and Takeda, 1967; Hurwitz and McGuffee, unpublished observations). It is accomplished by introducing a higher concentration of Cd^{2+} than that employed by Triggle *et al.* (1975) (from 1.8×10^{-3}M to 1×10^{-2}M) and by allowing a longer period of time for the divalent ions to build up a sufficient intracellular concentration to produce an increase in muscle tension. The slow increase in muscle tension that develops under these conditions is illustrated in Figure 2-a. If, however, 1×10^{-5}M acetylcholine is added to the Ca^{2+}-free medium in which the longitudinal muscle is immersed, the subsequent addition of 1×10^{-2}M Cd^{2+} to the bathing solution will lead to a much more rapid increase in the rate of development of tension. This finding is illustrated in Figure 2-b. The obvious inference is that acetylcholine induced a sharp increase in the rate of entry of Cd^{2+} into the longitudinal muscle cells. Moreover, as shown by the record presented in Figure 2-c, the introduction of 5×10^{-3}M Mn^{2+} will inhibit the rapid rate of entry of Cd^{2+} induced by acetylcholine but will not affect the rate of entry of Cd^{2+} which occurs in the absence of the cholinergic agent (Figure 2-d).

Based on these experimental findings, it would seem that Cd^{2+} can move across the plasma membrane of the longitudinal muscle by at least two different pathways. One does not require the presence of acetylcholine to become functional, the other becomes available for the transport of Cd^{2+} only when it is acted upon by acetylcholine (and presumably other excitatory agents). Manganese ion, which can block Ca^{2+} influx in smooth muscle (Osa, 1974; Prosser, 1974; Nonomura *et al.*, 1966), preferentially blocked the movement of Cd^{2+} that was coupled to the acetylcholine. This effect cannot be attributed to a blockade of cholinergic receptors. It is more likely the consequence of a blockade of specific sites or channels which permit the passage of Cd^{2+} across the smooth muscle membrane. Thus, the results obtained in these experiments appear to support the concept that the cholinergic agonist modifies selective areas of the membrane which are associated with the rapid transport of divalent ions, such as Ca^{2+} or Cd^{2+}, across the cell membrane.

A limited amount of information pertaining to the mode of operation of these specialized areas is also available. It is well known that substances may traverse biological membranes by a number of different mechanisms. Among these are the free diffusion of a substance down an electrochemical gradient through membrane pores, the transport of a substance down an electrochemical gradient via carrier molecules, the transport of a substance against an electrochemical gradient via a metabolically-dependent pump, etc. The manner in which the calcium transport system of the longitudinal muscle of guinea pig ileum moves Ca^{2+} into the cytoplasmic matrix is partially characterized by the data illustrated in Figure 3 (Hurwitz and Weissinger, unpublished

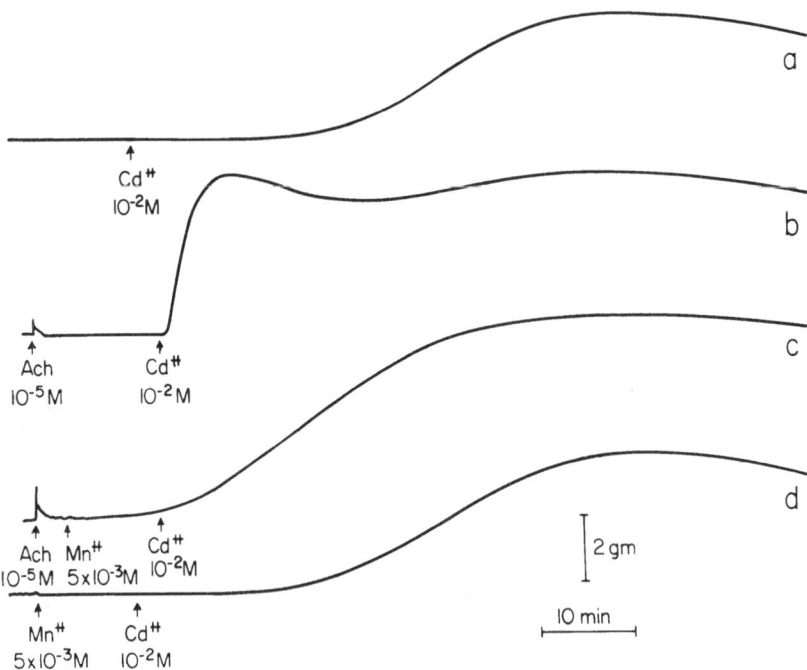

Figure 2. Cd^{2+}-induced contractions in the longitudinal muscle from guinea pig ileum immersed in a Ca^{2+}-free bathing medium. See text for further explanation. Ach = Acetylcholine.

observations). Figure 3 contains a series of dose-response curves in which the inverse of the magnitudes of a number of isometric contractile responses are plotted against the inverse of the extracellular Ca^{2+} concentration. Each of the three curves in the figure was generated by using a different acetylcholine concentration to initiate the response. In every case the experimental data showed that the magnitude of contraction in the ileal muscle varies as a hyperbolic function of the Ca^{2+} concentration in the extracellular medium. This relationship was then converted to the linear form shown in Figure 3 by plotting the data on a reciprocal plot.

Two characteristics of these dose-response curves are pertinent. First, the configurations of all three curves in the figure have an obvious resemblance to that of a simple saturation curve. Second, in at least two of the three curves, the saturation effect obtained cannot be attributed to a limitation in the capacity of the ileal muscle to develop a larger contraction. These experimental findings favor the suggestion that an acetylcholine-induced

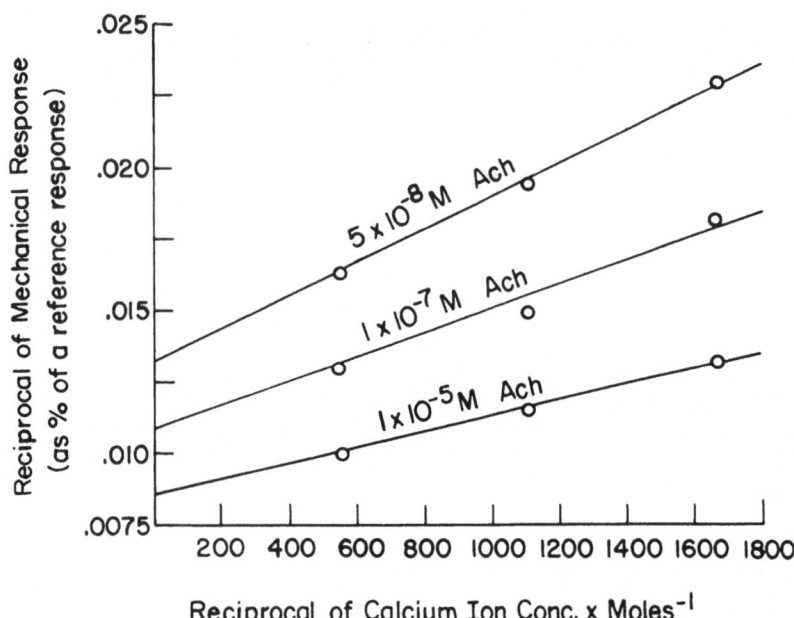

Figure 3. *Dose-response relationships representing the reciprocal of peak isometric tension versus the reciprocal of the extracellular Ca^{2+} concentration. Each of the three dose-response curves were obtained by employing the acetylcholine concentration shown in the figure. The smooth muscle preparation used in these experiments was the longitudinal muscle isolated from the guinea pig ileum.*

mechanical response of the ileal muscle is some function of a reversible complex that is formed between Ca^{2+} and a cellular component. Furthermore, this cellular component must necessarily be present in the muscle cell in some finite quantity. Previous work had indicated that the Ca^{2+} which can be mobilized for contraction in this longitudinal muscle came primarily from loosely held cellular stores and from the extracellular medium (Hurwitz and Joiner, 1970). These observations enhance the likelihood that the complex which appears to govern the magnitude of the mechanical response is made up of Ca^{2+} and units of the calcium transport system. The precise nature of the calcium transport system is not known. Consequently, one cannot say whether the formation of the complex involves the requisite adsorption of Ca^{2+} to the surface of membrane pores before these ions can diffuse across the membrane, an interaction between Ca^{2+} and carrier molecules which ferry the divalent ions across the membrane, an interaction between Ca^{2+} and some membrane component which can then release the divalent ions into the cytoplasmic matrix, or some other possible mechanism. In any case, the transport or release of Ca^{2+} into the cytoplasmic matrix during a smooth muscle contraction does not appear to involve the simple diffusion of the divalent ions through calcium channels.

An additional feature of the calcium transport system relates to the manner in which it is coupled to the agonist-receptor complex. In fast twitch striated muscle fibers the interaction between cholinergic receptors and agonist molecules does not elicit a mechanical response until the number of receptors complexed with the agonist is large enough to reach a threshold level (Woodbury et al., 1965). Moreover, the response elicited at threshold is not altered by inducing the formation of agonist-receptor complexes in excess of those needed to reach threshold (Woodbury, 1965). In many smooth muscle cells the situation appears to be quite different. The magnitude of the contractile response varies in a graded fashion with the number of receptors that interact with the agonist (Waud, 1968). As mentioned earlier, it also varies with the rate of entry of free calcium ions into the cytoplasmic matrix. Thus, one could surmise that variations in the extracellular concentration of the agonist will induce graded changes in the level of activation of the calcium transport system.

It is not yet possible to propose a model which would account for graded increases in the activation of the calcium transport system that presumably occur with incremental increases in the concentration of an agonist. One could speculate that the progressive saturation of the tissue receptors with molecules of agonist will lead ultimately to the conversion of an increasingly greater percentage of calcium transport or releasing sites from a nonfunctional to a functional state. Alternatively, an increase in the level of saturation of the tissue receptors could possibly raise all individual units of the calcium transport or releasing system from a lower to a higher functional level. In the latter case, one could view each individual calcium transport site as being some sort of carrier with a capacity, upon stimulation, to undergo an increase in turnover number. Either of these mechanisms or variations thereof would result in graded increases in Ca^{2+} movement in response to incremental increases in the concentration of the agonist.

The central point of the preceding discussion is the contention that a drug-induced shift of Ca^{2+} from storage sites to cytoplasmic matrix is carried out by a finite number of specialized areas that exist in various cellular membranes of smooth muscle cells. These calcium transport sites are normally nonfunctional unless they are made operational by two independent cellular reactions. One of these reactions involves a stepwise activation

of the calcium transport sites which is achieved in some unknown
manner by the interaction of an excitatory agent with specific
tissue receptors. The other involves the formation of a reversible complex between the Ca^{2+} present in storage depots and the
activated calcium transport sites. The rate of entry of free Ca^{2+}
into the cytoplasmic matrix and, ultimately, the magnitude of the
mechanical response, is dependent upon the percent of the total
number of calcium transport sites that have participated in both
types of activating cellular reactions. This relationship may be
represented in the following manner:

$$[\text{Response}] = f\left[s \cdot \frac{T_A}{T_M} \right] \qquad (1)$$

where [Response] refers to the magnitude of the muscle contraction,
s is a quantity which can vary from 0 to 1 and indicates the level
to which the calcium transport system is saturated (complexed)
with the Ca^{2+} , $T_M = 1$ and represents the maximum level to which
the calcium transport system can be stimulated by an infinitely
high concentration of an agonist, T_A is some value, usually less
than 1, such that T_A/T_M equals the fraction of the total transport
system that has been stimulated by some given concentration of an
agonist, and f refers to some complex function which relates the
magnitude of contraction to the fraction of calcium transport sites
that are actively engaged in moving Ca^{2+} into the cytoplasmic
matrix.

One may assume, as a first approximation, that the interaction
between Ca^{2+} and transport or releasing sites obeys simple saturation kinetics. The evidence for this assumption may be found in
Figure 3 where all three dose-response curves are seen to have the
typical configuration of a simple saturation curve. Thus, the expression which represents the relationship between the fractional
level of saturation of the calcium transport system, s, and the
extracellular Ca^{2+} concentration may be written as:

$$s = \frac{Ca_O}{K_c + Ca_O} \qquad (2)$$

where Ca_O is the extracellular Ca^{2+} concentration, and K_c is the
concentration of extracellular calcium at which the activated
transport system is at half maximal saturation, i. e., s = 0.5.
One could view the K_c as being an apparent dissociation constant
for the calcium-transport site complex that is formed. Because
the concentration of Ca^{2+} in the extracellular medium may be only
indirectly related to the actual Ca^{2+} concentration in immediate
contact with the transport or releasing system, K_c cannot be

considered a true dissociation constant. Nevertheless, it does denote the extracellular Ca^{2+} concentration at which the transport system is at half maximal saturation. By replacing s in equation 1 with its equivalent in equation 2 one obtains the expression:

$$[\text{Response}] = f \frac{T_A/T_M \ Ca_0}{K_c + Ca_0} \qquad (3)$$

This equation which relates the interaction between Ca^{2+} and calcium transport sites to the contractile response of the muscle has the same form as the well known equation (Response $= f \frac{\alpha \ R_T \ D)}{K_D + D}$ which relates the interaction between agonist molecules (D) and tissue receptors (R_T) to the contractile response.

For many years, considerable interest has been shown in the chemical characteristics of tissue receptors and in their affinities for various types of agonists and antagonists. The strong probability that a second distinct population of loci, namely the calcium transport sites, must combine reversibly with Ca^{2+} to produce a physiological response fosters a similar interest in these loci. As in the case with tissue receptors, it would be advantageous to obtain a quantitative determination of the extracellular concentration of the reactant, which in this instance is Ca^{2+}, that induces 50% saturation of the transport sites. This may be done by employing a method that is analogous to the one designed by Furchgott and co-workers (Furchgott and Bursztyn, 1967; Furchgott, 1966) for the determination of the dissociation constant for an agonist-receptor complex.

Furchgott and co-workers (Furchgott and Bursztyn, 1967; Furchgott, 1966) were able to estimate the dissociation constant (K_D) for the agonist-receptor complex by a procedure which necessitated performing control experiments and experiments in which the total population of active receptors (R_T) was reduced by introducing the poorly reversible inhibitor, dibenamine. Using a similar procedure in which the total population of activated calcium transport sites (T_A/T_M) was reduced by employing an agonist concentration that was lower than that used in control experiments, we were able to determine the dissociation constant or apparent dissociation constant (K_c) for the calcium-transport site complex.

In the acetylcholine-stimulated transport system of the longitudinal muscle from guinea pig ileum the K_c was found to be 8.2×10^{-4}M (Hurwitz and Weissinger, unpublished observations). In the norepinephrine stimulated transport system of the rabbit aorta, it was found to be 5×10^{-5}M (Hurwitz, unpublished observations). The difference in the relative affinities of the transport systems for Ca^{2+} in these two muscles suggest that calcium transport sites in various types of smooth muscle cells may differ widely in their basic physical-chemical properties.

INTERACTIONS AMONG CALCIUM TRANSPORT SYSTEM, MECHANICAL RESPONSE AND AGONIST-RECEPTOR COMPLEX

The determination of K_c also reveals the relationship that exists between the degree of saturation of the calcium transport system and the mechanical response. In the longitudinal muscle, when $1 \times 10^{-5}M$ acetylcholine was used to elicit the response, an extracellular concentration of Ca^{2+} which led to half maximal saturation of transport sites induced a contraction that was 69% of maximum. A similar nonlinear relationship was observed in the rabbit aorta. In the presence of $4.0 \times 10^{-6}M$ norepinephrine, half maximal saturation of the transport sites induced a contraction that was 82% of maximum. Previous work had suggested that the contractile response in smooth muscle may not be a linear function of the percent of total tissue receptors occupied by agonist molecules. The occupation of a relatively small percentage of the receptors often appears to be sufficient to generate a near maximal contraction (Nickerson, 1956). This concept is reinforced by the finding that a nonlinear relationship may also exist between the contractile response and the percent of total transport sites that complex with Ca^{2+}.

In addition, with the information presently available (Hurwitz, unpublished observations), it is possible to calculate the level of activation of the calcium transport system produced by various concentrations of the agonist-receptor complex. Here again a lack of proportionality appears to exist in the longitudinal muscle and to a lesser extent in the aortic muscle. For example, calculations made from the data in Figure 3 indicate that a concentration of $1 \times 10^{-8}M$ acetylcholine will activate 14.9% of the calcium transport or releasing sites in the longitudinal muscle. Data reported in the literature indicate that $1 \times 10^{-8}M$ acetylcholine will occupy one percent or less of the total cholinergic receptor population in this muscle (Sastry and Cheng, 1972; Rico, 1971). Thus it appears that in the longitudinal muscle the occupation of a very small percentage of the receptor population by an agonist is sufficient to activate a comparatively large fraction of the calcium transport sites. These findings negate speculations which picture the tissue receptor as being directly coupled to the calcium transport site on a one to one basis. One would anticipate that future research will probably uncover a complex coupling mechanism between these two components in the smooth muscle membrane.

SUMMARY

The observations that have been made to date would suggest that smooth muscle cells contain a finite population (or populations) of membrane sites which, upon activation, facilitate the flow of Ca^{2+} from calcium depots to the cytoplasmic matrix. The calcium transport sites may be located in the plasma membrane as well as in the membranes of intracellular organelles such as sarcoplasmic reticulum and mitochondria. Activation of the calcium transport sites may be accomplished by an interaction between agonist molecules and specific tissue receptors which seem to be linked to the transport sites in some complex fashion. The increase in calcium conductance which results from the activation of the transport sites is in many instances a graded response. Its level is related to the percent of tissue receptors that have interacted with the agonist. Moreover, it would appear that the transport of Ca^{2+} by these activated sites must be preceded by the formation of a reversible complex between the calcium transport sites and the calcium ions that are to be transported. Alternately, the activated calcium transport sites may consist of open channels which permit single file movement of calcium ions across the membrane into the cytoplasmic matrix where they elicit a contraction. In any case, the rate at which calcium ions enter the cytoplasmic matrix is governed by at least two factors. One is the degree to which the calcium transport sites have been activated by the agonist-receptor complex. The other is the degree to which the activated sites interact with Ca^{2+}. The rate of entry of Ca^{2+} into the cytoplasmic matrix constitutes one of the important factors which controls the level of accumulation of free Ca^{2+} in the immediate vicinity of the contractile apparatus. It is, therefore, a key determinant of the magnitude of the contraction which a smooth muscle cell develops in response to an excitatory drug.

Acknowledgements

This work was supported by National Institutes of Health Grant HL 16179.

REFERENCES

Andersson, R., 1972, Cyclic AMP and calcium ions in mechanical and metabolic responses of smooth muscles; influence of some hormones and drugs, *Acta Physiol. Scand. Suppl.* 382: 1.
Andersson, R., and Nilsson, K., 1972, Cyclic AMP and calcium in relaxation in intestinal smooth muscle, *Nature, New Biol.* 238: 119.

Appleton, T. C., 1974, A cryostat approach to ultrathin 'dry' frozen sections for electron microscopy: a morphological and x-ray analytical study, *J. Microsc.* 100: 49.

Batra, S. C., 1973, The role of mitochondrial calcium uptake in contraction and relaxation of the human myometrium, *Biochim. Biophys. Acta* 305: 428.

Carsten, M. E., 1969, Role of calcium binding by sarcoplasmic reticulum in the contraction and relaxation of uterine smooth muscle, *J. gen. Physiol.* 53: 414.

Christensen, A. K., 1969, A way to prepare frozen thin sections of fresh tissue for electron microscopy, *in* "Autoradiography of Diffusible Substances" (L. J. Roth and W. E. Stumpf, eds.), pp. 349-362, Academic Press, New York.

Christensen, A. K., 1971, Frozen thin sections of fresh tissue for electron microscopy, with a description of pancreas and liver, *J. Cell Biol.* 51: 772.

Daniel, E. E., 1965, Attempted synthesis of data regarding divalent ions in muscle function, *in* "Muscle" (W. M. Paul, E. E. Daniel, C. M. Kay, and G. Monckton, eds.), pp. 295-313, Pergamon Press, New York.

Debbas, G., Hoffman, L., Landon, E. J., and Hurwitz, L., 1975, Electron microscopic localization of calcium in vascular smooth muscle, *Anat. Rec.* 182: 447.

Devine, C. E., Somlyo, A. V., and Somlyo, A. P., 1972, Sarcoplasmic reticulum and excitation-contraction coupling in mammalian smooth muscles, *J. Cell Biol.* 52: 690.

Falk, G., and Landa, J. F., 1960, Mode of action of drugs on depolarized smooth muscle, *Pharmacologist* 2: 69.

Fitzpatrick, D. F., Landon, E. J., Debbas, G., and Hurwitz, L., 1972, A calcium pump in vascular smooth muscle, *Science* 176: 305.

Fuchs, F., 1974, Striated muscle, *Annu. Rev. Physiol.* 36: 461.

Furchgott, R. F., 1966, The use of β-halo-alkylamines in the differentiation of receptors and in the determination of dissociation constants of receptor-agonist complexes, *Adv. Drug Res.* 3: 21.

Furchgott, R. F., and Bursztyn, P., 1967, Comparison of dissociation constants and of relative efficacies of selected agonists acting on parasympathetic receptors, *Ann. N.Y. Acad. Sci.* 144: 882.

Heumann, H. G., 1969, Calciummakkumulierende strukturen in einen glatten wirbellosenmuskel, *Protoplasma* 67: 111.

Hinke, J. A. M., 1965, Calcium requirements for noradrenaline and high potassium ion concentration in arterial smooth muscle, *in* "Muscle" (W. M. Paul, E. E. Daniel, C. M. Kay, and G. Monckton, eds.), pp. 269-284, Pergamon Press, New York.

Hinke, J. A. M., Wilson, M. L., and Burnham, S. C., 1964, Calcium and the contractility of arterial smooth muscle, *Amer. J. Physiol.* 206: 211.

Hiraoka, M., Yamagishi, S., and Sano, T., 1968, Role of calcium ions in the contraction of vascular smooth muscle, *Amer. J. Physiol.* 214: 1084.

Hudgins, P. M., and Weiss, G. B., 1968, Differential effects of calcium removal upon vascular smooth muscle contraction induced by norepinephrine, histamine and potassium, *J. Pharmacol. Exp. Ther.* 159: 91.

Hurwitz, L., 1975, Some characteristics of the excitation-contraction coupling process in smooth muscle, *in* "Concepts of Membranes in Regulation and Excitation" (M. Rocha e Silva and G. Suarez-Kurtz, eds.), pp. 55-72, Raven Press, New York.

Hurwitz, L., and Joiner, P. D., 1969, Excitation-contraction coupling in smooth muscle, *Fed. Proc.* 28: 1629.

Hurwitz, L., and Joiner, P. D., 1970, Mobilization of cellular calcium for contraction in intestinal smooth muscle, *Amer. J. Physiol.* 218: 12.

Hurwitz, L., and Suria, A., 1971, The link between agonist action and response in smooth muscle, *Annu. Rev. Pharmacol.* 11: 303.

Hurwitz, L., Hubbard, W., and Little, S., 1972, The relationship between the drug-receptor interaction and calcium transport in smooth muscle, *J. Pharmacol. Exp. Ther.* 183: 117.

Hurwitz, L., Fitzpatrick, D. F., Debbas, G., and Landon, E. J., 1973, Localization of calcium pump activity in smooth muscle, *Science* 179: 384.

Imai, S., and Takeda, S., 1967, Actions of calcium and certain multivalent cations on potassium contracture of guinea-pig's taenia coli, *J. Physiol. (London)* 190: 155.

Jhamandas, K. H., and Nash, C. W., 1967, Effects of inorganic anions on the contractility of vascular smooth muscle, *Can. J. Physiol. Pharmacol.* 45: 675.

Jonas, L., and Zelck, U., 1974, The subcellular calcium distribution in the smooth muscle cells of the pig coronary artery, *Exp. Cell Res.* 89: 352.

Krishnamurty, V. S. R., and Grollman, A., 1976, The mechanism of contraction of rat aorta to various agonists, *Arch. Int. Pharmacodyn. Ther.* 220: 180.

Langer, G. A., 1968, Ion fluxes in cardiac excitation and contraction and their relationship to myocardial contractility, *Physiol. Rev.* 48: 708.

McGuffee, L. J., and Bagby, R. M., 1976, Ultrastructure, calcium accumulation, and contractile response in smooth muscle, *Amer. J. Physiol.* 230: 1217.

Nickerson, M., 1956, Receptor occupancy and tissue response, *Nature* 178: 697.

Nonomura, Y., Hotta, Y., and Ohashi, H., 1966, Tetrodotoxin and manganese ions: effects on electrical activity and tension in taenia coli of guinea pig, *Science* 152: 97.

Osa, T., 1974, Modification of the mechanical response of the smooth muscles of pregnant mouse myometrium and guinea pig ileum by cadmium and manganese ions, *Jpn. J. Physiol.* 24: 101.

Peachey,L. D., 1964, Electron microscopic observations on the accumulation of divalent cations in intramitochondrial granules, *J. Cell Biol.* 20: 95.

Popescu, L. M., and Diculescu, I., 1975, Calcium in smooth muscle sarcoplasmic reticulum *in situ*. Conventional and x-ray analytical electron microscopy, *J. Cell Biol.* 67: 911.

Prosser, C. L., 1974, Smooth muscle, *Annu. Rev. Physiol.* 36: 503.

Rico, J. M. G. T., 1971, The influence of calcium on the activity of full and partial muscarinic agonists, *Eur. J. Pharmacol.* 13: 218.

Sandow, A., 1965, Excitation-contraction coupling in skeletal muscle, *Pharmacol. Rev.* 17: 265.

Sastry, B. V. R., and Cheng, H. C., 1972, Dissociation constants of D- and L-lactoylcholines and related compounds at cholinergic receptors, *J. Pharmacol. Exp. Ther.* 180: 326.

Somlyo, A. P., and Somlyo, A. V., 1968, Vascular smooth muscle. I. Normal structure, pathology, biochemistry, and biophysics, *Pharmacol. Rev.* 20: 197.

Somlyo, A. V., and Somlyo, A. P., 1971, Strontium accumulation by sarcoplasmic reticulum and mitochondria in vascular smooth muscle, *Science* 174: 955.

Somlyo, A. P., Somlyo, A. V., Devine, C. E., Peters, P. D., and Hall, T. A., 1974, Electron microscopy and electron probe analysis of mitochondrial cation accumulation in smooth muscle, *J. Cell Biol.* 61: 723.

Stirling, C. E., and Kinter, W. B., 1967, High-resolution radioautography of galactose-^{3}H accumulation in rings of hamster intestine, *J. Cell Biol.* 35: 585.

Stumpf, W. E., and Roth, L. J., 1969, Autoradiography using drymounted freeze-dried sections, *in* "Autoradiography of Diffusible Substances" (L. J. Roth and W. E. Stumpf, eds.), pp. 69-80, Academic Press, New York.

Su, C., Bevan, J. A., and Ursillo, R. C., 1964, Electrical quiescence of pulmonary artery smooth muscle during sympathomimetic stimulation, *Circ. Res.* 15: 20.

Triggle, D. J., 1971, "Neurotransmitter-Receptor Interaction," Academic Press, New York.

Triggle, C. R., Grant, W. F., and Triggle, D. J., 1975, Intestinal smooth muscle contraction and the effects of cadmium and A23187, *J. Pharmacol. Exp. Ther.* 194: 182.

Van Breemen, C., and Daniel, E. E., 1966, The influence of high potassium depolarization and acetylcholine on calcium exchange in the rat uterus, *J. gen. Physiol.* 49: 1299.

Waud, D. R., 1968, Pharmacological receptors, *Pharmacol. Rev.* 20: 49.

Woodbury, J. W., 1965, Action potential: properties of excitable membranes, *in* "Neurophysiology" (T. C. Ruch, H. D. Patton, J. W. Woodbury, and A. L. Towe, eds.), pp. 26-72, W. B. Saunders Company, Philadelphia.

Woodbury, J. W., Gordon, A. M., and Conrad, J. T., 1965, Muscle, *in* "Neurophysiology" (T. C. Ruch, H. D. Patton, J. W. Woodbury, and A. L. Towe, eds.), pp. 113-152, W. B. Saunders Company, Philadelphia.

SECTION II

SUBCELLULAR SITES AND INTERACTIONS:

CALCIUM AND DRUGS

In this second section, emphasis is shifted to consideration of roles of Ca^{2+} in cellular processes at an even more molecular level than in the first part. There is an increased focus on chemical interrelationships between the actions of Ca^{2+} and those of both drug molecules and modifiers of drug action. Thus, there is an increased focus on specific Ca^{2+}-related actions and, at the same time, a comparative approach that transcends specialized and limited areas of research.

The first chapter of this section considers the mutual interactions and the roles of Ca^{2+} and cAMP in biochemically-based information transfer in diverse biological areas of research. The interrelationships between Ca^{2+} and cAMP are presented in terms of a communication system with feedback controls which offer logical mechanisms for signal termination and signal frequency variation. The next chapter in this section (Chapter 6) surveys the roles of prostaglandins as mediators of cellular processes and, more specifically, the relationships between prostaglandins and Ca^{2+} in both contraction and secretion. Some mechanisms of interactions of both prostaglandins and Ca^{2+} with cyclic nucleotides are also explored. The next chapter (Chapter 7) focuses upon the biochemical and subcellular mechanisms of Ca^{2+} regulation (and control of activator Ca^{2+}) in vascular smooth muscle. Characteristics of Ca^{2+} binding and Ca^{2+} pumps in vesicular preparations consisting of **sarcolemma and sarcoplasmic** reticulum membrane as well as mitochondrial membrane **fractions** are discussed. In the final chapter of this section (Chapter 8), the role of Ca^{2+} as a regulator of membrane permeability (with particular emphasis on

K^+ permeability in exocrine glands) is considered. The activation of K^+ channels by Ca^{2+} is an important aspect in the actions of secretagogues on exocrine glands and the relationship between drug-receptor interactions and Ca^{2+} influx.

A common interest in all four chapters in this section is the general importance of Ca^{2+} as a primary regulator of subcellular events in the cell. Thus, drug-mediated effects on these actions of Ca^{2+} would result in such profound changes as (a) alterations in cellular and subcellular membrane permeabilities and binding characteristics and (b) changes in accumulation and release of hormonal and neurohumoral agents from subcellular sites. The information included in Section II provides an overview of these varied Ca^{2+}-related regulatory actions as well as a methodological introduction to some of the techniques successfully employed to analyze these complex cellular interactions.

CHAPTER 5

EFFECTS OF CALCIUM ON ADENYLATE CYCLASE, AS PART OF

THE Ca^{2+}-cAMP FEEDBACK IN BIOLOGICAL COMMUNICATION

Gideon A. Rodan

Department of Oral Biology
University of Connecticut
School of Medicine and Dental Medicine

INFORMATION TRANSFER IN BIOLOGICAL SYSTEMS

Normal function of the organism depends on a continuous flow of intercellular and intracellular information, which coordinates all biological (biochemical) processes. A few common principles underlie the transfer of biological information: (1) the information is stored in the structure of macromolecules (nucleic acids, enzymes, contractile proteins and others); (2) the transfer of information is often triggered by the interaction of the macromolecule with a small molecule; (3) if the information transfer involves energy expenditure (work), it is done at the expense of existing potential energy, such as the ion gradients across nerve membranes, and is initiated by removal of inhibition; and (4) the information transfer frequently involves amplification (multiple copies of a template, many product molecules generated by one molecule of activated enzyme, etc.).

I shall deal here mainly with the second property, the interaction of the macromolecule with smaller molecules. This interaction is frequently electrostatic (Coulombic) and results in a change in the shape of the macromolecule. Very frequently the small charged molecule is the ion Ca^{2+}. Through evolution Ca^{2+} has been selected for this task because of its abundance in the earth crust and its ability to form ionic or coordination bonds of variable strength (k_{ass} 50 to 10^{10}) with a large number of organic anions (Table I). Since the binding affinity is dependent on the distance between the functional groups of the ligand, it may change during changes in the shape of the macromolecule and

TABLE I.   STRUCTURAL DEPENDENCY OF CALCIUM AFFINITY TO ORGANIC ANIONS

	pK_1	pK_2 (Remarks)	pK_3
Acetate[a] $C_2H_4O_2$	1.24		
Succinate[a] $C_4H_6O_4$	1.2	0.54	
Oxalate[a] $C_2H_2O_4$	2.69	1.66	
Citrate[a] $C_6H_8O_7$	3.55	2.10	1.05
EGTA[a] $C_{14}H_{24}O_{10}N_2$	10.97	6.70	
Troponin C (TNC)[b]	8.7	6.70 *(affinity enhanced by binding of TNI)*	
Sarcoplasmic reticulum ATPase[c]	6.5	*(ratio of Ca^{2+} to Mg^{2+} affinities is strongly reduced by phosphorylation)*	
Calcium dependent regulator (of adenylate cyclase)[d]	5.4		

[a] *Sillen, L. G., and Martell, A. E. (1971). Stability Constants of Metal Ion Complexes, Supplement No. 1, The Chemical Society, Burlington House, London.*

[b] *Potter, J. D., and Gergely, J. (1975), J. Biol. Chem. 210: 4628-4633.*

[c] *Maclennan, D. H., and Holland, P. C. (1975), Annu. Rev. Biophys. Bioeng. 4: 377-404.*

[d] *Wolff, D. G., Brostrom, C. O. (1974), Arch. Biochem. Biophys. 163: 349-358.*

provide cooperativity. Cooperativity can generate quantal (all or none) responses which are a more reliable vehicle of information, as witnessed by the evolutionary selection of the nervous system. In the context of Ca^{2+} interaction with macromolecules, it is interesting that another common mechanism of biochemical regulation is phosphorylation. This is a covalent attachment of the highly charged anion phosphate to the macromolecule, which can certainly

affect its affinity for Ca^{2+}. A classical example of the joint
requirement for Ca^{2+} and phosphorylation is the activation of the
glycogen phosphorylase system. In this catalytic "cascade" Ca^{2+}
enhances the activity of several enzymes which are activated by
phosphorylation. At the beginning of the chain is the activation
of protein kinase by the small molecule cAMP, generated as a
messenger in response to information signals received at the cell
surface.

It is probably no coincidence that the modulation of cAMP
and the control of Ca^{2+} fluxes (Rasmussen, 1970) have evolved as
the major mechanisms for transducing information at the plasma
membrane, the important informational interface between the intra
and extracellular domains. This is particularly relevant to the
action of drugs, many of which exert their effect through interaction with the cell surface (as is apparent from this volume).
In this chapter I shall explore the mutual interactions of Ca^{2+}
and cAMP and the role these effects may play in increasing the
effectiveness of information transfer.

INVOLVEMENT OF CALCIUM ION AND cAMP IN BIOLOGICAL REGULATION

In an increasing number of biological processes, Ca^{2+} and
cAMP are being identified as regulators of rate determining steps.
Together with cyclic GMP they constitute the triad of "second
messengers" which seem to control major biological events, such
as cell division, differentiation, secretion, contraction, changes
in metabolism and even cell death. The outcome of the interplay
between the messengers varies from system to system and the
molecular detail is only beginning to unravel. In general the
cyclic nucleotides enhance the catalytic activity of protein
kinases and phosphatases and thus control the phosphorylation
and dephosphorylation of proteins, a recognized biochemical
regulatory mechanism. Calcium ion, through its effect on macromolecular structure, controls the function of contractile proteins
and can modify enzyme activity either directly or indirectly
through control of the binding of regulatory proteins. Calcium
ion also has a pronounced effect on the permeability of biological
membranes (to Ca^{2+} itself and to other ions), and thus contributes to the control of membrane potentials and the ionic composition of the cytosol. Rasmussen (1970) recognized the generality
of the regulatory function of Ca^{2+} and postulated that along
with cAMP it serves as "second messenger" in biological communication. Considerable evidence supporting involvement of both
nucleotides and Ca^{2+} in biological regulation has continued to
accumulate (see Rasmussen *et al.*, 1975, and Berridge, 1975).
Examples in this volume include platelet secretion and aggregation
and the effect of opiate ligands on Ca^{2+} binding to

synaptic membranes. I shall describe a few additional examples
to illustrate the great diversity of effects of Ca^{2+} and cyclic
nucleotides and point to common features and the potential role
of their interaction.

Insulin Secretion

In adult pancreas islets stimulation of insulin secretion by
glucose is mediated by Ca^{2+} (Malaisse, 1973). This conclusion
is supported by the requirement for extracellular Ca^{2+} (Rubin,
1970), the inhibitory effects of the local anesthetic tetracaine
(Brisson et al., 1971), the enhanced influx of ^{45}Ca (Malaisse-
Lagae and Malaisse, 1971), and the membrane depolarization attributed to a Ca^{2+} current (Dean and Matthews, 1970a,b). High extracellular K^+ also stimulates insulin secretion in the presence of
Ca^{2+}, probably through an increase in Ca^{2+} permeability caused
by membrane depolarization (Hales and Miller, 1968). On the other
hand veratridine, a drug which increases membrane permeability
to Na^+, stimulates insulin secretion independently of extracellular
Ca^{2+} (Lowe et al., 1976). The influx of Na^+ supposedly mobilizes
Ca^{2+} from an intracellular source. There is conflicting evidence
on the relationship between changes in cAMP and the secretory
response triggered by Ca^{2+}. Glucose does not stimulate the islet
cell adenylate cyclase but, in several experiments, glucose incubation increased cellular cAMP by a yet unidentified mechanism
(for reviews see Montague and Howell, 1975). It is clear, however,
that substances which increase cellular cAMP through adenylate
cyclase stimulation (glucagon, pancreozymin, secretin, cortico-
tropin, prostaglandins E_1 and E_2) or phosphodiesterase inhibition
(methylxanthines, sulfonylureas), as well as exogenously added
dibutyryl cyclic AMP, enhance insulin secretion. This is a facili-
tatory effect (Malaisse, 1973) and requires a minimum level of
glucose. The mechanism for the role of cAMP in insulin secretion
is not yet understood. A cAMP dependent protein kinase is present
in the islet cells and a variety of proteins from cytosol, microsomes, secretory granules or plasma membranes can serve as substrate for phosphorylation, but their function is unknown (Montague
and Howell, 1972; Davis and Lazarus, 1973). To integrate the
effects of cAMP and Ca^{2+} into a comprehensive picture it was proposed that a minimum level of cAMP and a primary secretory stimulus
such as glucose are both necessary. It was suggested that cAMP
is required for maintaining an essential protein, possibly tubulin
(Lacy and Malaisse, 1973; Letterier et al., 1974) in the phosphorylated state, whereas the Ca^{2+} flux resulting from the perturbation
of the membrane by glucose activates the contractile event leading
to secretion (Montague and Howell, 1975). According to an alternative hypothesis (Rasmussen, 1975; Berridge, 1975), cAMP does
not play a direct role in secretion but acts by mobilizing Ca^{2+}

from intracellular Ca^{2+} stores. Further studies on the molecular
basis of the secretory process are needed; but an intimate functional relationship between Ca^{2+} and cAMP is fully evident at
this point.

Excitation of Photoreceptors

This is a totally different biological function from that
described above. The stimulus is not chemical and the response
does not involve intracellular translocation or secretion. There
are, however, common features between the excitation of photoreceptors and excitation-secretion coupling. There is direct
evidence from studies with aequorin in the Limulus ventral eye
that illumination causes an increase in intracellular Ca^{2+} concentration (Brown and Blinks, 1972). The Ca^{2+} is most probably
released from the disks and its amount is related to the amount
of bleaching. In addition there is a certain relationship between
photoreception and cAMP (Bitensky *et al.*, 1973). The time course
of cAMP changes suggests that the cyclic nucleotides do not initiate the early events associated with photoreception (Pannbacker,
1973). However, cAMP decreases substantially with increasing
light intensity and under these conditions more Ca^{2+} is required
to produce the same effect on the Na^+ conductance of the cell
membrane. Cyclic AMP thus seems to have a permissive or facilita-
tory effect. The drop in cyclic nucleotides (Bitensky *et al.*,
1973) and the rise in intracellular Ca^{2+} (Bader *et al.*, 1976)
were suggested to control the light-dark adaptation process.

In summary, we deal here with an extracellular signal which
elicits a burst of Ca^{2+} in the cytoplasm, a change in the cell
membrane potential and changes in cyclic nucleotides (which may
affect the sensitivity to further signals). This sequence is very
similar to that described previously for insulin secretion.

Fertilization and Cell Division

Cell division is a much more primitive biological process than
the communication systems described above, but it is obvious that
subjection of cell division to environmental control provided
tremendous selective advantage and was an essential step in the
evolvement of multicellular organisms. The indication that Ca^{2+},
cyclic nucleotides and changes in membrane potential are involved
in the control of cell proliferation supports the idea of a
general common mechanism for the transduction of extracellular
signals into intracellular messages.

Steinhardt *et al.* (1971) have shown that fertilization of sea urchin eggs is associated with membrane depolarization caused by a Na^+ current, followed by K^+ conductance hyperpolarization. These changes are followed by a burst of intracellular Ca^{2+} which, presumably, initiates cell division. In other systems, there is only limited information on the role of membrane depolarization in the control of cell division. The proliferation of nerve cells in culture was shown to be stimulated by electric currents, and electrically competent intercellular junctions were demonstrated during the embryonic state of nonexcitable tissues (Sheridan, 1966; Bennett and Trinkaus, 1970; Loewenstein, 1973) and were implicated in the control of cell division and differentiation. There is a lot more information on the potential role of Ca^{2+} in proliferation control, and according to some investigators Ca^{2+} is the final common pathway for the action of various effectors (Whitfield *et al.*, 1976; Berridge, 1975). Steinhardt *et al.* (1974) have shown that the calcium ionophore A23187 mimicks the effects of fertilization and leads to cell division. Ridgway *et al.* (1976) have made similar observations in fucoid cells where cell division is initiated by Ca^{2+} currents. In mammalian cells, initiation of cell division often requires the presence of Ca^{2+} in the extracellular fluid. This was best demonstrated under culture conditions for cells which retain proliferative potential, such as lymphoblasts and fibroblasts (Whitfield *et al.*, 1976; Berridge, 1975; Balk, 1971). Lymphoblast activation can be triggered by the calcium ionophore A23187; and many mitogens, such as lectins (concanavalin A, phytohemagglutinin), acetylcholine, polyamines and detergents require calcium in the medium for exerting their effect (Whitfield *et al.*, 1976). Indeed, exposure of lymphoblasts to phytohemagglutinin enhances Ca^{2+} influx into the cells. Interestingly, in certain fibroblast lines the extracellular Ca^{2+} requirement can be circumvented by malignant transformation (Balk *et al.*, 1973; Boynton *et al.*, 1974). It was speculated, in analogy to excitation-secretion coupling, that in those cases the "regulatory" Ca^{2+} is recruited from intracellular sources. The independence of the proliferative process from environmental control has been attributed to changes in plasma membrane observed in transformed cells (Wallach, 1976; Racker, 1976; Anderson and Pastan, 1975). These changes may render the cells perpetually "excited" by altering an inhibitory function fulfilled by the normal membrane. This function was proposed to be mediated by cAMP (Burk, 1968; Otten *et al.*, 1972; Anderson and Pastan, 1975).

The role of cyclic nucleotides in the control of growth and proliferation has been the subject of many investigations and is still debated (for recent reviews see Friedman, 1976; and Chlapowski *et al.*, 1975). Following the initial observation that cAMP (or its analogues) reduce cell growth, a substantial body of literature has shown that in cultured fibroblasts there is a negative correlation between cell proliferation and cAMP (or adenylate cyclase). Cells rendered quiescent by serum deprivation show a significant increase in cAMP levels, whereas release from quiescence by various means (Burger *et al*., Froechlich and Rachmeler, 1972; Moens *et al*., 1975) results in a drop in cAMP and is prevented by the addition of exogenous dibutyryl cAMP (Willingham *et al*., 1972). It was also shown that malignantly transformed cells have low levels of cAMP and adenylate cyclase (Anderson *et al*., 1973; Carchman *et al*., 1974; Otter *et al*., 1972).

There are, however, a large number of exceptions to the growth inhibitory role of cAMP, especially in nonmesenchymal tissues such as hepatoma (Thomas *et al*., 1973) or adrenocortical carcinoma (Ney *et al*., 1969). Cell replication involves many processes and multiple control points, probably regulated by different mechanisms. Normal fibroblasts, for example, seem to be blocked at a different stage of the cell cycle than are malignant fibroblasts. The timing and duration of the cyclic nucleotide changes is probably of great importance and contradictory findings may be due to lack of cell synchrony. In all systems where cAMP levels were followed during the cell cycle a significant drop was observed during mitosis (Friedman, 1976).

The molecular site (or sites) of cAMP action is not known. It is thought that both Ca^{2+} and cAMP may control the various intracellular motile events associated with cell replication, probably carried out by the microtubule-microfilament system. It is interesting to associate the lack of Ca^{2+} requirement and the low adenylate cyclase activity of the transformed cells with the opposite effects of Ca^{2+} and cAMP on tubulin assembly (Borisy *et al*., 1974; Willingham and Pastan, 1975). It has also been suggested that the effects of cAMP are secondary to its effects on Ca^{2+} (Berridge, 1975). Cyclic GMP is probably also involved in growth activation (Rudland *et al*., 1974; Hadden *et al*., 1972; Hadden *et al*., 1973) and its accumulation may be stimulated by Ca^{2+}.

From this very brief review it is apparent that although there are many unanswered questions regarding the control of various steps in cell division, it is not unlikely that the environmental feedback is channeled through a mechanism similar to excitation-secretion coupling, involving membrane depolarization, Ca^{2+} fluxes and cyclic nucleotide modulation.

THE KINETICS OF CELLULAR FLUCTUATIONS IN CALCIUM ION
AND cAMP LEVELS

For most cells there are no good methods for measuring the
intracellular levels of ionic calcium since microelectrodes are
unavailable and fluorescent indicators such as murexide and aequorin
are difficult to inject harmlessly, and very hard to calibrate
intracellularly (Baker *et al.*, 1971). From studies on squid axons
and by extrapolation from muscular physiology and the known cyto-
toxic effect of Ca^{2+} it is believed that the intracellular ionic
calcium concentration of all mammalian cells is between 10^{-7} and
10^{-6} M. In addition, a substantial amount of cellular Ca^{2+} is
stored in mitochondria and endoplasmic reticulum and can be released
or reaccumulated according to the physiological needs of the cell.
Rasmussen (1975) has postulated that a two- to five-fold elevation
in cytoplasmic free Ca^{2+} is a general mechanism for "cell activation" by external effectors. It is obvious that for cells capable
of repeated activation the Ca^{2+} change ought to be transient. In
muscle, Ca^{2+} removal is carried out by the highly efficient sarcoplasmic reticulum. In other cells this role may be played by
mitochondria, which prefer Ca^{2+} uptake to ATP generation if the
ambient Ca^{2+} is above 10^{-6} M (Rossi and Lehninger, 1964). It is
not yet known in detail what determines the duration of elevated
Ca^{2+} concentration in the cytoplasm. ATP availability is probably
important and there is evidence that cyclic nucleotides participate
in the control of Ca^{2+} removal (see below).

It has been proposed that the major role of cyclic nucleotides
is the regulation of intracellular Ca^{2+} (Berridge, 1975). In that
case cyclic nucleotide levels would be expected to change in the
same spiked pattern as Ca^{2+} does. However, regardless of their
mechanism of action, sudden temporary fluctuations would be the
most appropriate way to turn processes on or off; there is ample
documentation for this kinetic pattern for cyclic nucleotide
changes.

The importance of the timing and duration of cAMP elevations
was mentioned above with regard to cell division. It was found
for example that elevated cAMP levels may promote processes in
the G_1 phase of the cell cycle but block the cells in G_2 (pre
mitosis) (Friedman, 1976). There are numerous examples of short
lived pulse-like rises in cAMP in response to cell stimulation.
The cAMP elevation produced by exposure of liver cells to isoproterenol or epinephrine (above 10^{-7} M) peaks at 1 min and is completely gone at 10 min even though the stimulant is not removed
(Tolbert *et al.*, 1973).

A similar phenomenon, though on a different time scale, was observed upon incubation of human fat cells with epinephrine (10^{-5} M) and phentolamine (10^{-5} M). Cyclic AMP peaked at 30 min and returned to the basal level within 2 hours, whereas the release of glycerol initiated by the hormone was significantly enhanced and still going up at 4 hours (Burns *et al.*, 1972). In rat fat cells exposed to noradrenaline, cAMP rose sharply for 10 minutes, then decreased exponentially, and by 60 min had returned to the baseline. The fast decrease was partly explained by adenosine inhibition of adenylate cyclase. However, even in the presence of adenosine deaminase there was a gradual decrease in cAMP, which was probably not due to phosphodiesterase (PDE) since its rate was not altered by theophylline (Schwabe *et al.*, 1974). The findings listed above were obtained *in vitro* and illustrate a phenomenon observed in practically every system examined. Similar kinetic patterns for cAMP changes were also observed *in vivo*. It was shown in dogs that pentagastrin (i.v.) caused a sharp increase in cAMP secretion into the gastric juice, which peaked at about 15 min and dropped thereafter, although the pentagastrin infusion was continued for 60 min. Histamine infusion caused repeated pulses of cAMP secretion about 15 min apart. In both cases enhanced HCl secretion persisted after the drop in cAMP.

In the guinea pig heart cAMP was measured at very short time intervals after exposure to inotropic agents (isoprenaline, histamine or oxyfedrine) and was found to peak at 10 sec and drop to about 30% of peak value at 1 min. Brooker (1975) showed that during normal (nonstimulated) contraction cAMP levels also change periodically, peaking at the beginning of systole. He suggested that cAMP changes play a role in the regulation of the rhythmicity of the heartbeat. Sustained oscillations in cAMP were also observed in a very different biological system - the slime mold *Dictyostelium discoideum*. During the formation of the fruiting body by cell aggregation, cAMP pulses are released from cells located at the aggregation center at 6 to 9 min intervals. These pulses, amplified and propagated through the colony, act chemotactically on the other cells in the "field" (Gerisch and Wick, 1975).

As mentioned before, the higher reliability of binary all or none signals in communication has probably led to the evolvement of the kinetic patterns described above, which may be the evolutionary precursors of neural transmission. A general property of systems capable of generating pulses or oscillations is non-linearity (Glansdorf and Prigogine, 1971). This property can lead to signal amplification and "cascades" characteristic of biological regulation. In enzyme systems non-linearity can result from positive or negative cooperativity, product or substrate inhibition, and modulation by other substances (related by feedback to the

enzymatic activity). Such responses usually imply allosteric
properties. In the system of enzymes which control the level of
cAMP, there are many possibilities for such effects. Several seem
to involve Ca^{2+}. Calcium ion participates in the regulation of
both phosphodiesterase and adenylate cyclase and may itself be
subject to cAMP regulation. This interaction can create the
feed-back loops necessary for pulse generation and signal termination. The rest of this chapter will deal in some detail with
the cAMP-Ca^{2+} interrelationship with particular emphasis on the
effect of Ca^{2+} on adenylate cyclase.

EFFECTS OF cAMP ON CALCIUM TRANSLOCATION

The possibility that cAMP modulates intracellular Ca^{2+} translocation was suggested by the inotropic effects of catecholamines
which usually act via cAMP. The best evidence for cAMP stimulation
of Ca^{2+} transport was obtained in studies on heart microsomes
(Kirchberger et al., 1972; Tada et al., 1974). It was shown that
cardiac microsomes contain a cAMP dependent protein kinase (PK)
capable of phosphorylating the microsomal membranes (LaRaia et
al., 1973). Phosphorylation was also catalyzed by exogenous bovine
heart protein kinase and resulted in increased Ca^{2+}-ATPase activity
and a two-fold enhancement of Ca^{2+} uptake in the presence of oxalate (Kirchberger et al., 1972; Tada et al., 1974). The phosphorylated moiety was found to be a serine group of a 20,000 dalton
membrane protein called phospholamban (Tada et al. 1973; 1975).
The phosphorylation was hydroxylamine insensitive and was not
stimulated by Ca^{2+}, unlike the phosphoacyl intermediate of the
Ca^{2+}-ATPase. An endogenous phosphoprotein phosphatase required
for the cleavage of phosphate was also present in the cardiac
microsomes (LaRaia et al., 1973). Similarly, phosphorylation of
the cardiac sarcolemma by an endogenous cAMP-stimulated PK
(Andrew et al., 1973; Hui et al., 1976; Sulakhe and Drummond, 1974)
results in enhanced Ca^{2+} accumulation. Phosphorylase b kinase
was also found to stimulate the phosphorylation of sarcolemma
proteins and Ca^{2+} uptake in sarcolemma vesicles (Sulakhe et al.,
1976). The phosphorylated proteins of approximate molecular weights
of 95,000 and 130,000 had not yet been identified. Following phosphorylation the activities of the Mg^{2+}, Ca^{2+}-ATPase and the
ouabain-sensitive Na^+, K^+-ATPase were increased (Sulakhe et al.,
1976). The mechanism for Ca^{2+} uptake enhancement by phospholamban
is not known. There is no change in the stoichiometry of the
Ca^{2+}/ATP ratio of 2 (Tada et al., 1974). Since the Ca^{2+}-ATPase
is both necessary and sufficient for carrying out the microsomal
Ca^{2+} transport it would have to be the modulated moiety. In
cardiac microsomes the results of Tada et al. (1974) show a 30%
increase in the V_{max} and a reduction in the k_a for Ca^{2+} from 1.8

to 0.9 μM; the k_m for Mg-ATP was not estimated. In the sarcolemma, phosphorylation enhanced the V_{max} of the transport system and had no effect on the affinity for Ca^{2+} (Sulakhe et al., 1976). In other muscles dissociation between phospholamban phosphorylation and increased Ca^{2+} accumulation was observed (Schwartz et al., 1976), suggesting multiple cAMP involving mechanisms for the control of microsomal Ca^{2+} accumulation. In slow skeletal muscle which, like cardiac muscle, responds to catecholamines by an increased rate of relaxation, endogenous or exogenous cAMP-stimulated PK also phosphorylates a 22,000 dalton protein and enhances Ca^{2+} accumulation (Kirchberger and Tada, 1976; Schwartz et al., 1976). In fast skeletal muscle which responds to catecholamines by a decreased rate of relaxation, there are contradictory reports. Kirchberger and Tada (1976) found no evidence for phosphorylation or Ca^{2+} uptake enhancement. Schwartz et al. (1976) reported the absence of an endogenous PK but found that exogenous cAMP-stimulated PK phosphorylated a 95,000 dalton protein and enhanced Ca^{2+} uptake. There was no evidence for phospholamban phosphorylation. Phosphorylase b kinase, itself activated by cAMP-stimulated PK, catalyzed the phosphorylation of 95,000 dalton proteins and accumulation of Ca^{2+} in both slow and fast muscle. Schwartz et al. (1976) suggested that increased Ca^{2+} uptake may be related to enhanced glycogenolysis.

Although all the experiments described above demonstrated stimulation of Ca^{2+} uptake under nonphysiological conditions in the presence of oxalate, there is a strong case for the cAMP dependency of Ca^{2+} translocation in muscle, in view of the effects of catecholamines on muscle contraction. If one considers the SR as a specialized ER and the sarcolemma analogous to other plasma membranes the same relationship between cAMP and Ca^{2+} may be present in other cells. Calcium ion accumulating ability of ER microsomes has been demonstrated in several tissues but no reports on cAMP-PK effects have been published.

Other possibilities for effects of cAMP on Ca^{2+} translocation have been contemplated: effects on the Ca^{2+} permeability of biological membranes (Hasselbach et al., 1969), Ca^{2+} binding to phosphorylated proteins in the cytoplasm (Rasmussen et al., 1975) and changes in mitochondrial Ca^{2+} transport. So far there is only limited experimental evidence to document these effects and their physiological importance has not been established.

The modulation of Ca^{2+} translocation by cyclic nucleotides may play a significant role in cellular communication. In the case of muscle contraction for example, it may accelerate signal termination and possibly signal initiation. This role of cyclic nucleotides is of particular importance if Ca^{2+} is indeed the universal intracellular communication molecule (Rasmussen et al., 1975;

Berridge, 1975). At any rate, effects of cyclic nucleotides on Ca^{2+} concentration, coupled with the effects of Ca^{2+} on cyclic nucleotide concentrations discussed below, can generate the feedback relationships necessary for signal termination, pulses and oscillations. I shall next consider the effects of Ca^{2+} on cAMP catabolism and biosynthesis.

EFFECTS OF CALCIUM ON cAMP (3'-5' PHOSPHODIESTERASE ACTIVITY)

Cyclic AMP and cyclic GMP are catabolized through cleavage of the 3'-5' ester bond. Phosphodiesterase (PDE) activity is present in all cells both in soluble as well as in membrane bound form (Appleman et al., 1973). The phosphodiesterase preparations act on cAMP as well as cGMP, but there is evidence that the two functions are under separate genetic control, and the combined activity may be due to an enzyme mixture (Russell and Pastan, 1974). For each substrate the enzymatic activity exhibits a high k_s in the mM range and a low k_s in the μM range, which is probably the physiologically relevant one. Partial purification of the soluble enzyme has revealed multiple forms with different specificities and different kinetic properties towards cAMP and cGMP (Russell and Pastan, 1974). Reversible transitions between 22,000, 75,000 and 140,000 dalton enzymes were recently shown to occur as a function of enzyme and substrate concentration. The low molecular weight form, which was favored in the presence of dibutyryl cAMP (B_2 cAMP), had higher activity on cAMP (Richard and Cheung, 1976). This and other studies suggest that the various kinetic properties observed reflect the degree of association of the enzyme, which may be of regulatory significance. The situation is much clearer with respect to the regulation of phosphodiesterase activity by a Ca^{2+} dependent activator protein (PAF). This protein was first isolated from brain independently by Kakiuchi and Yamazaki (1970) and Cheung (1970, 1971) and was shown to be present in heart, liver and kidney of various species. PAF is a heat stable protein of about 20,000 dalton and is considerably similar in structure (Watterson et al., 1976), amino acid composition and physical properties to the Ca^{2+} binding subunit of troponin (Wang et al., 1975). The Ca^{2+} affinity of PAF is in the physiological range, k_m approx. 2 μM. Upon binding Ca^{2+} confers to PAF a more helical conformation. The binding of PAF to phosphodiesterase does not depend on Ca^{2+}, but only the Ca^{2+} modified PAF enhances phosphodiesterase activity. Several PAF molecules can bind to PDE in a cooperative manner (Hill coefficient = 2). In the various tissues examined PAF was found to be in excess of PDE, suggesting that the Ca^{2+} concentration is the rate limiting factor in the activation of phosphodiesterase. The association of the enzyme into different size aggregates, mentioned above, was not dependent on PAF. The effect of PAF is primarily on the V_{max} of the

enzymatic activity. The PAF dependent PDE activity could account
for most of the cGMP hydrolyzing activity at substrate concentrations below 1 μM. However, the activation of cAMP breakdown was
more pronounced at higher substrate concentrations. The physiological role of the Ca^{2+} dependent cyclic nucleotide catabolism
has not been established, but the existence of a protein which
in the presence of μM concentrations of Ca^{2+} stimulates phosphodiesterase over ten-fold is strongly suggestive of its regulatory
importance. It remains to be seen if it affects cAMP as well as
cGMP and under what circumstances it is most likely to participate
in the cyclic nucleotide and Ca^{2+} mediated information transfer.

EFFECTS OF CALCIUM ON cAMP (ADENYLATE CYCLASE)

I shall now consider the properties of the adenylate cyclase
enzyme which may contribute to the kinetic features of the cAMP
response described above namely, amplification, pulse generation
and oscillations.

Although the enzyme has not been purified from mammalian
tissues and its structure is not known there is ample evidence,
based on kinetic considerations, for its allosteric nature. First,
adenylate cyclase exhibits anomolous kinetics with respect to substrate. Numerous reports describing the activity of the enzyme
as a function of ATP concentration have shown sigmoidicity in the
rising phase of enzyme activity. This behavior is seen predominantly in the concentration range between 10^{-6} and 10^{-4} and was
reported for liver membranes (Birnbaumer *et al.*, 1972), rat
kidney membranes (Rajerison *et al.*, 1974), retroorbital tissue
(Winand and Kohn, 1975), leucocyte membranes (Stolc, 1977), and
many other tissues. Second, another prominent kinetic feature
of adenylate cyclase is substrate inhibition. A reduction in
adenylate cyclase activity at ATP concentrations above 1 mM has
been reported in fat cell membranes (Birnbaumer *et al.*, 1969;
Cooper *et al.*, 1976) in retroorbital tissue (Winand and Kohn,
1975), in leucocyte membranes (Stolc, 1977), in skeletal muscle
adenylate cyclase (Severson *et al.*, 1972), in renal cortex membranes
(Queener *et al.*, 1975), in brain and cardiac adenylate cyclase
(Garbers and Johnson, 1975), and in other tissues. Substrate
inhibition has been attributed by deHaen (1974) and later by Rodbell
(1975) and Rendell *et al.* (1975) to the effect of free (non MgATP
associated) ATP species. On that basis the stimulatory effects
of Mg^{2+} and Mn^{2+} were attributed to a reduction in ATP^{4-} or ATP^{3-}
concentrations. However, later studies dealing specifically with
the effects of bivalent metals on adenylate cyclase activity
(Garbers and Johnson, 1975; Londos and Rodbell, 1977; Londos and
Preston, 1977a) led to the conclusion that metals affect the
enzyme directly. Experiments in which all ionic species in the

assay mixture were fully accounted for by solution of the simultaneous equations describing the interactions between Mg^{2+}, ATP^{4-} and ATP^{3-} and the dissociation of ATP as a function of pH (submitted for publication), have shown that the decrease in adenylate cyclase activity at high $MgATP^{2-}$ concentrations can be attributed directly to the substrate (Figure 1). This view confirms fully the model proposed by Garbers and Johnson (1975) derived from the studies of brain and cardiac adenylate cyclase and their analysis of previous literature results. Like Garbers and Johnson (1975), we have observed these properties also in the presence of lubrol-PX which suggests that the anomolous "kinetics" persist when the membrane is disrupted and may pertain to the nature of the enzyme itself. Third, there is abundant evidence for heterotropic effects on adenylate cyclase. In addition to hormone activation, which always shows sigmoidal dose dependency (Severson *et al.*, 1972; Rajerison *et al.*, 1974; Schramm and Rodbell, 1975; Thompson *et al.*, 1976), practically all adenylate cyclase preparations from mammalian tissues respond to guanine nucleotides. The stimulatory effects of GTP analogs also exhibit cooperativity (Schramm and Rodbell, 1975; Rendell *et al.*, 1975; Krishna *et al.*, 1972) and frequently have interesting hysteric effects showing time dependent activation (Neer, 1976) or the persistence of the activated states after incubation with Gpp(NH)p (Schramm and Rodbell, 1975; Spiegel *et al.*, 1976). There is also mutual interaction between the effect of guanine nucleotides and those of hormones (Salomon *et al.*, 1975; Spiegel *et al.*, 1976; Schramm, 1975; Krishna *et al.*, 1972). Prostaglandins are another example of heterotropic effects. The effects of metals mentioned briefly above will be discussed in more detail with special reference to calcium.

Fourth, another general property of allosteric enzymes is that agents which resemble the substrate structurally elicit biphasic responses; they activate at low concentrations and inhibit at high concentrations. This is typically the case for the effects of adenosine on adenylate cyclase preparations from liver (Londos, 1977b), platelets (Haslam and Lynham, 1973), cartilage (Rodan *et al.*, 1977) and bone (Peck *et al.*, 1976). Finally, a diagnostic property of allosteric enzymes is the susceptibility of heterotropic effects to agents, such as mercurials, which affect conformation. Few such investigations have been conducted on adenylate cyclase, but it was shown that the inhibitory effect of Cu^{2+} on Mn^{2+}-stimulated bovine spermatozoal adenylate cyclase was prevented by 2, 3-dimercaptoproponal (Braun, 1975). It was also shown that inactivation of turkey erythrocyte adenylate cyclase by sodium arsenite was much more effective in the presence of 2, 3-dimercaptol and under these conditions minimal effects on beta receptor specific binding occurred (Spiegel *et al.*, 1976).

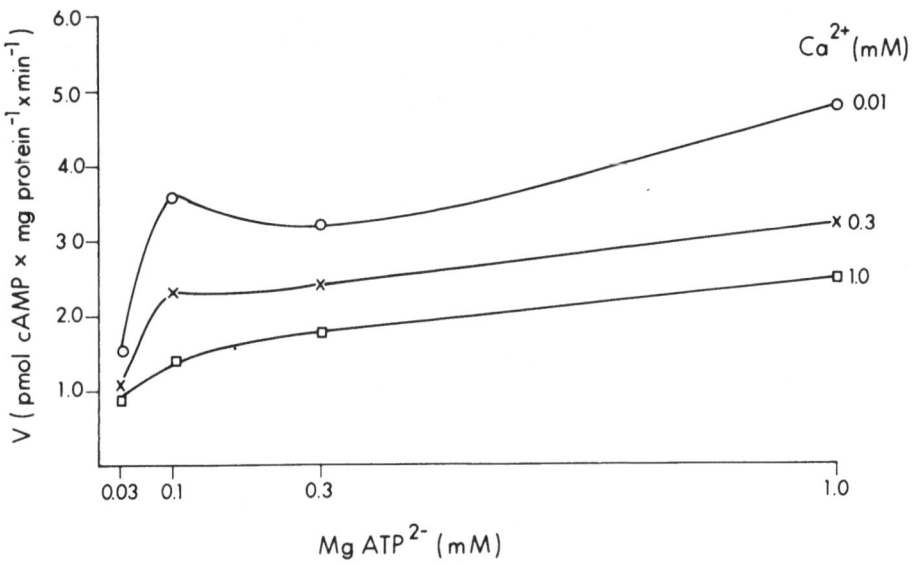

Figure 1.   Kinetic patterns of adenylate cyclase activity.   Enzymatic activity was measured by the method of Salomon, Y., Londos, C., and Rodbell, M., (1974, Anal. Biochem. 58: 541) on 17μg protein, measured according to Lowry, O. H., Rosebrough, N. J., Farr, A. L., and Randall, R. J., (1951, J. Biol. Chem 193: 265) from chick pectoralis sarcoplasmic reticulum prepared by the method of Severson, D. L., Drummond, G. J., and Sulakhe, P. V., (1972, J. Biol. Chem. 247: 2949).   The assay mixture contained 25 mM Tris-HCl, pH 7.6, 1 mM dithiothreitol, 1 mM cAMP, 0.1 mM EGTA, 5 mM $MgCl_2$, 65 mM KCl, 3×10^6 cpm ATP-α-^{32}P and an ATP regenerating system consisting of 5 mM creatine phosphate and 100 u/ml creatine phosphokinase. $MgCl_2$, $CaCl_2$ and Na_2ATP were adjusted to yield 5 mM Mg^{2+} and the concentrations of Ca^{2+} and $MgATP^{2-}$ shown in the figure.   The assay was started by the addition of the protein to preincubated assay mixture and incubated for 15 minutes at $37^{\circ}C$. Under the conditions described, the reaction was linear with time and protein concentration.

The allosteric properties of adenylate cyclase have been discussed by Goldbeter in the context of the oscillating pulses of cyclic AMP released in colonies of *Dictyostelium discoideum* (Goldbeter and Caplan, 1976; Goldbeter and Segel, 1977).   Changeux *et al.* (1967) have postulated that allosteric properties are inherent to the structure of biological membranes and may thus be responsible for the allosteric behavior of membrane bound enzymes. The effects of lipids (Orly and Schramm, 1975) and lypolytic treatments (Rodbell *et al.*, 1971; Puchwein *et al.*, 1974) have demonstrated the importance of the membrane environment in the control of adenylate cyclase activity. However, properties consistent with allosteric behavior have been observed in soluble forms of the enzyme (Neer, 1976; Pfeiffer and Helmreich, 1975) suggesting that the membrane only contributes to the modulation of an inherent allosteric structure.

The complex behavior of adenylate cyclase illustrated in Figure 1 had made it difficult in the past to define quantitatively the kinetic properties of the enzyme unless limited ranges of substrate concentrations were considered. Since the cooperative properties of the enzyme may be closely related to its functional role, substrate concentrations consistent with hyperbolic kinetics may not cover the physiologically relevant range. In collaboration with Dr. Ellis Golub, we have attempted to fit data similar to that presented in Figure 1 to a kinetic model which would describe the behavior of the enzyme for a wide range of substrate concentrations. The major kinetic features to be incorporated into the model were: slow takeoff (not shown in Figure 1), accelerated rise in activity, leveling off followed by a dropoff and (sometimes) a resurgence of activity at higher substrate concentrations. One could summarize this behavior as positive cooperativity followed by substrate inhibition, relieved at higher fractional saturation of the enzyme. We searched for a simple analytical expression to describe this behavior and used the following criteria: (i) Good fit to a large amount of experimental data, which we had collected, (ii) An expression which contains the smallest number of parameters, (iii) Internal consistency, evaluated by parameter variability among different experiments and parameter dependency on factors which modulate enzyme activity, and (iv) Adherence to general principles of enzyme activity.

The property which most strongly influenced the selection of the model was substrate inhibition. Substrate inhibition can be attributed either to covalent modification of the enzyme, for which there is little evidence, or to a reduction in catalytic activity of the enzyme complex resulting from the interaction of enzyme subunits. The latter assumption seemed logical on the basis of the allosteric properties of the enzyme described above. We assumed that when the number of protomers occupied by substrate increases beyond a certain point their catalytic activity decreases, and chose the classical expression of Adair (1925) to describe that behavior: $v = \Sigma \, i \times k_i \times S^i \times \Pi \, u_i \, / \, (n + n \, \Sigma \, S^i \times \Pi u_i)$, $i = 1, n$; where v is the apparent enzyme velocity; i, the order of the protomer; K_i, its catalytic activity; S, substrate concentration; u_i, the apparent substrate affinity of the i' th Protomer; and n, the number of interacting protomers in the enzyme complex. A two subunit enzyme, for example, is described by the equation:

$v = (k_1 u_1 S + 2k_2 u_1 u_2 S^2)/2(1 + u_1 S + u_1 u_2 S^2)$. Four interacting enzyme subunits would be required to generate the pattern presented in Figure 1. Assuming different values for each u_i and k_i that model would require eight independent parameters, too large a number to make it useful, since vast amounts of detailed data would be needed to obtain unique solutions by curve fitting procedures. To reduce the number of parameters, we searched for parameter dependency relationships between u_i's and k_i's of separate subunits. The search was based on statistical evaluation of the "goodness of fit" of 68 data sets obtained from assays at various $MgATP^{2-}$, Mg^{2+} and Ca^{2+} concentrations, run on membrane associated and lubrol solubilized enzymes from 3 types of tissue, muscle, embryonic bone and rat osteosarcoma. In the four subunit model necessary to describe Figure 1, substrate inhibition was attributed to a reduction in the catalytic activity of the enzyme complex in which 3 protomers were occupied by substrate. Protomer occupancy could also affect substrate binding, but independent determinations of such effects are impossible in the absence of pure enzyme. We assumed therefore the same intrinsic binding affinity for all protomers. According to this assumption, the fractional saturation of the enzyme is governed by statistical binding. The number of protomers occupied would simply be a function of substrate concentration and collision probability. The apparent binding affinity of sequential protomers, expressed relative to the affinity of the first protomer occupied, would be: $u_2 = 0.375 u_1$, $u_3 = 0.167 u_1$, $u_4 = 0.0625 u_1$. Substrate binding to all subunits was thus described by a single parameter "u". The sigmoidal increase in enzyme velocity with increasing substrate concentration, which is usually interpreted as positive cooperativity for substrate binding, was attributed, instead, to modulation of the catalytic activity; i.e. when two protomers are occupied by substrate each one assumes a higher activity $(k_2 > k_1)$. This model yielded excellent fits and revealed that $k_1 << k_2 >> k_3$. To further reduce the number of parameters we assumed that k_1 and k_3 were equal to zero. The expression became $v = (2k_2 \; 0.375 \; uS^2 + 4k_4 \; 0.039 \; uS^4)$ $/4(1 + uS + 0.037 \; uS^2 + 0.063 \; uS^3 + 0.0039 \; uS^4)$. The model was thus reduced to 3 parameters; u the apparent substrate affinity equivalent to $(k_m)^{-1}$ in the Michaelis - Menten model, and k_2 and k_4 equivalent to the V_{max} of the 2 and 4 protomer enzyme. If substrate affinity is low, or the substrate concentration range is limited, higher complexes may not contribute substantially to the observed enzymatic activity and the enzyme may behave as a three or two subunit complex.

The formalism described above generated the complete family of curves observed experimentally. The effects of variations in u or k_i on enzyme behavior were analyzed by computer simulation and are illustrated in Figures 2-6. It can be seen that the value of u will determine the substrate concentration at which maximal

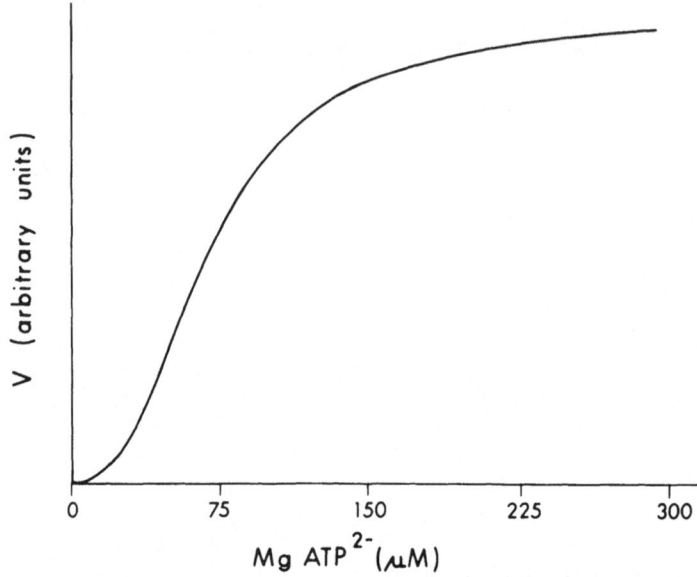

Figure 2. Simulation of adenylate cyclase activity using the Adair equation. MgATP^{2-} varied continuously between 0 and 0.3 mM. Substrate affinity u was set at 10^5 M^{-1}. Catalytic activities were set at 1000 (arbitrary units) for both K_2 and K_4. See text for detailed explanations.

activity occurs (Figures 3, 4, 5), whereas the value of k_2 determines the height of the peak. The ratio between k_2 and k_4 determines the extent of substrate inhibition (Figures 2, 3, 4, 5). For equal values of k_2 substrate inhibition was more pronounced for higher values of u. This model gave very good fits to a large amount of data and provided additional insight into the effects of metals on the behavior of the enzyme discussed in the next section.

The use of the Adair equation, as described above, is based on three assumptions: (i) quasi equilibrium (binding of substrate is fast relative to substrate conversion); (ii) existence of multiple interacting subunits; and (iii) subunit interaction affects the catalytic activity (catalytic cooperativity) and does not affect substrate binding. There is currently no independent information available to test these assumptions for adenylate cyclase. Quasi equilibrium is usually assumed for complicated enzyme mechanisms since it simplifies analysis and was supported in several cases by direct measurements of binding rates. There are exceptions however, and hysteretic properties sometimes observed for adenylate cyclase could be due to slow binding or

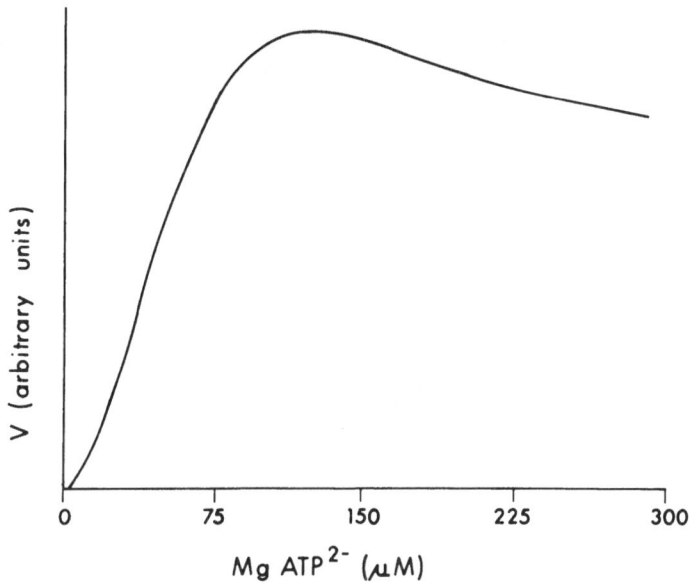

Figure 3. Simulation of adenylate cyclase activity using the Adair equation. MgATP^{2-} varied continuously between 0 and 0.3 mM. Substrate affinity u was set at 2 x 10^4 M^{-1}. Catalytic activities were set at 9000 (arbitrary units) for K$_2$ and 2000 for K$_4$.

release rates and would be better described by a steady state model.

The enzyme preparations used during the development of this model did not exhibit hysteretic properties. Random binding and non-interacting binding affinities are approximations which provide adequate description of the data, but probably do not fully hold. Availability of pure enzyme will make it possible to determine binding constants directly, make appropriate corrections to the model and distinguish between binding cooperativity and catalytic cooperativity. The attribution of substrate activation to positive catalytic cooperativity led to the interesting symmetrical model according to which the enzyme complex is active only if an even number of substrate molecules are bound to it.

Although the various properties discussed above may have intriguing structural implications, at this stage this model is only a convenient way of describing the kinetic properties of the enzyme. An important implication is the narrow range of substrate concentration for which maximum enzyme activity is seen; this would make the cyclic AMP responsiveness of a particular cell

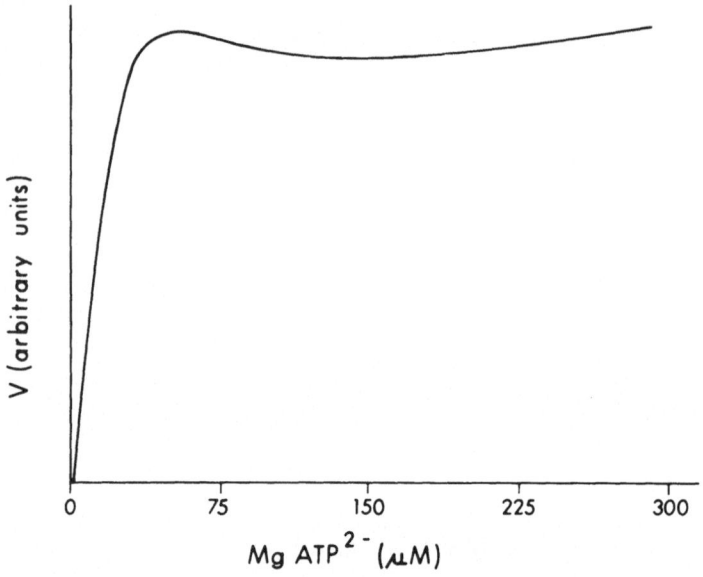

Figure 4.   Simulation of adenylate cyclase activity using the Adair equation. $MgATP^{2-}$ varied continuously between 0 and 0.3 mM.   Substrate affinity u was set at 10^5 M^{-1}.   Catalytic activities were set at 1000 (arbitrary units) for K_2 and 300 for K_4.

dependent on its ATP content. The ATP "window" is a function of u, which is also dependent on cation concentration.

It is generally accepted that $MgATP^{2-}$ is the substrate for enzyme activity. There is, however, some controversy on the effect of free metal bivalent cations on enzyme activity. It has been repeatedly observed that increased concentrations of Mg^{2+} or Mn^{2+}, in excess of those required to saturate the ATP present, stimulated significantly the enzymatic activity. Two alternative explanations were offered for this phenomenon: (i) The presence of a metal binding site, which when occupied modulates the catalytic activity of the enzyme (Birnbaumer *et al.*, 1969; Drummond and Duncan, 1970; Drummond *et al.*, 1971), and (ii) the removal of ATP anionic species ATP^{4-} and ATP^{3-} which compete with the substrate at the catalytic site (deHaen, 1974; Rendell *et al.*, 1975). The bulk of the evidence favors the former view (Garbers and Johnson, 1975; Londos and Preston, 1977; Steer and Levitzki, 1975; Blume and Foster, 1976). Moreover the effect of Mg^{2+} seems to be cooperative (Steer and Levitzki, 1975; 1977; Blume and Foster, 1976). The K_a for Mg^{2+} was found to be between 1 and 3 mM.

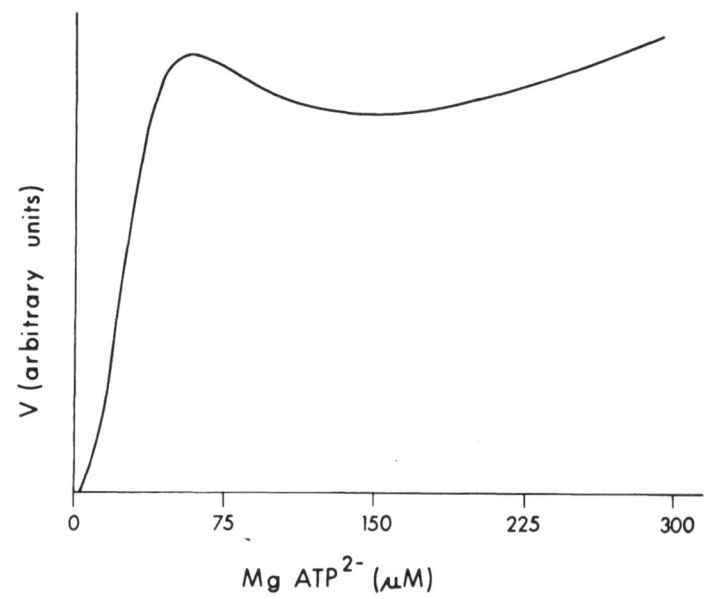

Figure 5. Simulation of adenylate cyclase activity using the Adair equation. MgATP^{2-} varied continuously between 0 and 0.3 mM. Substrate affinity u was set at 6 x 10^4 M^{-1}. Catalytic activities were set at 1500 (arbitrary units) for K$_2$ and 300 for K$_4$.

The inhibitory effect of Ca^{2+} concentrations above 10 μM was found to be a very general property of this enzyme (Perkins, 1973). However, few studies have dealt with the mechanism of Ca^{2+} inhibition. Steer and Levitzki (1975) analyzed the effect of Ca^{2+} on the epinephrine stimulated adenylate cyclase of turkey erythrocytes. The data are consistent with a separate allosteric binding site for bivalent cations competed for by Mn^{2+} and Ca^{2+}. The affinity for Ca^{2+} seems to be very high since substantial inhibition can be seen at 0.2 mM Ca^{2+} in the presence of 0.27 mM EGTA. The authors estimated that Ca^{2+} inhibition was cooperative, and calculated a Hill coefficient of 2. However, this figure is closer to 1 when the Ca^{2+} concentrations are corrected for EGTA binding. Calcium ion did not interfere with epinephrine stimulation. Nor did it affect the cooperative stimulation of MgCl$_2$ which was found to have a Hill coefficient of 3. The authors have also concluded that the enzyme has separate sites for MgATP^{2-} Mg^{2+} and a bivalent cation site competed for by Ca^{2+} which is inhibitory and Mn^{2+} which is stimulatory. The data strongly indicate that CaATP does not play a role in the inhibitory effects of Ca^{2+} on the enzyme.

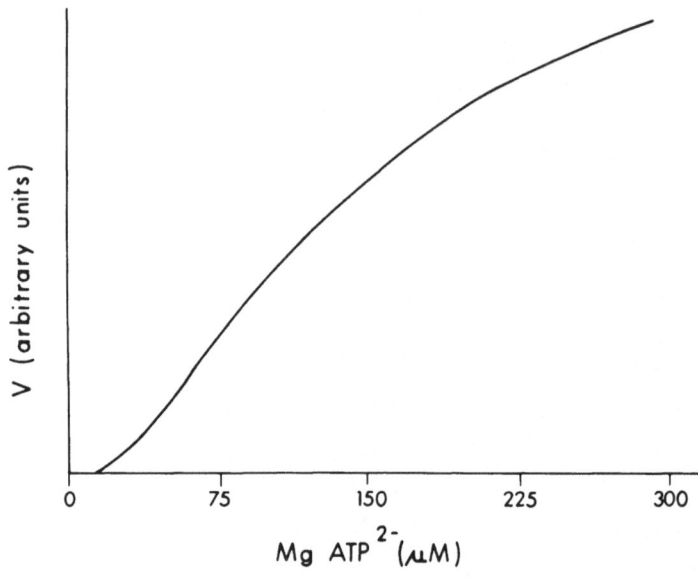

Figure 6. Simulation of adenylate cyclase activity using the Adair equation. MgATP^{2-} varied continuously between 0 and 0.3 mM. Substrate affinity u was set at 1 x 10^5 M^{-1}. Catalytic activities were set at 3000 (arbitrary units) for K$_2$ and 1000 for K$_4$.

Londos and Rodbell (1977), in studies of liver adenylate cyclase, found evidence for an allosteric metal binding site which can be occupied by Mg^{2+}, Mn^{2+} or Ca^{2+} competitively, Mn^{2+} and Mg^{2+} having stimulatory effects while Ca^{2+} was inhibitory. The concentrations of Mg^{2+} and Mn^{2+} required for half maximal activation were 4 mM and 0.3 mM, respectively. Similar findings were reported by Drummond *et al.* (1971) and Severson *et al.* (1972) who examined the adenylate cyclase of particulate fractions from cardiac and skeletal muscle. In skeletal muscle sarcolemma Mg^{2+}, Mn^{2+} and Co^{2+}, when present in excess of ATP concentrations were stimulatory. The k$_a$ for Mg^{2+} was estimated to be between 3 and 5 mM, Mn^{2+} 1 mM, and Co^{2+} 2 mM. Calcium ion inhibited the enzyme and had a k$_i$ of about 0.5 mM. The effect of the cations was mainly on the catalytic activity of the enzyme.

Blume and Foster (1976) studied the adenylate cyclase of neuroblastoma cells. They found that Mg^{2+} and Mn^{2+} in excess of ATP concentrations were stimulatory. The apparent k$_a$ for Mg^{2+} was about 2.5 mM and for Mn^{2+} 1 mM. Interestingly the affinity for these cations was strongly dependent on the presence of chloro-adenosine. The k$_a$ for Mg^{2+} decreased to 1 mM in the presence of this drug and that for Mn^{2+} decreased to 0.5 mM. Another interesting observation is that increasing concentrations of Mn^{2+} caused inhibition of catalytic activity similar to the substrate inhibition described earlier. The presence of 2-chloroadenosine shifted the concentrations at which the peak stimulation of Mn^{2+} was seen from 3.5 to 1 mM. Adenosine and Mn^{2+} acted cooperatively on the enzyme complex. Calcium ion was found to be a non-competitive inhibitor with respect to ATP with a k_i of approximately 0.45 mM. The binding of Ca^{2+} was cooperative and gave a Hill coefficient of 2. Calcium ion and Mn^{2+} appeared to compete for the same site since increasing Mn^{2+} concentrations removed the inhibitory effect of Ca^{2+}. However, Mg^{2+} seemed to bind to an additional site since, with increasing Mg^{2+} concentrations, the adenylate cyclase activity leveled off at lower levels when Ca^{2+} was present. Calcium ion had no effect on the cooperativity of adenosine activation; a Hill coefficient of 1 was calculated in the presence of various Ca^{2+} concentrations. Calcium ion interfered, however, with the interaction between Mg^{2+} and adenosine since, in the presence of 0.6 mM Ca^{2+}, the concentration of Mg^{2+} required to achieve 50% of maximal 2-chloroadenosine stimulation shifted from 0.7 mM to 2 mM.

In a recent paper Stolc (1977) studied the regulation of adenylate cyclase activity in human polymorphonuclear leucocytes. The findings were similar to those from other tissues. Magnesium ion was stimulatory at concentrations above those required to saturate ATP. The effect was cooperative and had a Hill coefficient of 2. Calcium ion inhibited the enzyme activity in a non-competitive way with respect to ATP and was non-cooperative, showing a Hill coefficient of approximately 1. The Hill number for ATP between 0.1 and 1 mM at excess Mg^{2+} was approximately 2 and was not affected by Ca^{2+}. Calcium ion also inhibited the Gpp(NH)p-stimulated enzyme in a non-competitive fashion. Gpp(NH)p had no effect on the Hill coefficient for Ca^{2+}. The k_i for Ca^{2+} was approximately 0.5 mM. In adrenal cortex adenylate cyclase, Glossmann and Gips (1976) demonstrated Ca^{2+} inhibition of adenylate cyclase with a k_i of approximately 0.4 mM and Mn^{2+} stimulation with a k_a of similar magnitude. The two cations seemed to compete for the same site.

The studies reviewed above are consistent with the existence of allosteric bivalent cation sites, the occupancy of which directly affects the catalytic activity of the enzyme. There is strong evidence for direct competition between the inhibitory effect of Ca^{2+} and the stimulatory effect of Mn^{2+}. The relationship between Ca^{2+} and Mg^{2+} is less clear, however, since there is evidence for both independent as well as competitive effects. Our studies were the first to fully account for the ionic composition of the media during adenylate cyclase assays and allow for controlled variation of individual constituents of the assay mixture by

solution of the equations describing the dissociation of ATP and
EGTA as a function of pH and the interactions of Ca^{2+} and Mg^{2+}
with ATP^{4-}, ATP^{3-}, $EGTA^{4-}$ and $EGTA^{3-}$. This made it possible to
study the effects of the free cations independent of their association with ATP at all concentrations, while keeping $MgATP^{2-}$ constant
and monitoring the changes in ATP^{4-} and ATP^{3-}, if any.

In a study on platelet adenylate cyclase (Rodan and Feinstein,
1976), Ca^{2+} was found to be a non-competitive inhibitor with respect
to $MgATP^{2-}$ with a k_i of approximately 0.3 mM and a Hill coefficient
smaller than 1. The effect of the interaction between Ca^{2+} and
Mg^{2+} was not examined. In a recent study we investigated the
microsomal adenylate cyclase from chick pectoralis muscle (submitted for publication). The data were consistent with uncompeti-
tive inhibition of Ca^{2+} relative to $MgATP^{2-}$ with a k_i of about
0.2 mM and a Hill coefficient of 1. Magnesium ion competitively
removed the Ca^{2+} inhibition on enzyme velocity and, in addition,
had stimulatory effects which were cooperative ($n_H = 2$) and unrelated to calcium. In an analogy with the model of Racker (1976)
for sarcoplasmic reticulum Ca^{2+}-ATPase, we interpreted these findings as evidence that binding of Ca^{2+} to the metal allosteric site
causes inhibition of catalytic activity and non-interaction between
subunits whereas binding of Mg^{2+} "energizes" the complex, is
stimulatory and is cooperative. The k_a for Mg^{2+} was 1.5 mM. In
studies of embryonic bone and osteosarcoma adenylate cyclase we
used the kinetic model described earlier which incorporates cooperativity for $MgATP^{2-}$. We found that Ca^{2+} inhibited the catalytic
activity with a k_i of about 0.2 mM. The binding of Ca^{2+} was non-
cooperative and Mg^{2+} competed directly for Ca^{2+} inhibition. The
apparent k_a for Mg^{2+} was about 2.5 mM. Magnesium ion also enhanced
the affinity for substrate. Our findings strongly support the
presence of cationic, regulatory sites in the adenylate enzyme
complex. The evidence also points to direct competition between
the inhibitory effects of Ca^{2+} on enzyme velocity and the stimulatory effects of Mg^{2+}. It is not clear yet if the cooperative
effects of Mg^{2+} on substrate affinity are due to its interaction
with the catalytic site or to changes in subunit interaction
caused by Mg^{2+} binding to the metal site.

In addition to its apparently direct effect on the enzyme,
Ca^{2+} is involved in the action of regulatory proteins which
modulate adenylate cyclase activity. Brostrom *et al.* (1976) in
studies of adenylate cyclase in glial tumor cells showed a biphasic effect of Ca^{2+}: stimulatory at low concentrations and inhibitory at higher concentrations. The Ca^{2+} effect was influenced
by a Ca^{2+} binding soluble protein called calcium dependent regulator
(CDR) which shifted the apparent affinity for Ca^{2+} to the left.
In the presence of CDR, Ca^{2+} concentrations above 0.1 μM (adjusted
with EGTA buffer) were inhibitory, whereas in the absence of CDR,

concentrations up to 30 μM were stimulatory in a concentration dependent manner. This biphasic behavior, with stimulatory effects at low Ca^{2+} concentrations, was observed in several systems, especially in the presence of target specific hormones: vasopressin stimulated adenylate cyclase from kidney medulla (Campbell et al., 1972), oxytocin stimulated bladder epithelium (Boeckart et al., 1972), adrenocorticotropic hormone stimulated adrenal gland (Lefkowitz et al., 1970; Glossman and Gips, 1976) isoproterenol stimulated parotid gland (Franks et al., 1974), and adrenocorticotropic stimulated adipocytes (Bar and Hechter, 1969). Many of these experiments were conducted with EGTA and, according to Glossman and Gips (1976), the effect of Ca^{2+} in removing EGTA inhibition may be non-specific. Other cations, such as Mn^{2+} did reproduce the low concentration stimulatory effects. However, this does not negate the possibility that in vivo adenylate cyclase is regulated by a Ca^{2+} dependent protein like phosphodiesterase.

In a recent study, Gnegy et al. (1976) have shown that membranes of rat caudate nucleus contain (i) calcium binding protein which activates phosphodiesterase and (ii) adenylate cyclase. They have further shown that, following phosphorylation by a cAMP-dependent protein kinase, the calcium binding protein was released from the membrane and the adenylate cyclase lost its responsiveness to dopamine. The adenylate cyclase itself was not phosphorylated. This study points to interesting feedback relationships. The protein released from the membrane when cytoplasmic cAMP increases seems to be essential for coupling the hormone receptor to adenylate cyclase. Once released it not only stimulates the breakdown of cAMP by phosphodiesterase but also contributes to signal termination at the membrane level. Dopamine activation would thus result in a short lived spike of cAMP (as discussed earlier) followed by a refractory period. Cytoplasmic cAMP and Ca^{2+} would determine the responsiveness of the membrane. Further studies are required to establish the generality of this phenomenon. In summary, it appears that local changes in the ionic concentration of calcium, magnesium and possibly manganese may play an important role in turning the adenylate cyclase enzyme on or off.

PHYSIOLOGICAL IMPLICATIONS

If the adenylate cyclase activity assayed in vitro indeed reflects the properties of the enzyme under native conditions, the rate of cAMP production would be strongly influenced by the local relative abundance of Ca^{2+}, Mg^{2+} or Mn^{2+}. The enzyme could be turned on by the release of Ca^{2+} from the membrane and it could be turned off by a rise in the Ca^{2+} to Mg^{2+} ratio. As an illustration, let us consider a hypothetical role for Ca^{2+}-cAMP

interaction during striated muscle contraction. Adenylate cyclase
was shown to be present in the cisternae of the sarcoplasmic
reticulum (SR) (Schulze *et al.*, 1972; Entman *et al.*, 1969; Schulze
and Wollenberger, 1976), the site of Ca^{2+} release during contraction. Let us assume that a certain level of cAMP is required to
maintain the SR membrane in a phosphorylated state which responds
to depolarization by Ca^{2+} release. The release of Ca^{2+} from the
membrane could generate a pulse of cAMP which would contribute
to the activation of the phosphorylase system. On the other hand,
if the Ca^{2+} sensitive site of adenylate cyclase faces the sarcoplasm, the enzyme would soon be inhibited, cAMP would fall and
the membrane would enter a refractory period as described by
Hodgkin and Horowicz (1960). Lüttgau (1963) has shown that re-
fractoriness in excitation-contraction coupling is enhanced by
Ca^{2+}. This may be a general scheme for Ca^{2+}-cAMP interaction in
systems where membrane perturbation leads to depolarization and
Ca^{2+} release. The modulation of adenylate cyclase by changes in
ion concentrations may have preceded, evolutionarily, the control
of the enzyme by hormones. Hammes and Rodbell (1976) have postulated that hormone activation may result from a change in the
affinity for metal. Van Cauter *et al.* (1976) have recently analyzed a cross inhibition model in which one agonist stimulates the
formation of two mediators which inhibit each other's accumulation.
This situation may well apply to the interaction of Ca^{2+} and cAMP.
Incorporation of a Ca^{2+} dependent regulatory protein into the
system would add additional fine tuning. In essence the interaction of Ca^{2+} and cAMP seems to have evolved into a sophisticated
binary communication system which can control the responsiveness
to membrane perturbation as well as the nature (cAMP or Ca^{2+})
shape (pulses) and duration of the generated signal.

SUMMARY AND CONCLUSIONS

Calcium ion fluxes and phosphorylation are frequently involved
in the control of biological processes. Some phosphorylations
are regulated by cAMP-dependent protein kinase. In many systems
cAMP and Ca^{2+} serve jointly as cellular messengers of intercellular
communication. The detailed relationship between the two has not
been fully elucidated and may vary from system to system. Three
examples are presented to illustrate joint involvement of Ca^{2+}
and cAMP: Insulin secretion, excitation of photoreceptors, and
control of cell division. A general feature of message transmission,
Ca^{2+} or cAMP mediated, is the spiked nature of the signal. Binary
(all or none) messages have higher reliability and are probably
precursors of the way information is transferred in the nervous
system. It has been suggested that the mutual effects of cAMP and
Ca^{2+} on each other's concentration may contribute to this kinetic
pattern. In certain specialized systems, such as the sarcoplasmic

reticulum of cardiac or striated muscle, cAMP-dependent phosphorylation was shown to enhance Ca^{2+} accumulation. On the other hand,
Ca^{2+} has a major effect on cAMP. On the catabolic side, the breakdown of cAMP by phosphodiesterase is enhanced by a Ca^{2+} binding
protein similar in structure to troponin C. On the anabolic side
Ca^{2+} affects the generation of cAMP by adenylate cyclase in several
ways. Adenylate cyclase has many properties of allosteric enzymes.
The enzyme exhibits sigmoidal kinetics, substrate inhibition, heterotropic modulation, biphasic effects for substrate analogs such as
adenosine, and hysteretic responses to guanine nucleotides. The
kinetic behavior of the enzyme is adequately described by a four
term Adair equation which assumes statistical binding of substrate
to four protomers and catalytic cooperativity. According to this
model it appears that the complex is catalytically reactive only
when an even number of protometers are occupied by substrate. This
model was used to examine the effect of the bivalent cations, Mg^{2+}
and Ca^{2+}, on the plasma membrane adenylate cyclase from a variety
of tissues. In these studies the ionic composition of the enzyme
assay mixture was fully defined and controlled by solving the simultaneous equation describing the dissociations of the various anions
as a function of pH and the associations of the individual anionic
and cationic species. EGTA was present in the assay as a cation
buffer. The findings supported previous studies which indicated
the existence of a regulatory cationic site which can bind Ca^{2+},
Mg^{2+} or Mn^{2+}. The binding of Ca^{2+} is inhibitory and has a k_i of
0.2 to 0.4 mM. Manganese ion can compete with Ca^{2+}, has similar
affinity and is stimulatory. The effect of Mg^{2+} is more complex.
It can remove the Ca^{2+} inhibition but seems to have an additional
stimulatory effect and its binding is cooperative. Those apparent
kinetic differences do not necessarily imply a different site and
may be due to different effects of Mg^{2+} binding. Recent reports
indicate that in addition to these seemingly direct effects of the
metal on the enzyme, calcium can affect enzymatic activity via a
Ca^{2+} binding protein in a manner similar to its effect on phosphodiesterase.

These interactions of Ca^{2+} and cAMP have several physiological
implications. Adenylate cyclase can be turned on or off through
changes in the relative local abundancy of Ca^{2+} and Mg^{2+}. Membrane
perturbation by hormones or other external agents could affect cellular cAMP and Ca^{2+} in different ways: it may stimulate adenylate
cyclase via receptor enzyme coupling and raise cAMP levels; it may
(in addition) increase Ca^{2+} influx, which would restrict the cAMP
message to a brief pulse; or it may increase Ca^{2+} influx without
stimulating adenylate cyclase, which would result in a decrease in
cellular cAMP. Combination of the two signals and the feedback relationship between them enriches the information potential of this
communication system by offering a mechanism for signal termination
and making possible spikes, oscillations, or messages based on
signal frequency.

REFERENCES

Adair, G. S., 1925, The hemoglobin system. VI. The oxygen dissociation curve of hemoglobin, *J. Biol. Chem.* 63: 529.

Anderson, W. B., Johnson, G. S., and Pastan, I., 1973, Transformation of chick embryo fibroblasts by wild-type and temperature-
sensitive Rous sarcoma virus alters adenylate cyclase activity,
Proc. Nat. Acad. Sci. U. S. A. 70: 1055.

Anderson, W. B., and Pastan, I., 1975, Altered adenylate cyclase
activity: Its role in growth regulation and malignant transformation of fibroblases, *in* "Advances in Cyclic Nucleotide Research",
Vol. 5, (G. L. Drummond, P. Greengard and G. A. Robison, eds.),
pp. 681-689, Raven Press, New York.

Andrew, C. G., Roses, A. D., Almon, R. R., and Appel, S. H., 1973,
Phosphorylation of muscle membranes: identification of a membrane-
bound protein kinase, *Science* 182: 927.

Appleman, M. M., Thompson, W. J., and Russell, T. R., 1973, Cyclic
nucleotide phosphodiesterase, *in* "Advances in Cyclic Nucleotide
Research", Vol. 3, (P. Greengard and G. A. Robison, eds.), pp.
65-98, Raven Press, New York.

Bader, C. R., Baumann, F., and Bertrand, D., 1976, Role of intracellular calcium and sodium in light adaptation in the retina
of the honey bee drone, *J. gen. Physiol.* 67: 475.

Baker, P. F., Hodgkin, A. L., and Ridgway, E. B., 1971, Depolarization and calcium entry in squid giant axons, *J. Physiol.*
(London) 218: 709.

Balk, S. D., 1971, Calcium as a regulator of the proliferation of
normal but not of transformed, chicken fibroblasts in a plasma-
containing medium, *Proc. Nat. Acad. Sci. U. S. A.* 68: 271.

Balk, S. D., Whitfield, J. F., Youdale, T., and Braun, A. C.,
1973, Roles of calcium, serum, plasma and folic acid in the
control of cell proliferation of normal and Rous sarcoma virus-
infected chicken fibroblasts, *Proc. Nat. Acad. Sci. U. S. A.*
70: 675.

Bär, H. P., and Hechter, O., 1969, Adenyl cyclase and hormone
action I. Effects of adrenocorticotropic hormone, glucagon,
and epinephrine on the plasma membrane of rat fat cells, *Proc.*
Nat. Acad. Sci. U. S. A. 63: 350.

Bennett, M. V. L., and Trinkaus, J. P., 1970, Electrical coupling
between embryonic cells by way of extracellular space and
specialized junctions, *J. Cell Biol.* 44: 592.

Berridge, M. J., 1975, The interaction of cyclic nucleotides and
calcium in the control of cellular activity, *in* "Advances in
Cyclic Nucleotide Research", Vol. 6, (P. Greengard and G. A.
Robison, eds.), pp. 1-98, Raven Press, New York.

Birnbaumer, L., Pohl, S. L., and Rodbell, M., 1969, Adenyl cyclase
in fat cells. I. Properties and the effects of adrenocorticotropin and fluoride, *J. Biol. Chem.* 244: 3468.

Birnbaumer, L., Pohl, S. L., and Rodbell, M., 1972, The glucagon-sensitive adenylate cyclase system in plasma membranes of rat liver, *J. Biol. Chem.* 247: 2038.

Bitensky, M. W., Miki, N., Marcus, F. N., and Keirns, J. J., 1973, The role of cyclic nucleotides in visual excitation, *Life Sciences* 13: 1451.

Blume, A. J., and Foster, C. J., 1976, Mouse neuroblastoma cell adenylase cyclase: Regulation by 2-chloroadenosine, prostaglandin E_1, and the cations Mg^{2+}, Ca^{2+} and Mn^{2+}, *J. Neurochem.* 26: 305.

Boeckart, J., Roy, C., and Jard, S., 1972, Oxytocin-sensitive adenylate cyclase in frog bladder epithelia cells. Role of calcium, nucleotides, and other factors in hormonal stimulation, *J. Biol. Chem.* 247: 7073.

Borisy, G. G., Olmsted, J. B., Marum, J. M., and Allen, C., 1974, Microtubule assembly *in vitro*, *Fed. Proc.* 33: 167.

Boynton, A. L., Whitfield, J. F., Isaacs, R. J., and Morton, H. J., 1974, Control of 3T3 cell proliferation by calcium, *In Vitro* 10: 12.

Braun, T., 1975, The effect of divalent cations on bovine spermatozoal adenylate cyclase activity, *J. Cyclic Nucleotide Res.* 1: 271.

Brisson, G. R., Camu, F., Malaisse-Lagae, F., and Malaisse, W. J., 1971, Effects of a local anesthetic upon calcium uptake and insulin secretion by isolated isles of langerhans, *Life Sciences* 10: 445.

Brooker, G., 1975, Implications of cyclic nucleotide oscillations during the myocardial contraction cycle, *in* "Advances in Cyclic Nucleotide Research", Vol. 5, (G. I. Drummond, P. Greengard and G. A. Robison, eds.), pp. 435, Raven Press, New York.

Brostrom, M. A., Brostrom, C. A., Breckenridge, B. M., and Wolff, D. J., 1976, Regulation of adenylate cyclase from glial tumor cells by calcium and a calcium-binding protein, *J. Biol. Chem.* 251: 4744.

Brown, J. E., and Blinks, J. R., 1972, Changes in $[Ca^{2+}]$ of *Limulus* ventral photoreceptors measured with aequorin, *Biological Bulletin* 143: 456.

Burger, M. M., Bombik, B. M., Breckenridge, B. M., and Sheppard, J. R., 1972, Growth control and cyclic alteration of cyclic AMP in the cell cycle, *Nature, New Biol.* 239: 161.

Burk, R. R., 1968, Reduced adenyl cyclase activity in a polyoma virus transformed cell line, *Nature* 219: 1272.

Burns, T. W., Langley, P. E., and Robison, G. A., 1972, Studies on the role of cyclic AMP in human lipolysis, *in* "Advances in Cyclic Nucleotide Research", Vol. 1, (P. Greengard, R. Paoletti, and G. A. Robison, eds.), pp. 63-85, Raven Press, New York.

Campbell, B. J., Woodward, G., and Borberg, V., 1972, Calcium-mediated interactions between the antidiuretic hormone and renal plasma membranes, *J. Biol. Chem.* 247: 6167.

Carchman, R. A., Johnson, G. S., Pastan, I., and Scolnick, E. M., 1974, Studies on the levels of cyclic AMP in cells transformed by wild-type and temperature-sensitive kirsten sarcoma virus, *Cell* 1: 59.

Changeux, J. P., Thiery, J., Tung, Y., and Kittel, C., 1967, On the cooperativity of biological membranes, *Proc. Nat. Acad. Sci. U. S. A.* 57: 335.

Cheung, W. Y., 1970, Cyclic 3',5'-nucoeotide phosphodiesterase; Demonstration of an activator, *Biochem. Biophys. Res. Commun.* 38: 533.

Cheung, W. Y., 1971, Cyclic 3',5'-nucleotide phosphodiesterase: Evidence for and properties of a protein activator, *J. Biol. Chem.* 246: 2859.

Chlapowski, F. J., Kelley, L. A., and Butcher, R. W., 1975, Cyclic nucleotides in cultured cells, *in* "Advances in Cyclic Nucleotide Research", Vol. 6, (P. Greengard, and G. A. Robison, eds.), pp. 245-338, Raven Press, New York.

Cooper, B., Partilla, J. S., and Gregerman, R. I., 1976, Human fat cell adenylate cyclase. Enzyme characterization and guanine nucleotide effects on epinephrine responsiveness in cell membranes *Biochem. Biophys. Acta* 445: 246.

Davis, B., and Lazarus, N. R., 1973, Insulin release from pancreatic islets: Properties of a membrane bound phosphokinase from cod and mouse islets, "Proceeding of 8th Congress of the International Diabetes Federation", *Excerpter Medica ICS* 280: 7.

Dean, P. M., and Matthews, E. K., 1970a, Glucose-induced electrical activity in pancreatic islet cells, *J. Physiol. (London)* 210: 255.

Dean, P. M., and Matthews, E. K., 1970b, Electrical activity in pancreatic islet cells: Effect of ions, *J. Physiol. (London)* 210: 265.

deHaen, C., 1974, Adenylate cyclase. A new kinetic analysis of the effects of hormones and fluoride ion, *J. Biol. Chem.* 249: 2756.

Drummond, G. I., and Duncan, L., 1970, Adenyl cyclase in cardiac tissue, *J. Biol. Chem.* 245: 976.

Drummond, G. I., Severson, D. L., and Duncan, L., 1971, Adenyl cyclase. Kinetic properties and nature of fluoride and hormone stimulation, *J. Biol. Chem.* 246: 4166.

Entman, M. L., Levey, G. S., and Epstein, S. E., 1969, Mechanism of action of epinephrine and glucagon on the canine heart: evidence for increase in sarcotubular calcium stores mediated by cyclic 3', 5'-AMP, *Circulation* 25: 429.

Franks, D. J., Perrin, L. S., and Malamud, D., 1974, Calcium ion: A modulator of parotid adenylate cyclase activity, *FEBS Lett.* 42: 267.

Friedman, D. L., 1976, Role of cyclic nucleotides in cell growth and differentiation, *Physiol. Rev.* 56: 652.

Froechlich, J. E., and Rachmeler, M., 1972, Effect of adenosine
3', 5'-cyclic monophosphate on cell proliferation, *J. Cell Biol.*
55: 19.

Garbers, D. L., and Johnson, R. A., 1975, Metal and Metal-ATP
interactions with brain and cardiac adenylate cyclase, *J. Biol.
Chem.* 250: 8449.

Gerisch, G., and Wick, U., 1975, Intracellular oscillations and
release of cyclic AMP from *Dictyostelium* cells, *Biochem. Biophys.
Res. Commun.* 65: 364.

Glansdorf, P., and Prigogine, I., 1971, "Thermodynamics Theory of
Structure Stability and Fluctuations", Wiley Interscience,
New York.

Glossmann, H., and Gips, H., 1976, Adrenal cortex adenylate cyclase,
Naunyn-Schmied. Arch. Pharmacol. 292: 199.

Gnegy, M. E., Uzunov, P., and Costa, E., 1976, Regulation of dopamine stimulation of striatal adenylate cyclase by an endogenous
Ca^{++} binding protein, *Proc. Nat. Acad. Sci. U. S. A.* 73: 3887.

Goldbeter, A., and Caplan, S. R., 1976, Oscillatory enzymes, *Annu.
Rev. Biophys. Bioeng.* 5: 449.

Goldbeter, A., and Segel, L. A., 1977, Unified mechanism for relay
and oscillation of cyclic AMP in *Dictyostelium discoideum*, *Proc.
Nat. Acad. Sci. U. S. A.* 74: 1543.

Hadden, J. W., Hadden, E. M., Haddox, M. K., and Goldberg, N. S.,
1972, Guanosine 3':5'-cyclic monophosphate: a possible intracellular mediator of mitogenic influences in lymphocytes, *Proc.
Nat. Acad. Sci. U. S. A.* 69: 3024.

Hadden, J. W., Hadden, E. M., Meetz, G., Good, R. A., Haddox, M.
K., and Goldberg, N. D., 1973, Cyclic GMP in cholinergic and
mitogenic modulation of lymphocyte metabolism and proliferation,
Fed. Proc. 32: 1022.

Hales, C. N., and Miller, R. D. G., 1968, Cations and secretion
of insulin from rabbit pancreas in vitro, *J. Physiol. (London)*
199: 177.

Hammes, G. G., and Rodbell, M., 1976, Simple model for hormone-
activated adenylate cyclase systems, *Proc. Nat. Acad. Sci. U.
S. A.* 73: 1189.

Haslam, R. J., and Lynham, J. A., 1973, Activation and inhibition
of blood platelet adenylate cyclase by adenosine or by 2-chloro-
adenosine, *Life Sciences* 11: 1143.

Hasselbach, W., Fiehn, W., Makinose, M., and Migala, A. J., 1969,
Calcium fluxes across isolated sarcoplasmic membranes in the
presence and absence of ATP, *in* "The Molecular Basis of Membrane
Function", (D. C. Tosteson, ed.), pp. 299-316, Prentice Hall,
Englewood Cliffs, New Jersey.

Hodgkin, A. L., and Horowitz, P., 1960, Potassium contractures
in single muscle fibres, *J. Physiol. (London)* 153: 386.

Hui, C. W., Drummond, M., and Drummond, G. I., 1976, Calcium
accumulation and cyclic AMP-stimulated phosphorylation in plasma
membrane-enriched preparations of myocardium, *Arch. Biochem.
Biophys.* 173: 415.

Kakiuchi, S., and Yamazaki, R., 1970, Calcium dependent phosphodiesterase activity and its activating factor isolated from
brain: Studies on cyclic 3':5'-nucleotide phosphodiesterase,
Biochem. Biophys. Res. Commun. 41: 1104.

Kirchberger, M. A., Tada, M., Repke, D. I., and Katz, A. M., 1972,
Cyclic adenosine 3',5'-monophosphate-dependent protein kinase
stimulation of calcium uptake by canine cardiac microsomes,
J. Mol. Cell. Cardiol. 4: 673.

Kirchberger, M. A., and Tada, M., 1976, Effects of adenosine
3',5'-monophosphate dependent protein kinase in sarcoplasmic
reticulum isolated from cardiac and slow and fast contractory
skeletal muscles, *J. Biol. Chem.* 251: 725.

Krishna, G., Harwood, J. P., Barber, A. J., and Jamieson, G. A.,
1972, Requirement for guanosine triphosphate in the prostaglandin
activation of adenylate cyclase of platelet membranes, *J. Biol.
Chem.* 247: 2253.

Lacy, P. E., and Malaisse, N. J., 1973, Microtubules and beta cell
secretion, *Recent Prog. Hormone Res.* 29: 199.

LaRaia, P. J., Zerling, L. J., and Morkin, E., 1973, Phosphoryla-
tion-dephosphorylation of cardiac microsomes: A possible mechanism for control of calcium uptake by cyclic-AMP, *Fed. Proc.* 32:
346.

Lefkowitz, R. J., Roth, J., and Pastan, I., 1970, Effects of calcium on ACTH stimulation of the adrenal. Separation of hormone
binding from adenyl cyclase activation, *Nature* 228: 864.

Letterier, J. F., Rappaport, L., and Nunez, J., 1974, Phosphorylation and aggregation and neurotubulin and "associated" protein
kinase, *Mol. Cell. Endocrinol.* 1: 65.

Loewenstein, W. R., 1973, Membrane junctions in growth and differentiation, *Fed. Proc.* 32: 60.

Londos, C., and Preston, M. S., 1977a, Activation of the hepatic
adenylate cyclase system by divalent cations: A reassessment,
J. Biol. Chem. 252: 5957.

Londos, C., and Preston, S. M., 1977b, Regulation by glucagon and
divalent cations of inhibition of hepatic adenylate cyclase by
adenosine, *J. Biol. Chem.* 252: 5951.

Londos, C., and Rodbell, M., 1977, Adenylate cyclase: Actions and
interactions of regulatory ligands, *in* "Drug action at the
molecular level", (G. C. K. Roberts, ed.), pp. 235-247, McMillan
Press, London.

Lowe, D. A., Richardson, B. P., Taylor, P., and Donatsch, P.,
1976, Increasing intracellular sodium triggers calcium release
from bound pools, *Nature* 260: 337.

Lüttgau, H. C., 1963, The action of calcium ions on potassium
contractures of single muscle fibers, *J. Physiol. (London)*
168: 679.

Malaisse-Lagae, F., and Malaisse, W. J., 1971, Stimulus-secretion
coupling of glucose-induced insulin release. III. Uptake of
^{45}calcium by isolated islets of Langerhans, *Endocrinology* 88: 72.

Malaisse, W. J., 1973, Insulin secretion: Multifactorial regulation for a single release process, *Diabetologia* 9: 167.

Moens, W. A., Vokaer, A., and Kran, R., 1975, Cyclic AMP and cyclic GMP concentrations in serum- and density-restricted fibroblast cultures, *Proc. Nat. Acad. Sci. U. S. A.* 72: 1063.

Montague, W., and Howell, S. L., 1972, The mode of action of 3'5'-cyclic monophosphate in mammalian islets of Langerhans. Preparation and properties of islet cell protein phosphokinase, *Biochem. J.* 129: 551.

Montague, W., and Howell, S. L., 1975, Cyclic AMP and the physiology of the islets of Langerhans, *in* "Advances in Cyclic Nucleotide Research", Vol. 6, (P. Greengard and G. A. Robison, eds.), pp. 201-244, Raven Press, New York.

Neer, E. J., 1976, Two soluble forms of guanosine 5'-(β,γ-imino)-triphosphate and fluoride-activated adenylate cyclase, *J. Biol. Chem.* 251: 5831.

Ney, R. L., Hochella, N. J., Grahame-Smith, D. G., Dexter, R. N., and Butcher, R. W., 1969, Abnormal regulation of adenosine 3',5'-monophosphate and corticosterone formation in an adrenocortical carcinoma, *J. Clin. Invest.* 48: 1733.

Orly, J., and Schramm, M., 1975, Fatty acids as modulators of membrane functions: catecholamine activated adenylate cyclase of the turkey erythrocyte, *Proc. Nat. Acad. Sci. U. S. A.* 9: 3433.

Otten, J., Johnson, G. S., and Pastan, I., 1971, Cyclic AMP levels in fibroblasts: Relationships to growth rate and contact inhibition of growth, *Biochem. Biophys. Res. Commun.* 44: 1192.

Otten, J., Bader, J., Johnson, G. S., and Pastan, I., 1972, A mutation in a Rous sarcoma virus gene that controls adenosine 3',5'-monophosphate levels and transformation, *J. Biol. Chem.* 247: 1632.

Pannbacker, R. G., 1973, Control of guanylase cyclase activity in the rod outer segment, *Science* 182: 1138.

Peck, W. A., Carpenter, J. G., and Schuster, R. J., 1976, Adenosine-mediated stimulation of bone cell adenylate cyclase activity, *Endocrinology* 99: 901.

Perkins, J. P., 1973, Adenyl cyclase, *in* "Advances in Cyclic Nucleotide Research", Vol. 3., (P. Greengard and G. A. Robison, eds.), pp. 1-64, Raven Press, New York.

Pfeuffer, T., and Helmreich, E. J. M., 1975, Activation of pigeon erythrocyte membrane adenylate cyclase by guanylnucleotide analogues and separation of a nucleotide binding protein, *J. Biol. Chem.* 250: 867.

Pichard, A. -L., and Cheung, W. Y., 1976, Cyclic 3':5'-nucleotide phosphodiesterase: Interconvertible multiple forms and their effects on enzyme activity and kinetics, *J. Biol. Chem.* 251: 5726.

Puchwein, G., Pfeuffer, T., and Helmreich, E. J. M., 1974, Un-coupling of catecholamine activation of pigeon erythrocyte membrane adenylate cyclase by filipin, *J. Biol. Chem.* 249: 3232.

Queener, S. F., Fleming, J. W., and Bell, N. H., 1975, Solubilization of calcitonin-responsive renal cortical adenylate cyclase, *J. Biol. Chem.* 250: 7586.

Racker, E., 1976, "A New Look at Mechanisms in Bioenergetics," Academic Press, New York.

Rajerison, R., Marchetti, J., Roy, C., Bockaert, J., and Jard, S., 1974, The vasopressin-sensitive adenylate cyclase of the rat kidney, *J. Biol. Chem.* 249: 6390.

Rasmussen, H., 1970, Cell communication, calcium ion, and cyclic adenosine monophosphate, *Science* 170: 404.

Rasmussen, H., Jensen, P., Lake, W., Friedmann, N., and Goodman, D. B. P., 1975, Cyclic nucleotides and cellular calcium metabolism, *in* "Advances in Cyclic Nucleotide Research", Vol. 5, (G. I. Drummond, P. Greengard and G. A. Robison, eds.), pp. 375-394, Raven Press, New York.

Rendell, M., Salomon, Y., Lin, M., Rodbell, M., and Berman, M., 1975, The hepatic adenylate cyclase system. III. A mathematical model for the steady state kinetics of catalysis and nucleotide regulation, *J. Biol. Chem.* 250: 4235.

Ridgway, E. B., Gilkey, J. C., and Jaffe, L. F., 1976, Free calcium increases explosively in activated medaka eggs, *J. Cell Biol.* 70: 227a.

Rodan, G. A., and Feinstein, M. B., 1976, Interrelationships between Ca^{2+} and adenylate and guanylate cyclases in the control of platelet secretion and aggregation, *Proc. Nat. Acad. Sci. U. S. A.* 73: 1829.

Rodan, G. A., Bourret, L. A., and Cutler, L. S., 1977, Membrane changes during cartilage maturation. Increase in 5'-nucleotidase and decrease in adenosine inhibition of adenylate cyclase, *J. Cell Biol.* 72: 493.

Rodbell, M., Krans, H. M., Pohl, S. L., and Birnbaumer, L., 1971, The glucagon-sensitive adenyl cyclase system in plasma membranes of rat liver. III. Binding of glucagon: Method of assay and specificity, *J. Biol. Chem.* 246: 1861.

Rodbell, M., 1975, On the mechanism of activation of fat cell adenylate cyclase by guanine nucleotides, *J. Biol. Chem.* 250: 5826.

Rossi, C. S., and Lehninger, A. L., 1964, Stoichiometry of respiratory stimulation, accumulation of Ca^{++} and phosphate, and oxidative phosphorylation in rat liver mitochondria, *J. Biol. Chem.* 239: 3971.

Rubin, R. P., 1970, The role of calcium in the release of neurotransmitter substances and hormones, *Pharmacol. Rev.* 22: 389.

Rudland, P. S., Seeley, M., and Seifert, W., 1974, Cyclic GMP and Cyclic AMP. Levels in normal and transformed fibroblasts, *Nature* 251: 417.

Russell, T. R., and Pastan, I., 1974, Cyclic adenosine 3': 5'-
monophosphate phosphodiesterase activities are under separate
genetic control, *J. Biol. Chem.* 249: 7764.

Salomon, Y., Lin, M. C., Londos, C., Rendell, M., and Rodbell, M.,
1975, The hepatic adenylate cyclase system. I. Evidence for
trsnsition states and structural requirements for guanine
nucleotide activation, *J. Biol. Chem.* 250: 4239.

Schramm, M., 1975, The catecholamine-responsive adenylate cyclase
system and its modification by 5'-guanylylimidodiphosphate, *in*
"Advances in Cyclic Nucleotide Research", Vol. 5, (G. I. Drummond,
P. Greengard, and G. A. Robison, eds.), pp. 105-115, Raven Press,
New York.

Schramm, M., and Rodbell, M., 1975, A persistent active state of
the adenylate cyclase system produced by the combined actions
of isoproterenol and guanylyl imidodiphosphate in frog erythrocyte membranes, *J. Biol. Chem.* 250: 2232.

Schulze, W., Krause, E. -G., and Wollenberger, A., 1972, Cytochemical demonstration and localization of adenyl cyclase in
skeletal and cardiac muscle, *in* "Advances in Cyclic Nucleotide
Research", Vol. 1, (P. Greengard, R. Paoletti, and G. A. Robison,
eds.), pp. 249-260, Raven Press, New York.

Schulze, W., and Wollenberger, A., 1976, Zur Lokalisation der
adenylatzyklase im roten und weissen skelettmuskel: Eine
zytochemische Untersuchung, *Acta Biol. Med. Germ.* 35: 837.

Schwabe, U., Schönhöfer, P. S., and Ebert, R., 1974, Facilitation
by adenosine of the action of insulin on the accumulation of
adenosine 3':5'-monophosphate, lipolysis, and glucose oxidation
is isolated fat cells, *Eur. J. Biochem.* 46: 537.

Schwartz, A., Entman, M. L., Koniike, K., Lane, L. K., Van Winkle,
B., and Bornet, E. P., 1976, The rate of calcium uptake into
sarcoplasmic reticulum of cardiac and skeletal muscle: effccts
of cyclic AMP-dependent protein kinase and phosphorylase b
kinase, *Biochim. Biophys. Acta* 426: 57.

Scvcrson, D. L., Drummond, G. I., and Sulakhe, P. V., 1972, Adenylate cyclase in skeletal muscle, *J. Biol. Chem.* 247: 2949.

Sheridan, J. D., 1966, Electrophysiological study of special
connections between cells in the early chick embryo, *J. Cell
Biol.* 31: C1.

Spiegel, A. M., Brown, E. M., and Aurbach, G. D., 1976, Inhibition
of adenylate cyclase by arsenite and cadmium: evidence for a
vicinal dithiol requirement, *J. Cyclic Nucleotide Res.* 2: 393.

Steer, M. L., and Levitzki, A., 1975, The control of adenylate
cyclase by calcium in turkey erythrocyte ghosts, *J. Biol. Chem.*
250: 2080.

Steinhardt, R. A., Lundin, L., and Mazia, D., 1971, Bioelectric
responses of the echinoderm egg to fertilization, *Proc. Nat. Acad.
Sci. U. S. A.* 68: 2426.

Steinhardt, R. A., and Epel, D., 1974, Activation of sea-urchin eggs by a calcium ionophore, *Proc. Nat. Acad. Sci. U. S. A.* 71: 1915.

Stolc, V., 1977, Mechanism of regulation of adenylate cyclase activity in human polymorphonuclear leukocytes by calcium, guanosyl nucleotides, and positive effectors, *J. Biol. Chem.* 252: 1901.

Sulakhe, P. V., and Drummond, G. I., 1974, Protein kinase-catalyzed phosphorylation of muscle sarcolemma, *Arch. Biochem. Biophys.* 161: 448.

Sulakhe, P. V., Leung, N. L., and St. Louis, P. J., 1976, Stimulation of calcium accumulation in cardiac sarcolemma by protein kinase, *Can. J. Biochem.* 54: 438.

Tada, M., Kirchberger, M. A., Iorio, J. A., and Katz, A. M., 1973, Phosphorylation of a low molecular weight component (phospholamban) in cardiac sarcoplasmic reticulum catalyzed by a cyclic AMP-dependent protein kinase, *Circulation* 48: (Suppl. IV.): 25.

Tada, M., Kirchberger, M. A., Repke, D. I., and Katz, A. M., 1974, The stimulation of calcium transport in cardiac sarcoplasmic reticulum by adenosine 3', 5'-monophosphate dependent protein kinase, *J. Biol. Chem.* 249: 6174.

Tada, M., Kirchberger, M. A., and Katz, A. M., 1975, Phosphorylation of a 22,000 dalton component of the cardiac sarcoplasmic reticulum by adenosine 3',5'-monophosphate dependent protein kinase, *J. Biol. Chem.* 250: 2640.

Thomas, E. W., Murad, F., Looney, W. B., and Morris, H. P., 1973, Adenosine 3',5'-monophosphate and guanosine 3',5'-monophosphate: concentrations in Morris hepatomas of different growth rates, *Biochim. Biophys. Acta* 297: 564.

Thompson, W. J., Johnson, D. G., and Williams, R. H., 1976, Hormonal regulation of pancreatic islet adenyl cyclase, *Biochemistry* 15: 1658.

Tolbert, M. E. M., Butcher, F. R., and Fain, J. N., 1973, Lack of correlation between catecholamine effects on cyclic adenosine 3':5'monophosphate and gluconeogenesis in isolated rat liver cells, *J. Biol. Chem.* 248: 5686.

Van Cauter, E., Hardman, J. G., and Dumont, J. E., 1976, Implications of cross inhibitory interactions of potential mediators of hormone and neurotransmitter action, *Proc. Nat. Acad. Sci. U. S. A.* 73: 2982.

Wang, J. H., Teo, T. S., Ho, H. C., and Stevens, F. C., 1975, Bovine heart protein activator of cyclic nucleotide phosphodiesterase, *in* "Advances in Cyclic Nucleotide Research", Vol. 5, (G. I. Drummond, P. Greengard, and G. A. Robison, eds.), pp. 179-194, Raven Press, New York.

Wahrman, J. P., Winand, R., and Luzzati, D., 1973, Effect of Cyclic AMP on growth and morphological differentiation of an established myogenic cell line, *Nature (New Biol.)* 245: 112.

Wallach, D. F. H., 1976, Some biochemical anomalies that can contribute to the malignant behavior of cancer cells, *J. Mol. Med.* 1: 97.

Watterson, D. M., Harrelson, Jr., W. G., Keller, P. M., Sharief, F., and Vanaman, T. C., 1976, Structural similarities between the Ca^{2+} dependent regulatory proteins of 3':5'-cyclic nucleotide phosphodiesterase and actomyosin ATPase, *J. Biol. Chem.* 251: 4501.

Whitfield, J. R., MacManus, J. P., Rixon, R. H., Boynton, A. C., Youdale, T., and Swierenga, S., 1976, The positive control of cell proliferation by the interplay of calcium ions and cyclic nucleotides: A Review, *In Vitro* 12: 1.

Willingham, M. C., Johnson, G. S., and Pastan, I., 1972, Control of DNA synthesis and mitosis in 3T3 cells by cyclic AMP, *Biochem. Biophys. Res. Commun.* 48: 743.

Willingham, M. C., and Pastan, I., 1975, Cyclic AMP and cell morphology in cultured fibroblasts. Effects on cell shape, microfilament and microtubule distribution, and orientation to substratum, *J. Cell Biol.* 67: 146.

Winand, R. J., and Kohn, L. D., 1975, Stimulation of adenylate cyclase activity in retroorbital tissue membranes by thyrotropin and an exophthalmogenic factor derived from thyrotropin, *J. Biol. Chem.* 250: 6522.

CHAPTER 6

PROSTAGLANDINS, CALCIUM, AND CYCLIC NUCLEOTIDES

IN STIMULUS-RESPONSE COUPLING

Ronald P. Rubin and Suzanne G. Laychock

Departments of Pharmacology
Medical College of Virginia,
Virginia Commonwealth University
Richmond, Virginia 23298 and
Vanderbilt University, School of Medicine
Nashville, Tennessee 37232

INTRODUCTION

There is now little doubt that muscle contraction and secretory activity involve fundamentally similar processes, with an
increase in free Ca^{2+} within the cytosol providing the critical
link between membrane activation by a stimulus and the specific
tissue response (Rubin, 1974a; Douglas, 1975a). On the one hand,
Ca^{2+} is instrumental in initiating muscle myofilament contraction
while, on the other hand, Ca^{2+} facilitates the fusion of secretory
granule membranes with the cell membrane of exocytotic tissues.
The fact that Ca^{2+} is a mediator in these two basic biological
processes has prompted speculation that they share a similar molecular basis involving a contractile event (Poisner, 1970; Kuo and
Coffee, 1976; Trifaro and Ulpian, 1976).

The central role of Ca^{2+} in contraction and secretion makes
the physiological regulation of this cation a potentially prime
target for other putative mediators and pharmacologic agents.
Since the Ca^{2+} responsible for activation of both processes may
originate from extracellular or intracellular sources, certain
stimulants will enhance plasma membrane permeability and allow an
influx of extracellular cation, while others will release Ca^{2+}
from intracellular binding sites such as the sarcoplasmic reticulum, the mitochondria, or the plasma membrane itself. Secondary
to a mobilization of Ca^{2+}, the cation exerts its effects through
interactions with other putative mediators of cell function such
as the prostaglandins (PGs) and cyclic nucleotides. Conversely,

135

inhibitors of secretion and contraction may elicit their effects by decreasing membrane permeability to the cation; by facilitating its intracellular binding or active sequestration from the cytoplasm; or by inhibiting some secondary cellular phenomenon vital to the Ca^{2+} stimulated response.

The primary emphasis of this presentation will be placed upon the possible relations between PGs and Ca^{2+}, with attention directed toward the role of cyclic nucleotides only as they have been implicated to interact with PGs and Ca^{2+} in excitation-contraction and stimulus-secretion coupling. A more extensive analysis of the interaction of cyclic AMP (cAMP) and Ca^{2+} is presented in another chapter of this volume. The general theme of Ca^{2+}-drug interaction has been reviewed previously (Rubin, 1974b), but more recent pharmacologic studies have provided additional salient information pertaining to stimulus-response coupling; the contributions of these studies as well as their limitations will be discussed.

ROLE OF PROSTAGLANDINS IN CELL FUNCTION

As a preface to the discussion of PG-Ca^{2+} interactions, a brief account of the metabolism of PGs and their role as putative mediators will show that the ubiquitous PGs have been implicated in a variety of cellular processes, although a specific physiological function for one or another of the PGs has yet to be irrefutably defined. PGs are synthesized and released by diverse agents - many of which have the capacity to perturb membranes (Ramwell and Rabinowitz, 1972; Ferreira and Vane, 1974). Biosynthesis is catalyzed by a complex enzyme system known as PG synthetase (Flower, 1974), which has been found in most tissues and utilizes arachidonic acid as substrate. A major pathway which has been elaborated in blood platelets is catalyzed by a membrane bound cyclo-oxygenase complex, which converts arachidonic acid to labile intermediates called endoperoxides (PGG_2 and PGH_2); these intermediates are then further metabolized either to PGs or to thromboxanes (TXA_2 or TXB_2) (Samuelsson, 1976). However, the primary stimulus in PG synthetic events apparently acts not by directly enhancing the activity of the PG-synthesizing enzymes, but by providing more of the available precursor substrate from membrane phospholipids (Kunze and Vogt, 1971). Bartels *et al.* (1971) have shown that perfusion with phospholipase A increases the release of prostaglandins from perfused frog intestine. Furthermore, evidence is now accumulating that hormones are capable of stimulating phospholipase A_2 activity (Haye *et al.*, 1976; Laychock *et al.*, 1977a; Rillema and Wild, 1977), and this stimulation is associated with the release of arachidonic acid from acidic phospholipids (Haye *et al.*, 1976). Thus, the critical enzyme system is probably phospholipase A_2, which frees arachidonic acid from position 2 of a phosphoglyceride thereby providing substrate for the cyclo-oxygenase prostaglandin pathway. In a later section, altered phospholipase activity will be discussed as a critical event during membrane activation.

In order to assign a key regulatory role to PGs in the events which occur following membrane activation and culminate in the cellular response, the following criteria - which have been applied to establishing cAMP as a cellular intermediate (Robison *et al.*, 1971) - should be satisfied: (a) the primary stimulus should be able to augment PG synthesis by stimulating rate-limiting enzymes concerned with PG synthesis; (b) PGs should mimic the physiologic effect of the primary stimulus; and (c) the administration of drugs which interfere with PG metabolism should alter the response to the primary stimulus.

Recently, many attempts have been made to correlate alterations in PG synthesis with the physiological response to a stimulus. Our own investigations using the adrenal gland as a model for hormonal stimulus-secretion phenomena have attested to the role of PGs as cellular intermediates in ACTH-induced steroid production and release according to the specified criteria. In the intact perfused feline adrenal gland, the rise in PG release produced by ACTH precedes the facilitation of steroid production and release (Laychock *et al.*, 1977b) (Figure 1). This *in situ* observation was supported by the response to ACTH of dispersed cat adrenocortical cells, which show an increase in PGE and PGF synthesis and release upon exposure to the tropic hormone (Laychock and Rubin, 1976). The biochemical events involved in this hormone-induced activation of PG synthesis appear to involve an activation of adrenocortical phospholipase A_2 and the enhanced conversion of arachidonic acid to PGs (Laychock and Rubin, 1975; 1976; Laychock *et al.*, 1977a). PGs also increase steroid synthesis in isolated cortical cells, where PGE_2 is more potent than cAMP and as potent as the dibutyryl derivative of cAMP in stimulating steroidogenesis (Warner and Rubin, 1975). Although ACTH is more potent than PGE_2 as a steroidogenic agent, the dose-response curves of the two agents suggest similar modes of action, and the steroid synthesis profiles resulting from stimulation by either agent are indistinguishable (Warner and Rubin, 1975).

PGs are also synthesized and released in response to stimulatory agents in such tissues as the thyroid gland, the heart, kidney, platelets and isolated smooth muscle preparations (Smith *et al.*, 1974; Haye *et al.*, 1976; McGiff *et al.*, 1976; Needleman, 1976). While the effects of PGs on these tissues vary with species of PG employed, they generally manifest potent vasoconstrictor, vasodepressor, cardiotonic and release reactions (cf. Horton, 1969)

and potentiate or inhibit contractile activity induced by chemical
or electrical stimulation (Clegg *et al.*, 1966; Altura and Altura,
1976). However, since the PG concentrations used to stimulate are
generally within the μmol range, whereas the endogenous PG concentrations are in the pmol to nmol range, interpreting such experiments within the scope of physiological mechanisms appears tenuous.
An alternative approach to this problem is to utilize inhibitors
of PG synthesis and thus determine a response in the absence of
alterations in PG metabolism. Under these conditions effects on
contraction and secretion are variable. For example, whether PG
synthetase inhibitors potentiate, inhibit, or have no effect on
responses appears to depend upon the specific tissue involved
(Altura and Altura, 1976), and the concentration of inhibitor
(Laychock and Rubin, 1976). Such variable effects may be due to
the differential inhibition of various prostaglandins. Thus, endoperoxides (PGG_2 and PGH_2), which are PG precursors, have potent
actions of their own, and it has been claimed that when all detectable PGE and PGF synthesis is inhibited, there still may be considerable endoperoxide synthesis to account for the observed effects
in the presence of PG synthesis inhibitors (Gorman, 1975). Further
complicating the interpretation of the effects of PG synthetase
inhibitors is their potential for altering cellular events distinct
from PG synthesis (Flower, 1974). Indomethacin, for example, has
been implicated as an inhibitor of Ca^{2+} uptake in smooth muscle
(Northover, 1971), although the participation of PGs in this action
was not defined. All of the existing data are difficult to interpret in light of our as yet incomplete understanding of the specific
roles of individual PGs in cellular function; so that the general-
ization that PGs are obligatory intermediates in secretion and
contraction will require additional analysis.

CALCIUM AND PROSTAGLANDIN METABOLISM

     If PGs function as intermediates in the sequence of events
associated with secretion and contraction, then their role must
somehow be related to that of the critical cations involved in
these processes. In searching for a clue as to the nature of the
interaction between Ca^{2+} and PGs, an effect of this cation on
phospholipase immediately comes to mind, since this enzyme appears
to be a key factor regulating PG biosynthesis by providing free
precursor fatty acids (Kunze and Vogt, 1971).

     In contrast to the lysosomal enzyme, phospholipase A_2 isolated
from mitochondria, microsomes, and plasma membranes is active at
neutral or basic pH and is Ca^{2+} dependent (McMurray and Magee,
1972; Brockerhoff and Jensen, 1974). In fact, the Ca^{2+} requirement for non-lysosomal phospholipase is absolute; the enzyme becoming completely inactive if Ca^{2+} is omitted and chelating

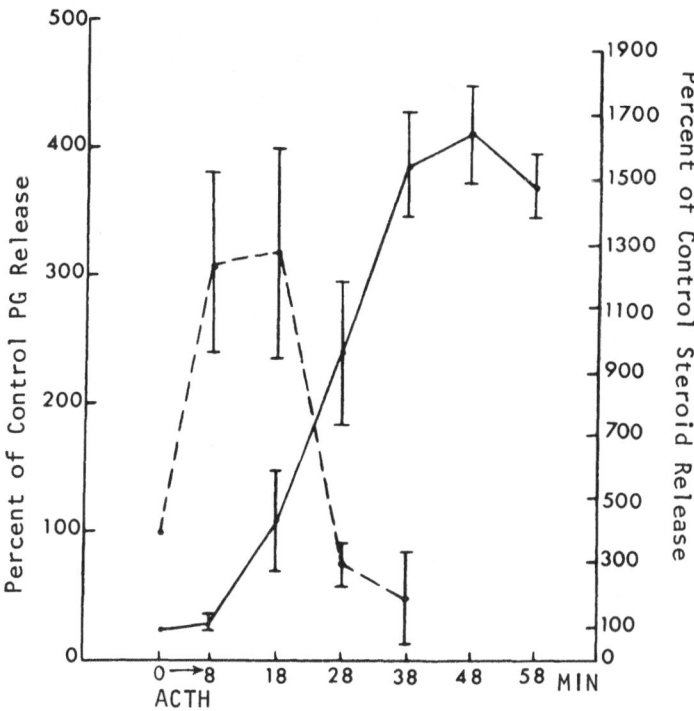

Figure 1.   Time course of $PGF_{2\alpha}$ (broken line) and corticosteroid release (solid line) from the perfused cat adrenal gland.   Values are expressed as percent of basal values obtained from saline perfusate collected during a 10 min interval immediately prior to the 8 min exposure to ACTH (50 μU/ml) (Laychock et al., 1977b).

agent added (McMurray and Magee, 1972).   Since phospholipase A_2 regulates PG synthesis by providing free precursor fatty acids, one might expect to find alterations in PG formation during Ca^{2+} deprivation.   Accordingly, Ca^{2+} deprivation results in an inhibition of PG synthesis in seminal vesicles (Kunze et al., 1974) and the adrenal cortex (Laychock et al., 1977b) (Figure 2).   In addition, the adrenal cortex has phospholipase A_2 activity which at neutral pH is activated by ACTH and exhibits a dependency upon Ca^{2+} (Laychock et al., 1977a).   Thus, in the adrenal cortex for example, Ca^{2+} lack may be responsible for inhibiting phospholipase activity; this will lead to inhibition of PG synthesis caused by the diminished liberation of arachidonic acid from phospholipids.   An ACTH-induced increase in the activity of a microsomal ATP-dependent Ca^{2+} pump (S. Laychock, private communication) may provide the cationic requirement for enhanced phospholipase activity in this tissue.   In support of the schema outlined for adrenocortical phospholipase-PG regulation are studies in the

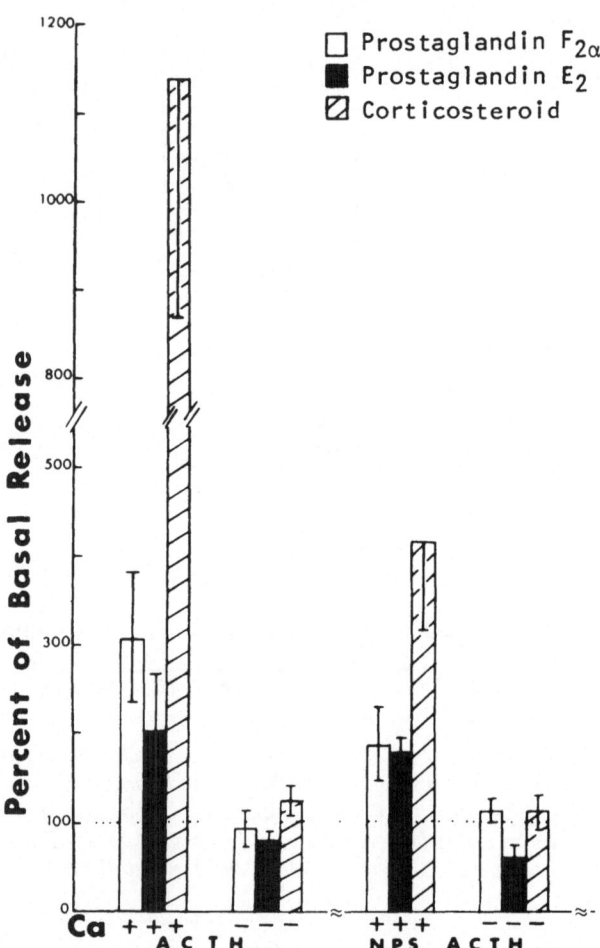

*Figure 2. The effects of calcium deprivation on PG and steroid
release from isolated cat adrenocortical cells induced by ACTH
and NPS-ACTH. Cells were incubated for 60 min in normal or Ca^{2+}-
free medium containing EGTA (0.4 mM) in the presence or absence
of ACTH (0.6 nM (250 µU) or NPS-ACTH (3200 mM). Each vertical bar
represents a mean value (±S.E.M.) from 3 or more preparations, expressed as percent of basal values obtained in the presence of
Ca^{2+} (Laychock et al., 1977b).*

thyroid gland where phospholipase activation and subsequent PG
synthesis are also Ca^{2+} dependent (Haye *et al.*, 1976).   In addition, both platelet and renal PG formation is enhanced by the
divalent cation ionophore A23187 (Knapp *et al.*, 1977; Oelz *et al.*,
1977); these studies further support a role for Ca^{2+} in the regulation of PG synthetase activity *vis a vis* phospholipase activation

and subsequent arachidonate release. Thus, Ca^{2+} is implicated as a modulator of PG synthesis in that it contributes to the availability of free fatty acids for PG synthesis. Alternatively, the release of unsaturated fatty acids mediated by Ca^{2+} activated phospholipase may effect an increase in membrane permeability to Ca^{2+} (Seiler and Hasselbach, 1971) or may stimulate a Ca^{2+}-activated ATPase serving to translocate Ca^{2+} (Knowles et al., 1976; Repke et al., 1976).

Phospholipase activity and prostaglandin synthesis are also altered by local anesthetics, which compete with and displace membrane bound Ca^{2+} from fixed negative sites of membrane phospholipids (Papahadjopoulos, 1972), and inhibit PG synthesis by antagonizing in a competitive manner (Kunze et al., 1976) the stimulant effects of Ca^{2+} on phospholipase A_2 activity (Scherphof et al., 1972; Waite and Sisson, 1972) (Figure 3). The inhibition of phospholipase activity by local anesthetics, which is roughly the same order of potency as that of local anesthetic activity in nerve (Kunze et al., 1974; 1976) (Table I) appears to be a consequence of interference with Ca^{2+} binding, although it is not clear whether the interference occurs at an enzyme or substrate site (Hendrickson and van Dam-Mieras, 1976). Thus, drugs such as local anesthetics which interfere with binding of Ca^{2+} to membranes may exert inhibitory effects on phospholipase A_2 activity and phospholipid and PG metabolism. In addition, these molecular actions of local anesthetics may help to account for their ability to inhibit secretory (cf. Rubin, 1974a) and contractile activity (Feinstein and Paimre, 1969). Thus, an important clue as to the nature of the role of Ca^{2+} in cell fusion reactions of secretory systems, such as exocytosis, and in contractile events may be sought in defining more precisely the molecular processes associated with phospholipase A_2 activity, phospholipid turnover, and prostaglandin synthesis. However, the critical position of Ca^{2+} in secretion and contraction can be specifically attributed to its functional role in regulating PG formation only if one accepts the rather tenuous premise that PGs are obligatory mediators of these cellular responses.

CALCIUM AND PROSTAGLANDIN ACTION

In addition to data favoring a key role for Ca^{2+} in PG biosynthesis, one can also marshal evidence for the concept that this cation is also an important factor in enabling PGs to express their cellular effects. PG receptors have been demonstrated in a number of tissues, including the liver (Smigel et al., 1974), corpus luteum (Rao, 1975), and the adrenal cortex (Dazord et al., 1974). PG receptor interactions are not affected by severe Ca^{2+} deprivation in subcellular fractions of bovine adrenal tissue

*TABLE I.   EFFECTS OF LOCAL ANESTHETICS (5 mM) ON PHOSPHOLIPASE A$_2$
ACTIVITY IN RELATION TO THE LIPID SOLUBILITIES OF THESE DRUGS[a]*

Drug	log P[b]	Percentage Inhibition of Phospholipase A$_2$ activity in human seminal plasma
Chlorpromazine	5.3	100
Dibucaine	4.4	100
Tetracaine	3.7	86
Lidocaine	2.3	12
Cocaine	2.3	6
Procaine	1.9	1

[a]*Data taken from Kunze et al., 1976.*
[b]*Partition coefficient of octanol/water.*

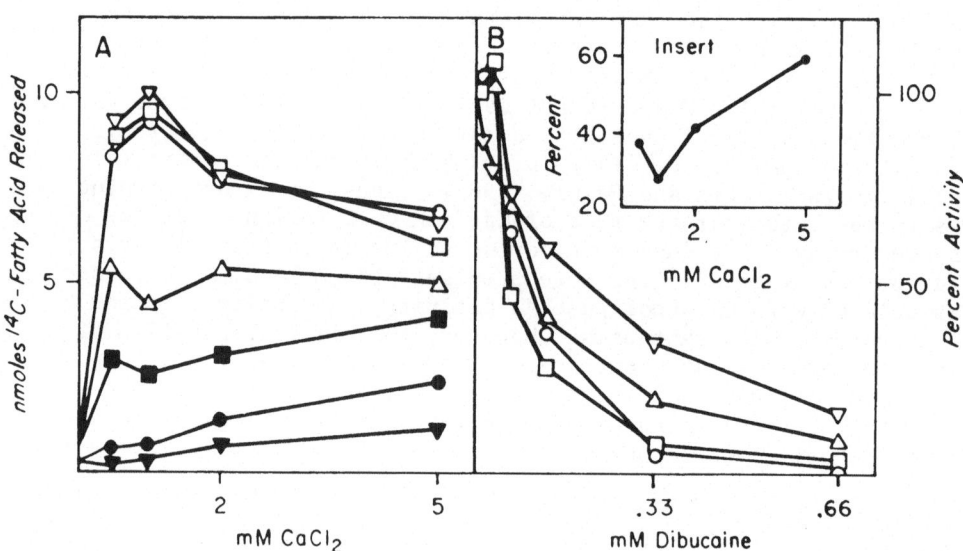

*Figure 3. The competition between the local anesthetic dibucaine
and Ca^{2+} on the activity of phospholipase A$_2$ isolated from rat
liver mitochondria.   In part A the designations are for dibucaine
concentrations (mM): 0 (○), 0.013 (□), 0.033 (▽), 0.066 (△),
0.132 (■), 0.33 (●), 0.66 (▼).   The designations in B are for
calcium concentrations (mM): 0.5 (○), 1.0 (□), 2.0 (△) and 5.0
(▽).   The percent activity with 0.132 mM dibucaine is plotted
versus calcium concentration in the insert (Waite and Sisson, 1972).*

(Dazord *et al.*, 1974), although PGF_2 binding to high affinity receptors in luteal cell membranes appears to manifest a dependency upon Ca^{2+} (Rao, 1975).

A cellular action of PGs mediated through an alteration in Ca^{2+} metabolism has been suggested in one form or another by a number of investigators (cf. Strong and Bohr, 1967; Ramwell and Shaw, 1970). The stimulant actions of PGs in muscle preparations (cf. Altura and Altura, 1976) and secretory organs (Rubin, 1974a) depend upon the external Ca^{2+} concentration. Thus, PGE elicits spiking and contraction of myometrial smooth muscle, which is modified by changes in the Ca^{2+} concentration of the medium (Clegg *et al.*, 1966; Harbon *et al.*, 1975). PGE not only elicits an inotropic effect in isolated cardiac muscle but also produces a concomitant increase in ^{45}Ca exchange (Klaus and Piccinini, 1967). Additionally, $PGF_{2\alpha}$ evokes a concomitant increase in drug induced contraction and radiocalcium uptake in arterial and venous smooth muscle preparations (Greenberg *et al.*, 1973). The basis of the ability of PGs to facilitate Ca^{2+} movements across cell membranes may relate to their proposed actions as ionophores to form lipid-soluble complexes with the cation (Eagling *et al.*, 1972); alternatively, PGs may alter cell permeability by displacing Ca^{2+} from superficial membrane-binding sites (Ramwell and Shaw, 1970; Silver and Smith, 1975). Unsaturated fatty acids appear necessary for Ca^{2+}-dependent ATPase activity (Seiler and Hasselbach, 1971; Meissner and Fleischer, 1972), thus PGs may enhance Ca^{2+} transport by modulating the activity of this enzyme system.

PGs enhance the response of myometrial smooth muscle to electrical or chemical stimulation. The lack of effect of alterations in extracellular Ca^{2+} on this enhanced response supports an intracellular locus of PG action which is dependent upon the availability of intracellular cation (Clegg *et al.*, 1966). The additional findings of Carsten (1974) that the contractile stimuli, PGE_2 and $PGF_{2\alpha}$, inhibit ATP-dependent Ca^{2+} binding and enhance Ca^{2+} release from sarcoplasmic reticulum preparations isolated from the uterine smooth muscle (Figure 4) suggest that physiological concentrations of PGs modulate cellular activity by mobilizing the active form of Ca^{2+} from intracellular binding sites. The manner in which PGs mediate the release phenomenon may be ascribed to their ionophoretic properties (Carsten and Miller, 1977), although alternative modes of PG action may also contribute to the mobilization of intracellular cation *in vivo*.

In summarizing the effects of PGs on biological systems, it should be noted that PGs may be inhibitory agents as well as stimulatory ones. For example, PGE relaxes arterial smooth muscle (Horton, 1969) and inhibits norepinephrine release (Hedqvist, 1970). In an attempt to reconcile the antagonistic effect of PGs on smooth

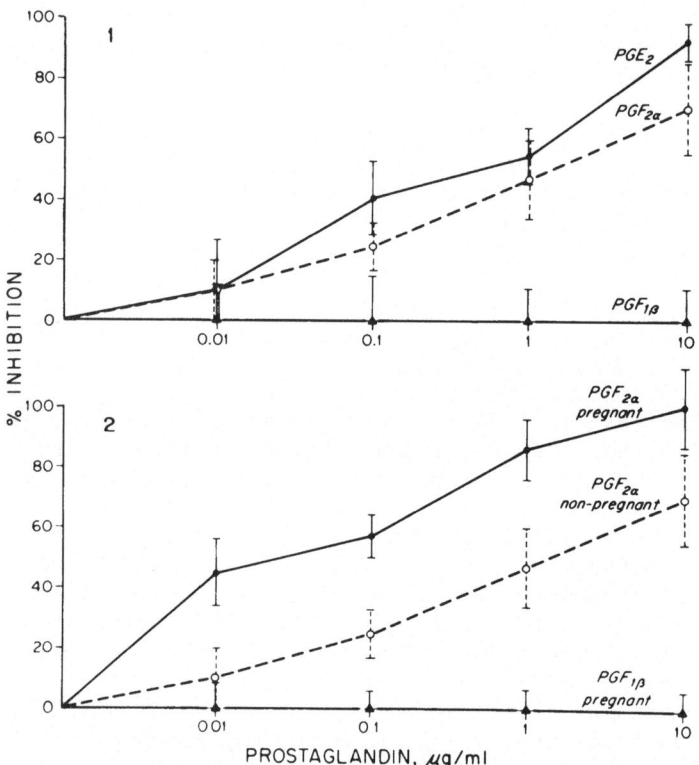

Figure 4. Inhibition of ATP-dependent Ca^{2+} *binding by various PGs in subcellular fractions isolated from non-pregnant and pregnant bovine uteri (Carsten, 1973).*

muscle, Strong and Bohr (1967) offered the hypothesis that the stimulant effects of PGs are due to the enhanced cationic permeability of the membrane or due to decreased Ca^{2+} binding to intracellular organelles. The inhibitory effects of PGs, on the other hand, would be due to a decrease in free cytosol Ca^{2+} levels as a result of enhanced intracellular binding to organelles such as the mitochondria. Under certain conditions, PGs render isolated mitochondria permeable to Ca^{2+} in a manner reminiscent of the ionophore A23187 (Kirtland and Baum, 1972; Malmstrom and Carafoli, 1975). Despite its obvious attractiveness, this theory, which implicates PGs as modulators of Ca^{2+} activity at both extra- and intracellular loci, will remain speculative at least until it has been ascertained whether PGs act primarily as intracellular messengers or as blood-borne mediators with primary effects on the plasma membrane.

PROSTAGLANDINS AND CYCLIC NUCLEOTIDES

The ability of PGs to mimic the actions of hormones and neurotransmitters in certain tissues, and to inhibit their actions in others might not only be related to a direct action on Ca^{2+} availability but to effects mediated through cAMP. Indeed, PGs are capable of stimulating the adenylate cyclase-cAMP system in a number of tissues (Ramwell and Rabinowitz, 1972), even in a dose-dependent manner (Dalton and Hope, 1974), thereby providing evidence for the view that PGs act as second messengers, with cAMP acting as a third messenger (Kuehl, 1974). Calcium ion is an important regulator of adenylate cyclase activity (cf. Rubin, 1974a; Halkerston, 1975); so PGs, by producing changes in cellular Ca^{2+} levels could affect adenylate cyclase activity and thereby modulate cAMP levels. However, Ca^{2+} deprivation fails to prevent the stimulatory effect of PGE on cAMP accumulation in the pituitary (Borgeat *et al.*, 1972) and adrenal cortex (Dazord *et al.*, 1974), thereby weakening the possibility that the critical action of Ca^{2+} is mediated through PG-induced alterations in cAMP. Nevertheless, the PG-induced increase in cyclic nucleotide levels could contribute to alterations in intracellular Ca^{2+} metabolism (Will *et al.*, 1976), resulting in an enhanced cation availability for contractile and secretory events.

Other alternatives for the interaction of PGs, Ca^{2+} and cAMP deserve to be considered in an attempt to correlate the actions of the three putative mediators. The fact that inhibition of PG synthesis does not alter the increase in cAMP accumulation initiated by the primary hormone (Kuehl *et al.*, 1974; Rigler *et al.*, 1976) suggests that a PG-induced alteration in cAMP synthesis may not be involved in contractile-secretory phenomena. Perhaps a Ca^{2+}-induced change in adenylate cyclase activity results in altered cAMP levels and leads to alterations in PG metabolism.

Alternatively, the contractile and secretory activity of cAMP, PGs and Ca^{2+} may, indeed, occur independently of an effect of one agent upon another (Figure 2). The hypothesis that cAMP and PG formation occur in parallel rather than in series is buttressed by the fact that NPS-ACTH, a weak steroidogenic analogue of ACTH, is able to augment PG synthesis in the adrenal cortex with no discernible increase in cAMP (Laychock *et al.*, 1977b). Moreover, NPS-ACTH-induced steroid release - though Ca^{2+}-dependent - is not blocked in the absence of PG synthesis. Thus, the obligatory role of Ca^{2+} in this release reaction does not appear to reside in the actions of either PGs or cAMP. In this context, it has previously been proposed that secretory and contractile stimulatory agents influence distinct control mechanisms for Ca^{2+} availability and cAMP accumulation in cells (Schramm and Selinger, 1975). Hormonal or neurotransmitter substances may, on the one hand, stimulate a receptor responsible for adenylate cyclase activation, and on the other hand, bind to a receptor responsible for intracellular Ca^{2+} mobilization. The dual-receptor mechanism would seem to apply to the adrenal cortex where receptors of differing affinity for ACTH have been identified (Lefkowitz *et al.*, 1971; McIlhinney and Schulster, 1974) and demonstrated to exhibit a differential response to ACTH and its NPS-analogue in terms of cAMP generation (Moyle *et al.*, 1973). Thus, it is conceivable that as a consequence of receptor activation, both ACTH and NPS-ACTH enhance Ca^{2+} availability and phospholipase activity but only ACTH is able to activate adenylate cyclase; this, of course, would imply a dissociation between events regulating cAMP and PG metabolism involving the activation of two distinct receptor systems. In other secretory systems dual receptors for 5-hydroxytryptamine (deGroat and Lally, 1973) and histamine also appear to exist (Black *et al.*, 1972).

The relationship between cyclic GMP (cGMP), Ca^{2+} and PG metabolism in the course of events culminating in cell contraction or a secretory response is even less clear. It has been well documented that guanylate cyclase activity can be enhanced by Ca^{2+} (Hardman *et al.*, 1971; Rodan and Feinstein, 1976) and that some tissues require Ca^{2+} for stimulation of cGMP synthesis (Schultz and Hardman, 1975; Ferrendelli *et al.*, 1976). More recently, A23187 has been proven to be a pharmacologic asset in demonstrating that enhanced influx of Ca^{2+} ions into thyroid slices (Van Sande *et al.*, 1975), rat parotid gland (Butcher, 1975) and umbilical artery segments (Clyman *et al.*, 1975) or enhanced calcium efflux from isolated pancreatic acinar cells (Christophe *et al.*, 1976) culminate in increased levels of cellular cGMP. Thus, it appears that alterations in intracellular Ca^{2+} levels brought about by a stimulatory agent may secondarily induce changes in guanylate cyclase activity; however, the enhancement of guanylate cyclase activity by Ca^{2+} may be mediated by an intermediate messenger such as fatty acids (Wallach and Pastan, 1976; Asakawa *et al.*, 1976) or PGs (Kuehl, 1974; Rubin *et al.*, 1977). Therefore, it is not surprising that enhanced phospholipase activity and arachidonic acid are capable of stimulating guanylate cyclase activity (Fujimoto and Okabayashi, 1975; Glass *et al.*, 1977). Regarding the hypothesis that increases in cAMP and cGMP levels are antagonistic in some biological systems (Goldberg *et al.*, 1973), it is possible that the PG endoperoxides are regulatory compounds responsible for enhancing guanylate cyclase activity and for antagonizing adenylate cyclase activity (Gorman, 1975; Miller and Gorman, 1976). However, the role of cGMP in contraction and secretion phenomena remains tentative.

PERSPECTIVE

It is unfortunately not possible to draw any firm conclusions from the rather diffuse data presented in this overview and it is apparent that an argument can be made for a number of potential sites of Ca^{2+} interaction with the PGs. The experiments which employ exogenous PGs as stimulating agents reveal that Ca^{2+} is needed for full expression of the effects of PGs. A primary site of Ca^{2+} action in the intact cell must also be associated with one or more of the early events taking place at the cell membrane as a consequence of the interaction of the primary stimulating agent with its receptor. This conclusion is supported by findings in the adrenal cortex that when ACTH-receptor interaction is bypassed using the corticosteroid precursor, pregnenolone, as the steroido-genic agent, PG synthesis is not enhanced and the Ca^{2+} require-ment for steroid production and release is essentially obviated (Laychock and Rubin, 1977). More specifically, at least a portion of the critical role of Ca^{2+} may be exerted through effects on PG synthesis by regulating the activity of the plasmalemmal phos-pholipase A_2, the enzyme responsible for providing substrate pre-cursor for PG synthesis.

The induction of cAMP synthesis by hormonal activation of adenylate cyclase also requires Ca^{2+} in certain systems (cf. Rubin et al., 1972; Halkerston, 1975) but not others (Rasmussen and Tenenhouse, 1968; Steiner et al., 1970); and the action of exo-genous cAMP requires the presence of Ca^{2+} in some secretory systems (cf. Rubin, 1974a) but not others (Haksar and Peron, 1972; Warner and Rubin, 1975). But since evidence presented herein favors the conclusion that PG and cAMP are not inextricably linked and that these substances play only modulatory roles, Ca^{2+} may exert direct actions on certain physiological functions such as secretion with-out necessarily having a cellular intermediate interposed. For example, if surface membrane events are bypassed by various experi-mental manipulations, the mere addition of Ca^{2+} to the adrenal medulla (Douglas and Rubin, 1961), somatic motor nerve ending (Miledi, 1973), or the mast cell (Douglas, 1975b) causes an immediate explosive discharge of secretory product; thus providing support for an active and direct role for Ca^{2+} in stimulus-secretion coupling. A similar sequence of events may exist for activation of the contractile elements in certain muscle cells (Podolsky and Constantin, 1965; Sandow, 1965). Such experiments give credence to the supposition that PGs - and perhaps cAMP as well - function merely to modulate the direct actions of Ca^{2+} either by enhancing the availability of free cellular Ca^{2+} or by sensitizing the appropriate Ca^{2+} "receptor" to the action of this cation. Never-theless, the gaps in our knowledge underscore the need to continue the search for additional clues regarding the nature of the inter-action of Ca^{2+} with PGs and cAMP, because this approach may provide

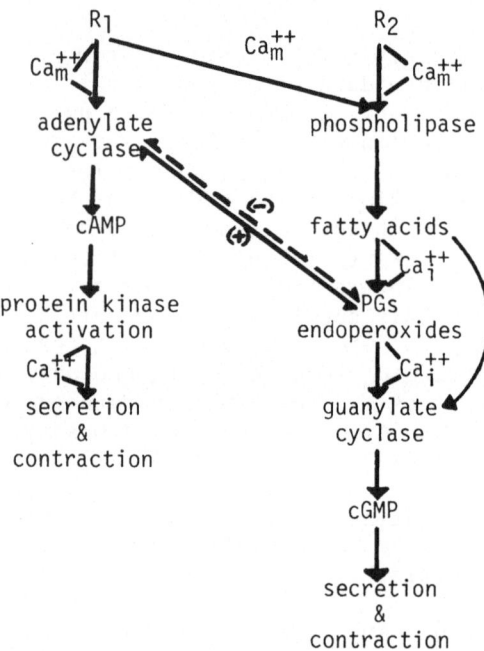

Figure 5. Hypothetical scheme of possible sites of interaction between Ca^{2+}, prostaglandins and the cyclic nucleotides.

the key to the understanding of the fundamental role of Ca^{2+} in contraction and secretion.

Perhaps, as a final attempt to meaningfully arrange the three putative mediators of contractile and secretory phenomena in a sequence of events compatible with most of their effects on biological systems, a schematic representation of the interactions of Ca^{2+}, PGs, and cyclic nucleotides is deemed appropriate. As Figure 5 indicates, two receptor mechanisms (R_1 and R_2) may exist for the activation of adenylate cyclase and phospholipase activity, respectively. Both receptors, however, may induce alterations in membrane calcium (Ca_m^{++}). The activation of adenylate cyclase will result in an increase in cAMP, followed by alterations in protein kinase activity, translocation of Ca^{2+}, and subsequent secretory or contractile phenomena. The enhanced phospholipase activity in response to receptor stimulation and membrane-associated calcium mobilization (Ca_m^{++}) may result in a more complex pattern of cellular activity. As a direct result of phospholipase activation, fatty acids will be liberated. The fatty acids themselves may have a multiplicity of actions, including the mobilization of intracellular calcium (Ca_i^{++}) with an increase in the free form of the cation; an increase in PG and endoperoxide synthesis from arachidonic acid; and the more direct stimulatory effect of a number of fatty acids upon guanylate cyclase activity. In turn, the PG compounds may also alter intracellular calcium binding (Ca_i^{++}) and stimulate guanylate cyclase activity. Free intracellular Ca^{2+} made more readily available might participate in PG synthesis and guanylate cyclase activation, as well as in other related cellular events. The PGs and endoperoxides are also candidates as mediators in the synthesis of cAMP and cGMP. The PG compounds may not only behave as stimulators (solid line in figure) and inhibitors (dashed line) of adenylate cyclase activity, but in some systems the adenylate cyclase activity and cAMP levels may modulate cyclo-oxygenase activity and resultant PG synthesis (Malmsten *et al.*, 1976). But it must be kept in mind that regardless of the putative mediators synthesized, the receptors remain key regulatory sites by conferring specificity to the response.

REFERENCES

Asakawa, T., Scheinbaum, I., and Ho, R., 1976, Stimulation of guanylate cyclase by several fatty acids, *Biochem. Biophys. Res. Commun.* 73: 141.

Altura, B. M., and Altura, B. T., 1976, Vascular smooth muscle and prostaglandins, *Fed. Proc.* 35: 2360.

Bartels, J., Kunze, H., Vogt, W., and Wille, G., 1970, Prostaglandin: liberation from and formation in perfused frog intestine, *Naunyn-Schmied. Arch. Pharmacol.* 266: 199.

Black, J. W., Duncan, W. A., Durant, C. J., Ganellin, C. R., and Parsons, E. M., 1972, Definition and antagonism of histamine H2-receptors, *Nature* 236: 385.

Borgeat, P., Chavancy, G., Dupont, A., Labrie, F., Arimura, A., and Schally, A. V., 1972, Stimulation of adenosine 3':5'-cyclic monophosphate accumulation in anterior pituitary gland *in vitro* by synthetic luteinizing hormone-releasing hormone, *Proc. Nat. Acad. Sci. U. S. A.* 69: 2677.

Brockerhoff, H., and Jensen, R. G., 1974, "Lipolytic Enzymes," pp. 194-265, Academic Press, New York.

Butcher, F. R., 1975, The role of calcium and cyclic nucleotides in α-amylase release from slices of rat parotid: studies with the divalent cation ionophore, *Metab.* 24: 409.

Carsten, M. E., 1974, Prostaglandins and oxytocin: their effects on uterine smooth muscle, *Prostaglandins* 5: 33.

Carsten, M. E., and Miller, J. D., 1977, Effects of prostaglandins and oxytocin on calcium release from a uterine microsomal fraction. Hypothesis for ionophoretic action of prostaglandins, *J. Biol. Chem.* 252: 1576.

Christophe, J. P., Frandsen, E. K., Conlon, T. P., Krishna, G., and Gardner, J. D., 1976, Action of cholecystokinin, cholinergic agents, and A-23187 on accumulation of guanosine 3':5' monophosphate in dispersed guinea pig pancreatic acinar cells, *J. Biol. Chem.* 251: 4640.

Clegg, P. C., Hall, W. J., and Pickles, V. R., 1966, The action of ketonic prostaglandins on the guinea pig myometrium, *J. Physiol. (London)* 183: 123.

Clyman, R. I., Blacksin, A. S., Sandler, J. A., Manganiello, V. C., and Vaughan, M., 1975, The role of calcium in regulation of cyclic nucleotide content in human umbilical artery, *J. Biol. Chem.* 250: 4718.

Dalton, C., and Hope, W. C., 1974, Cyclic AMP regulation of prostaglandin biosynthesis in fat cells, *Prostaglandins* 6: 227.

Dazord, A., Morera, A. M., Bertrand, J., and Saez, J. M., 1974, Prostaglandin receptors in human and ovine adrenal glands: binding and stimulation of adenyl cyclase in subcellular preparations, *Endocrinology* 95: 352.

deGroat, W. C., and Lally, P. M., 1973, Interaction between picrotoxin and 5-hydroxytryptamine in the superior cervical ganglion of the cat, *Brit. J. Pharmacol.* 48: 233.

Douglas, W. W., 1975a, Secretomotor control of adrenal medullary secretion: Synaptic, membrane, and ionic events in stimulus-secretion coupling, *in* "Handbook of Physiology," Vol. 6, Sect. 7 (H. Blaschko, G. Sayers, and A. D. Smith, eds.), pp. 367-388, Williams and Wilkins, Baltimore.

Douglas, W. W., 1975b, Stimulus-secretion coupling in mast cells: regulation of exocytosis by cellular and extracellular calcium, *in* "Calcium Transport in Contraction and Secretion" (E. Carafoli, F. Clementi, W. Drabikowski, and E. Margreth, eds.), pp. 167-174, North-Holland, Amsterdam.

Douglas, W. W., and Rubin, R. P., 1961, The role of calcium in the secretory response of the adrenal medulla to acetylcholine, *J. Physiol. (London)* 159: 40.

Eagling, E. M., Lovell, H. G., and Pickles, V. R., 1972, Interaction of prostaglandin E$_1$ and calcium in the guinea pig myometrium, *Brit. J. Pharmacol.* 44: 510.

Feinstein, M. B., and Paimre, M., 1969, Pharmacological action of local anesthetics on excitation-contraction coupling in striated and smooth muscle, *Fed. Proc.* 28: 1643.

Ferreira, S. H., and Vane, J. R., 1974, New aspects of the mode of action of nonsteroid antiinflammatory drugs, *Annu. Rev. Pharmacol.* 14: 57.

Ferrendelli, J. A., Rubin, E. H., and Kinscherf, D. A., 1976, Influence of divalent cations on regulation of cyclic GMP and cyclic AMP levels in brain tissue, *J. Neurochem.* 26: 741.

Flower, R. J., 1974, Drugs which inhibit prostaglandin biosynthesis, *Pharmacol. Rev.* 26: 33.

Fujimoto, M., and Okabayashi, T., 1975, Proposed mechanisms of stimulation and inhibition of guanylate cyclase with reference to the actions of chlorpromazine, phospholipases and Triton X-100, *Biochem. Biophys. Res. Commun.* 67: 1332.

Glass, D. B., Gerrard, J. M., Townsend, D., Carr, D. W., White, J. G., and Goldberg, N. D., 1977, The involvement of prostaglandin endoperoxide formation in the elevation of cyclic GMP levels during platelet aggregation, *J. Cyclic Nucleotide Res.* 3: 37.

Goldberg, N. D., O'Dea, R. F., and Haddox, M. K., 1973, Cyclic GMP, *in* "Advances in Cyclic Nucleotide Research," Vol. 3 (P. Greengard and G. A. Robison, eds.), pp. 155-223, Raven Press, New York.

Gorman, R. R., 1975, Prostaglandin endoperoxides: possible new regulators of cyclic nucleotide metabolism, *J. Cyclic Nucleotide Res.* 1:1.

Greenberg, S., Kadowitz, P. J., Diecke, F. P., and Long, J. P., 1973, Effects of prostaglandin $F_{2\alpha}$ ($PGF_{2\alpha}$) on arterial and venous contractility and ^{45}Ca uptake, *Arch. Int. Pharmacodyn. Ther.* 205: 381.

Haksar, A., and Peron, F. G., 1972, Comparison of the Ca^{++} requirement for the steroidogenic effect of ACTH and dibutyryl cyclic AMP in rat adrenal cell suspensions, *Biochem. Biophys. Res. Commun.* 47: 445.

Halkerston, I. D., 1975, Cyclic AMP and adrenocortical function, *in* "Advances in Cyclic Nucleotide Research," Vol. 6 (P. Greengard and G. A. Robison, eds.), pp. 99-136, Raven Press, New York.

Harbon, S., Vesin, M. F., and Dokhac, L., 1975, The effects of epinephrine and prostaglandins on cAMP formation and binding to its intracellular receptors, *in* "Smooth Muscle Pharmacology and Physiology" (M. Worcel and G. Vassort, eds.), pp. 83-100, INSERM, Paris.

Hardman, J. G., Beavo, J. A., Gray, J. P., Chrisman, T. D., Patterson, W. D., and Sutherland, E. W., 1971, The formation and metabolism of cyclic GMP, *Ann. N. Y. Acad. Sci.* 185: 27.

Haye, B., Champion, S., and Jacquemin, C., 1976, Stimulation by TSH of prostaglandin synthesis in pig thyroid, *in* "Advances in Prostaglandin and Thromboxane Research" (B. Samuelsson and R. Paoletti, eds.), pp. 29-34, Raven Press, New York.

Hedqvist, P., 1970, Antagonism by calcium of the inhibitory action of prostaglandin E_2 on sympathetic neurotransmission in the cat spleen, *Acta. Physiol. Scand.* 80: 269.

Hendrickson, H. S., and van Dam-Mieras, M. C. E., 1976, Local anesthetic inhibition of pancreatic phospholipase A_2 action on lecithin monolayers, *J. Lipid Res.* 17: 399.

Horton, E. W., 1969, Hypotheses on physiological roles of prostaglandins, *Physiol. Rev.* 49: 122.

Kirtland, S. J., and Baum, H., 1972, Prostaglandin E_1 may act as a calcium ionophore, *Nature* 236: 47.

Klaus, W., and Piccinini, F., 1967, Uber die Wirkung von Prosta-glandin E_1 auf den Ca-Haushalt Isolierter Meerschweinchenherzen, *Experientia* 23: 556.

Knapp, H. R., Oelz, O., Roberts, L. J., Sweetman, B. J., Oates, J. A., and Reed, P. W., 1977, Ionophores stimulate prostaglandin and thromboxane biosynthesis, *Proc. Nat. Acad. Sci. U. S. A.* 74: 4251.

Knowles, A. F., Eytan, E., and Racker, E., 1976, Phospholipid-protein interactions in the Ca^{2+}-adenosine triphosphatase of sarcoplasmic reticulum, *J. Biol. Chem.* 251: 5161.

Kuehl, F., 1974, Prostaglandins, cyclic nucleotides and cell function, *Prostaglandins* 5: 325.

Kuehl, F. A., Oien, H. G., and Ham, E. A., 1974, Prostaglandins and prostaglandin synthetase inhibitors: actions on cell func-tion, *in* "Prostaglandin Synthetase Inhibitors" (H. F. Robinson and J. R. Vane, eds.), pp. 53-65, Raven Press, New York.

Kunze, H., Bohn, E., and Vogt, W., 1974, Effects of local anesthe-tics on prostaglandin biosynthesis *in vitro*, *Biochim. Biophys. Acta* 360: 260.

Kunze, H., Nahas, N., Traynor, J. R., and Wurl, W., 1976, Effects of local anesthetics on phospholipases, *Biochim. Biophys. Acta* 441: 93.

Kunze, H., and Vogt, W., 1971, Significance of phospholipase A for prostaglandin formation, *Ann. N. Y. Acad. Sci.* 180: 123.

Kuo, I. C., and Coffee, C. J., 1976, Purification and characteri-zation of a troponin-C-like protein from bovine adrenal medulla, *J. Biol. Chem.* 251: 1603.

Laychock, S. G., Franson, R. C., Weglicki, W. B., and Rubin, R. P., 1977a, Identification and partial characterization of phospho-lipases in isolated adrenocortical cells: the effects of ACTH and calcium, *Biochem. J.* 164: 753.

Laychock, S. G., and Rubin, R. P., 1975, ACTH-induced prostaglandin biosynthesis from ^{3}H-arachidonic acid by adrenocortical cells, *Prostaglandins* 10: 529.

Laychock, S. G., and Rubin, R. P., 1976, Indomethacin-induced alterations in corticosteroid and prostaglandin release by iso-lated adrenocortical cells of the cat, *Brit. J. Pharmacol.* 57: 273.

Laychock, S. G., and Rubin, R. P., 1977, Regulation of steroido-genesis and prostaglandin formation in isolated adrenocortical cells: the effects of pregnenolone and cycloheximide, *J. Steroid Biochem.* 8: 663.

Laychock, S. G., Warner, W., and Rubin, R. P., 1977b, Further studies on the mechanisms controlling prostaglandin biosynthesis in the cat adrenal cortex: the role of calcium and cyclic AMP, *Endocrinology* 100: 74.

Lefkowitz, R. J., Roth, J., and Pastan, I., 1971, ACTH-receptor interaction in the adrenal: A model for the initial step on the action of hormones that stimulate adenyl cyclase, *Ann. N. Y. Acad. Sci.* 185: 195.

Malmsten, C., Granstrom, E., and Samuelsson, B., 1976, Cyclic AMP inhibits synthesis of prostaglandin endoperoxide (PGG_2) in human platelets, *Biochem. Biophys. Res. Commun.* 68: 569.

Malmstrom, K., and Carafoli, E., 1975, Effects of prostaglandins on the interaction of Ca^{2+} with mitochondria, *Arch. Biochem. Biophys.* 171: 418.

McGiff, J. C., Malik, K. U., and Terragno, N. A., 1976, Prostaglandins as determinants of vascular reactivity, *Fed. Proc.* 35: 2382.

McIlhinney, R. A. J., and Schulster, A., 1974, Characterization of adrenocortical receptors for adrenocorticotrophin, *J. Endocrinol.* 61: 43.

McMurray, W. C., and Magee, W. L., 1972, Phospholipid metabolism, *Annu. Rev. Biochem.* 41: 129.

Meissner, G., and Fleischer, S., 1972, The role of phospholipid in Ca^{2+}-stimulated ATPase activity of sarcoplasmic reticulum, *Biochim. Biophys. Acta.* 255: 19.

Miledi, R., 1973, Transmitter release induced by injection of calcium ions into nerve terminals, *Proc. R. Soc. London, Ser. B.* 183: 421.

Miller, O. V., and Gorman, R. R., 1976, Modulation of platelet cyclic nucleotide content by PGE_1 and the prostaglandin endoperoxide PGG_2, *J. Cyclic Nucleotide Res.* 2: 79.

Moyle, W. R., Kong, Y. C., and Ramachandran, J., 1973, Steroidogenesis and cyclic adenosine 3',5'-monophosphate accumulation in rat adrenal cells. Divergent effects of adrenocorticotropin and its o-nitrophenyl sulfenyl derivative, *J. Biol. Chem.* 248: 2409.

Needleman, P., 1976, The synthesis and function of prostaglandins in the heart, *Fed. Proc.* 35: 2376.

Northover, B. J., 1971, Mechanism of the inhibitory action of indomethacin on smooth muscle, *Brit. J. Pharmacol.* 41: 540.

Oelz, O., Knapp, H. R., Roberts, L. J., Sweetman, B. J., Oates, J. A., and Reed, P. W., 1977, Calcium ionophores stimulate thromboxane and prostaglandin formation by platelets, *Prostaglandins* 13: 1013.

Papahadjopoulos, D., 1972, Studies on the mechanism of action of local anesthetics with phospholipid model membranes, *Biochim. Biophys. Acta.* 265: 169.

Podolsky, R. J., and Costantin, L. L., 1964, Regulation by calcium of the contraction and relaxation of muscle fibers, *Fed. Proc.* 23: 933.

Poisner, A. M., 1970, Release of transmitters from storage: A contractile model, *Adv. Biochem. Psychopharmacol.* 2: 95.

Ramwell, P. W., and Rabinowitz, I., 1972, Interaction of prostaglandins and cyclic AMP, *in* "Effects of Drugs on Cellular Control Mechanisms" (B. R. Rabin and R. B. Freedman, eds.), pp. 207-235,

MacMillan, Baltimore.

Ramwell, P. W., and Shaw, J. E., 1970, Biological significance of the prostaglandins, *Recent Prog. Horm. Res.* 26: 139.

Rao, Ch. V., 1975, Cationic dependency of high affinity prostaglandin $F_{2\alpha}$ receptors in bovine corpus luteum cell membranes, *Biochem. Biophys. Res. Commun.* 67: 1242.

Rasmussen, H., and Tenenhouse, A., 1968, Cyclic adenosine monophosphate, Ca^{++}, and membranes, *Proc. Nat. Acad. Sci. U. S. A.* 59: 1364.

Repke, D. I., Spivak, J. C., and Katz, A. M., 1976, Reconstitution of an active calcium pump in sarcoplasmic reticulum, *J. Biol. Chem.* 251: 3169.

Rigler, G. L., Peake, G. T., and Ratner, A., 1976, Effects of follicle-stimulating hormone and luteinizing hormone on ovarian cyclic AMP and prostaglandin E *in vivo* in rats treated with indomethacin, *J. Endocrinol.* 70: 285.

Rillema, J. A., and Wild, E. A., 1977, Prolactin activation of phospholipase A activity in membrane preparations from mammary glands, *Endocrinology* 100: 1219.

Robison, G. A., Butcher, R. W., and Sutherland, E. W., 1971, "Cyclic AMP," pp. 36-47, Academic Press, New York.

Rodan, G. A., and Feinstein, M. B., 1976, Interrelationships between Ca^{2+} and adenylate and guanylate cyclases in the control of platelet secretion and aggregation, *Proc. Nat. Acad. Sci. U. S. A.* 73: 1829.

Rubin, R. P., 1974a, "Calcium and The Secretory Process," pp. 25-149, Plenum Press, New York.

Rubin, R. P., 1974b, The role of calcium in drug action, *in* "Drug Interactions" (P. L. Morselli, S. Garattini, and S. N. Cohen, eds.), pp. 163-172, Raven Press, New York.

Rubin, R. P., Jaanus, S. D., and Carchman, R. A., 1972, The role of calcium and adenosine cyclic 3'5' phosphate in the action of adrenocorticotrophin, *Nature* 240: 150.

Rubin, R. P., Laychock, S. G., and End, D. W., 1977, On the role of cyclic AMP and cyclic GMP in steroid production by bovine cortical cells, *Biochim. Biophys. Acta.* 496: 329.

Samuelsson, B., 1976, New trends in prostaglandin research, *in* "Advances in Prostaglandin and Thromboxane Research" (B. Samuelsson and R. Paoletti, eds.), Vol. 1, pp. 1-6, Raven Press, New York.

Sandow, A., 1966, Excitation-contraction coupling in skeletal muscle, *Pharmacol. Rev.* 17: 265.

Scherphof, G. L., Scarpa, A., and van Toorenenbergen, A., 1972, The effect of local anesthetics on the hydrolysis of free and membrane-bound phospholipids catalyzed by various phospholipases, *Biochim. Biophys. Acta.* 270: 226.

Schramm, M., and Selinger, Z., 1975, The functions of cyclic AMP and calcium as alternative second messengers in parotid gland and pancreas, *J. Cyclic Nucleotide Res.* 1: 181.

Schultz, G., and Hardman, J. G., 1975, Regulation of cyclic GMP levels in the ductus deferens of rats, *in* "Advances in Cyclic Nucleotide Research," vol. 5 (P. Greengard and G. A. Robison, eds.), p. 339-351, Raven Press, New York.

Seiler, D., and Hasselbach, W., 1971, Essential fatty acid deficiency and the activity of the sarcoplasmic calcium pump, *Eur. J. Biochem.* 21: 385.

Silver, M. J., and Smith, J. B., 1975, Prostaglandins as intracellular messengers, *Life Sci.* 16: 1635.

Smigel, M., Fröhlich, J. C., and Fleischer, S., 1974, Characterization of prostaglandin E receptor in membrane and its use in the assay of prostaglandin E, *in* "Methods in Enzymology 32, Part B" (S. Fleischer and L. Packer, eds.), pp. 109-123, Academic Press, New York.

Smith, J. B., Ingerman, C. M., Kocsis, J. J., and Silver, M. J., 1974, Studies on platelet aggregation: Synthesis of prostaglandins and effects of synthetase inhibitors, *in* "Prostaglandin Synthetase Inhibitors" (H. J. Robinson and J. R. Vane, eds.), pp. 229-240, Raven Press, New York.

Steiner, A. L., Peake, G. T., Utiger, R. D., Karl, I. E., and Kipnis, D. M., 1970, Hypothalamic stimulation of growth hormone and thyrotropin release *in vitro* and pituitary 3'5'-adenosine cyclic monophosphate, *Endocrinology* 86: 1354.

Strong, C. G., and Bohr, D. F., 1967, Effect of prostaglandins E_1, E_2, A and $F_{2\alpha}$ on isolated vascular smooth muscle, *Amer. J. Physiol.* 213: 725.

Trifaro, J. M., and Ulpian, C., 1976, Isolation and characterization of myosin from the adrenal medulla, *Neuroscience* 1: 483.

Van Sande, J., Decoster, C., and Dumont, J. E., 1975, Control and role of cyclic 3',5'-guanosine monophosphate in the thyroid, *Biochem. Biophys. Res. Commun.* 62: 168.

Waite, M., and Sisson, P., 1972, Effect of local anesthetics on phospholipases from mitochondria and liposomes. A probe into the role of calcium ion in phospholipid hydrolysis, *Biochemistry* 11: 3098.

Wallach, D., and Pastan, I., 1976, Stimulation of guanylate cyclase of fibroblasts by free fatty acids, *J. Biol. Chem.* 251: 5802.

Warner, W., and Rubin, R. P., 1975, Evidence for a possible prostaglandin link in ACTH-induced steroidogenesis, *Prostaglandins* 9: 83.

Will, H., Schirpke, B., and Wollenberger, A., 1976, Stimulation of Ca^{2+} uptake by cyclic AMP and protein kinase in sarcoplasmic reticulum-rich and sarcolemma-rich microsomal fractions from rabbit heart, *Acta. Biol. Med. Germ.* 35: 529.

CHAPTER 7

REGULATION OF CALCIUM BY VASCULAR SMOOTH

MUSCLE CELLULAR COMPONENTS

Julius C. Allen

Baylor College of Medicine
Houston, Texas 77030

INTRODUCTION

In the case of smooth muscle in general and vascular smooth muscle in particular, the number of contractile or relaxing agents is quite large and all of them must ultimately, in some way, affect the interaction of Ca^{2+} with the regulatory component of the contractile protein apparatus. The specific nature of this interaction, the components of the regulatory proteins, and the specific mechanisms regulating Ca^{2+} in smooth muscle are, essentially, unknown. Consequently, this chapter will not try to elucidate specific Ca^{2+} involvement in drug actions, but will try to review recent biochemical data which have attempted to define the various mechanisms of Ca^{2+} regulation in this tissue. To date, no unifying hypothesis can be drawn regarding the mechanism(s) of regulation as can be done for other muscle tissue.

SARCOLEMMA AND SARCOPLASMIC RETICULUM

It is clear that Ca^{2+} interaction with contractile proteins initiates contraction in smooth muscle as it does in both cardiac and skeletal muscle. However, despite this acknowledged role of Ca^{2+}, both the control of available Ca^{2+} (activator Ca^{2+}) which interacts with the contractile proteins and the nature of the Ca^{2+} receptor on the contractile proteins has not been clarified in this type of muscle. While this paper emphasizes the control of activator Ca^{2+}, it should be noted that mechanisms of contractile protein regulation in smooth muscle are such that, at the moment, the reasonable suggestion involves a myosin-linked control

157

rather than a troponin-linked system as in other muscle types.
To date, there are few reports in the literature suggesting the
existence of relaxing proteins in smooth muscle as we know them
in cardiac and skeletal muscle (Carsten, 1969; Ebashi, 1975, 1977).
Using chicken gizzard, Driska and Hartshorne (1975) and Sobieszek
and Bremel (1975) indicated that on SDS (sodium dodecyl sulfate)
gel electrophoresis, no components appeared similar to those of
skeletal muscle troponin. These workers concluded that it seemed
unlikely that a protein such as troponin could be involved in the
regulation of the ATPase activity of gizzard actomyosin. Bremel
(1974) suggested that myosin itself serves a regulatory function
in gizzard actomyosin, basing his conclusion on experiments with
protein isolated from skeletal muscle. His hypothesis was that
control sites are located only on the myosin molecule. Thus,
addition of unregulated actin would not influence the Ca^{2+} sensitivity of gizzard actomyosin (since there would be no dilution
of the regulatory component) and the addition of the skeletal
muscle myosin or certain of its fragments would reduce Ca^{2+}
sensitivity of actomyosin. The reason for the latter result is
that skeletal myosin does not possess the same control mechanism
as gizzard myosin and the gizzard actin (which activates the
myosin magnesium ATPase activities) is not regulated. This theory,
while current for regulation of smooth muscle contraction, however,
is by no means universally accepted. For example, Ebashi (1975,
1977) has recently reported the isolation of troponin from gizzard
smooth muscle as well. A complete current discussion can be
found in Stephens (1977). The reason for this brief discussion
of possible contractile protein regulatory systems in smooth
muscle is only to develop a more complete story concerning regulation of activator Ca^{2+}. The mechanism for control of Ca^{2+} is
clearly unknown and the nature of the specific interactions with
contractile proteins also remains to be elucidated.

   In the last few years, a significant amount of work has been
carried out attempting to clarify the mechanism of subcellular
regulation of Ca^{2+} in vascular smooth muscle. Figure 1 represents
possible areas controlling the total intracellular free Ca^{2+}
($[Ca_i]$) at any given instant. This concentration determines
whether or not Ca^{2+} binding sites on the Ca^{2+} regulatory protein
will be occupied. If they are occupied, i.e., $[Ca_i]$ is high
enough ($> 10^{-7}$ M) contraction will ensue. If they are vacant,
the actomyosin reaction will be prevented and the muscle will
relax. While this free intracellular Ca^{2+} is obviously the
immediate source of Ca^{2+} available for interaction with the
regulatory site, the mechanism of the regulation of its pool
size is, in fact, what must be determined experimentally. Concentration of free Ca^{2+} will depend on equilibrium of Ca^{2+} binding and release in each of five possible Ca^{2+}-containing areas:
plasma membrane and associated surface vesicles, sarcoplasmic

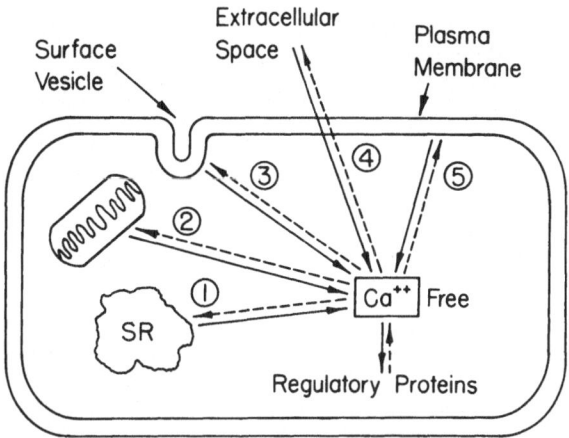

Figure 1. Schematic diagram of the various subcellular areas which can control intracellular "free Ca²⁺". This "free Ca²⁺" or "activator Ca²⁺" is that which is available to interact with the regulatory proteins to effect contraction. The respective lines represent binding and release of Ca²⁺ to each of the possible regulatory areas: (1) sarcoplasmic reticulum (2) mitochondria (3) surface vesicles (4) extracellular space (5) cell membrane.

reticulum, mitochondria, and the extracellular space. Thus, free available intracellular Ca^{2+} will be the sum of Ca^{2+} movements of each independent (or interdependent) source.

It is well known that cardiac muscle requires external Ca^{2+} for contractility and that skeletal muscle can utilize internal stores of Ca^{2+} for contraction. However, among the smooth muscle types, there are those which resemble skeletal muscle and can utilize internal Ca^{2+}, and those that are like cardiac muscle which require external Ca^{2+}. Indeed, even in vascular smooth muscle, both types exist. For example, portal vein, renal artery and coronary artery are dependent on extracellular Ca^{2+}, whereas the aorta and the femoral and carotid arteries are less dependent on extracellular Ca^{2+}. Clearly, because of these different characteristics, regulation of free Ca^{2+} available for interaction with contractile protein as indicated in Figure 1, may differ among the types of smooth muscle. Indeed, Devine *et al.* (1973) have found a correlation between the percentage volume of sarcoplasmic reticulum contained in various smooth muscles and the ability to contract in response to external Ca^{2+}. It was suggested that those muscles which have a higher sarcoplasmic reticulum volume, can utilize this organelle as a source of activator Ca^{2+}, whereas those muscles which have a lower volume of sarcoplasmic reticulum must utilize external Ca^{2+} or, perhaps, another source of Ca^{2+} to activate the contractile proteins. The main pulmonary artery had the largest percentage of sarcoplasmic reticulum volume and was much more capable of responding in the absence of external Ca^{2+} (and in the presence of EGTA) than any of the other arteries tested. To date, no functional correlation has been presented regarding subcellular fraction Ca^{2+} binding characteristics and Ca^{2+} requirements of types of vascular smooth muscle.

The first demonstration of a Ca^{2+} pump associated with a vesicular fraction of vascular smooth muscle, presumably the sarcoplasmic reticulum, was by Hurwitz and coworkers in 1972 (Fitzpatrick *et al.*, 1972), although Carsten (1969) and Batra and Daniel (1971) had published earlier data obtained from uterine microsomes. Since that time, a number of different laboratories have isolated microsomal material which demonstrates Ca^{2+} sequestering abilities. However, it is difficult to designate these various fractions as either cell membrane or sarcoplasmic reticulum membrane until purification studies are carried out.

These fractions are clearly heterogeneous and, in all probability, consist of membranes from various sources (at least from sarcoplasmic reticulum and cell membrane). Because of work carried out with cardiac and skeletal muscle sarcoplasmic reticulum fractions that demonstrate particular types of ATP-dependent Ca^{2+} binding, many workers have suggested that, in the particular sources of vascular smooth muscle studied, the fractions indeed constitute sarcoplasmic reticulum and, further, that the sarcoplasmic reticulum may well be the chief source of Ca^{2+} binding and release in these various muscles.

The reported Ca^{2+} binding characteristics of sarcoplasmic reticulum membranes seem to be reasonably consistent and will be summarized here. ATP stimulates Ca^{2+} binding. There is a stimulation of this Ca^{2+} binding by oxalate and the ATPase activities present are also stimulated by Ca^{2+} and oxalate. There seems to be little mitochondrial contamination as evidenced by low cytochrome oxidase activity, and relatively small amounts of cell membrane activity as evidenced by 5'-nucleotidase, ouabain sensitive ATPase and potassium phosphatase activities. However, there are significant complications in attempting to clarify what organelle systems really constitute the various isolated fractions that are being studied. This is because this same aortic fraction has now been shown to contain a Na^+, K^+-ATPase activity, as well as Ca^{2+} binding characteristics. Furthermore, one questions the integrity of the membrane systems studied, in view of the fact that some aortic fractions must be specifically treated with SDS in order to demonstrate Na^+, K^+-ATPase activity. If the SDS treatment is really affecting the vesicles by altering permeability characteristics, then simple studies of organelle yield, binding sensitivity or capacity are not valid for use in suggesting that one organelle exerts predominant control of Ca^{2+} in a given vascular smooth muscle type.

Hurwitz and coworkers (1973) have attempted to correlate the biochemistry of subcellular fractions from smooth muscles and the ability of the muscles to contract in the absence of external Ca^{2+}. These workers isolated a microsomal fraction of guinea pig longitudinal smooth muscle and layered it on density gradient. For comparison, they isolated the same fraction from rabbit aorta and also layered it on sucrose density gradient. In the gastrointestinal muscle preparation, the results suggested that Ca^{2+} uptake capacity corresponded to a fraction with Na^+, K^+-ATPase activity, which obviously is a marker for enzymatic activity of the cell membrane. The aortic material possessed Ca^{2+} uptake capability in a fraction not containing cell membrane. The cell membrane marker was 5'-nucleotidase, since these workers suggested that Na^+, K^+-ATPase was not found in the rabbit aorta (but see later). They further suggested that these data are consistent with the observed physiologic response, i. e., that drug induced contraction of aorta does not require external Ca^{2+} and utilizes intracellular Ca^{2+} and that guinea pig longitudinal muscle from the gut does require external Ca^{2+} and (hence) Ca^{2+} binding would occur more readily in a cell membrane fraction. The characteristics reported in this paper may be subject to an altered interpretation in view of the fact that our laboratory has now been able to demonstrate Na^+, K^+-ATPase activity in rabbit aortic microsomes.

Originally, we were able to show a large Ca^{2+} binding capacity of isolated microsomes from canine aortic smooth muscle (Allen, 1977). Our values ranged up to 100 nmoles Ca^{2+}/mg protein. In that preparation, however, we were unable to demonstrate any specific Na^+, K^+-ATPase activity. If we treated the Ca^{2+} binding microsomal preparation isolated from canine aorta with SDS for 20 minutes at room temperature, a ouabain inhibited ATPase activity could be seen. The peculiar thing about this ouabain sensitive activity was that, in order for it to be demonstrated, EGTA had to be added. This resulted in a stimulation of the ATPase activity which was then inhibited by ouabain. The ouabain sensitive ATPase activity ranged up to 15-20 μmoles P_i/mg/hr. A possible explanation for these data is that Ca^{2+} is inhibiting the Na^+, K^+-ATPase and the addition of large quantities of EGTA chelates the Ca^{2+}, thus increasing the ATPase activity which can then be inhibited by the glycoside.

We then looked at rat and rabbit aortic preparations and found that they contained a large EGTA stimulated ATPase activity in these membrane fractions and that the EGTA stimulation, as in canine microsomes, was inhibited by ouabain. Therefore, the suggestion made previously by others, that rat and rabbit aortic tissue has very little, if any, Na^+, K^+-ATPase activity, is no longer tenable. It should also be pointed out that earlier, Hess and Ford (1974) clearly showed that a microsomal fraction from bovine aorta that had Ca^{2+} accumulating capabilities also had a significant Na^+, K^+-ATPase activity. The isolation procedure for that preparation was somewhat different from ours, but the data certainly indicate the presence of both Ca^{2+} binding fraction and Na^+, K^+-ATPase activity. Quite recently, Wei *et al.* (1976a) have shown a ouabain sensitive Na^+, K^+-ATPase activity in a density gradient fraction from rat mesenteric arteries. However, these workers were unable to show any ouabain sensitive activity from rat aortic tissue. The reasons for this are not clear.

The mechanism of the effect of SDS on the microsomal fraction may be similar to that suggested by Besch *et al.* (1976) quite recently for cardiac microsomes. This suggestion was that the preparation utilized was vesicular in nature, and the ouabain binding sites, perhaps even the sodium or potassium activation sites, were shielded from the specific reagent because of the nature of the vesicles. Thus, SDS "opened" the vesicles up and allowed ouabain to reach the internal binding site.

Clearly there are problems in defining the nature of the different vesicular preparations which various laboratories are using to study Ca^{2+} binding properties of vascular smooth muscle. Thus far, we have discussed the Ca^{2+} binding characteristics of preparations that also demonstrate Na^+, K^+-ATPase activity. The studies of Wei *et al.* (1976b) show that Ca^{2+} binding to a cell membrane fraction is not stimulated by oxalate. They demonstrated ATP dependent Ca^{2+} binding to both plasma membrane (as determined by 5'-nucleotidase and ouabain sensitive Na^+, K^+-ATPase) and sarcoplasmic reticulum. However, only the binding to the latter fraction could be stimulated by oxalate (6.92 to 14.63 µmoles Ca^{2+}/g/10 min). Values of Ca^{2+} binding to the sarcolemmal fraction remained the same in the presence of 5 mM oxalate.

The preparation used by Hess and Ford (1974) and mentioned earlier, yields data that contradicts this suggestion that Ca^{2+} binding to sarcolemma is not oxalate sensitive and that to sarcoplasmic reticulum is. In addition, our laboratory has shown Ca^{2+} binding to an aortic microsomal fraction which is *not* stimulated by oxalate (Allen, 1977). This fraction also contains Na^+, K^+-ATPase. It is very difficult to compare various studies which

are performed on different membrane fractions isolated from smooth
muscle since no one fraction is really specific for either cell
membrane or sarcoplasmic reticulum membrane. Consequently, it
is critical to more rigorously define the various fractions being
used before we apply specific Ca^{2+} binding characteristics as
relating to an *in situ* muscle situation.

Stauber and Schottelius (1975) have begun attempts to study
smooth muscle organelles isolated from hog carotid artery by
isopycnic zonal centrifugation techniques used previously by
DeDuve and coworkers (1972). These workers have shown that a
plasma membrane fraction (5'-nucleotidase used as a marker) can
be partially separated from other organelles in the sucrose
gradient and that it does have some Ca^{2+} binding capabilities.
The sarcoplasmic reticulum fraction showed Ca^{2+} uptake ability,
but the Ca^{2+} ATPase activity reflected multiple sources of enzyme
activity (such as mitochondrial, plasma and sarcoplasmic reticulum
membranes) and, therefore, the sarcoplasmic reticulum could not
be specifically defined. It is clear that, at present, both
sarcoplasmic reticulum and sarcolemmal membrane preparations may
well bind Ca^{2+}. But the assignment of functional roles of each
with respect to regulation of activator Ca^{2+} (Figure 1) awaits
clarification.

Some of the suggestions regarding Ca^{2+} sequestration by
smooth muscle microsomes and its regulatory role have been somewhat premature because of the lack of homogeneity of the various
fractions studied. For example, a number of workers have suggested
that c-AMP can stimulate Ca^{2+} uptake into the microsomal vesicles
of smooth muscle and, thereby, provide some biochemical and
mechanistic basis for the relaxation effect of β-adrenergic agents
on vascular smooth muscle (Andersson, 1977; Webb and Bhalla, 1976a).
The suggestion is that relaxation occurs because stimulation of
adenyl cyclase causes an increase in c-AMP which, in turn, directly increases Ca^{2+} binding to the sarcoplasmic reticulum subsequent
to phosphorylation associated with the sarcoplasmic reticulum.
At the present time, the quantitative aspects of such c-AMP involvement seem somewhat unlikely. There are large variations in
c-AMP content (0.6 - 13.3 nmol/g tissue) in vascular smooth
muscle (Namm, 1976; Diamond, 1977). Whether such variations
depend on experimental techniques or actually reflect tissue
differences is not clear at present.

In addition, only relatively large concentrations of c-AMP
(10^{-5} M, 10^{-6} M) stimulate Ca^{2+} binding or uptake into vascular
smooth muscle microsomal preparations, and about 20 nm Ca^{2+}/mg
pro. has been the highest stimulation of Ca^{2+} binding achieved
with vascular smooth muscle microsomes (Andersson, 1977). Total
tissue c-AMP has been known to increase 2-3 times after the

administration of high concentrations of β-adrenergic agents. Consequently, these quantitative aspects make it somewhat difficult to assign such a role to sarcoplasmic reticulum. Even assuming a maximum catalyzing role of protein kinase, levels of c-AMP are 2-3 orders of magnitude below those necessary for direct involvement. Also, whereas other laboratories have shown that c-AMP increases Ca^{2+} uptake into microsomal fractions from vascular smooth muscle, this laboratory (Allen, 1977) has been unable to detect any increase in Ca^{2+} sequestration by aortic microsomes (despite the significant protein kinase dependent c-AMP stimulated phosphorylation of proteins in the fraction). Suggestions which have previously been offered for cardiac and skeletal muscle regarding the actual biochemical mechanism involved cannot yet be advanced for vascular smooth muscle.

Some additional recent work regarding the role of altered Ca^{2+} binding capabilities of membranes in the development of hypertension is of interest. A short comment should be made regarding these isolated fractions and their possible involvement in hypertensive situations. Some workers have attempted to characterize Ca^{2+} binding to vascular smooth muscle microsomal material in control and hypertensive animals. Interpretation of these data is difficult, again primarily because of lack of homogeneity of different fractions, difference in alterations that may occur, and the different characteristics of fractions isolated from various types of smooth muscle. Indeed, we feel that such designations are premature at best. One critical experiment which adds to the complexity of the problems involved has been the isolation and characterization of subcellular fractions of both mesenteric arteries and aorta of spontaneously hypertensive rats by Wei *et al*. (1976c, 1977). They found that ATP dependent Ca^{2+} uptake by the plasma membrane fraction from spontaneously hypertensive rats was higher than that from normotensive rats. However, the ATP dependent Ca^{2+} uptake by the plasma membrane fraction from SHR was decreased as compared to that of the normotensive strain. These workers felt that this qualitative difference in the response of various membranes may reflect differences in the mechanism controlling contraction and relaxation of both large and small vessels. In addition, Webb and Bhalla (1976b) have presented data suggesting that a sarcoplasmic reticulum membrane fraction, rather than a cell membrane fraction, is altered in hypertension. Clearly, such mechanisms must be defined before we can even begin to predict what may happen in a diseased artery vs. a normal artery. Furthermore, the role of Ca^{2+} in any mechanism of drug action in different arteries and in arteries altered by disease must be viewed with care until the mechanism regulating contractility is defined for that particular artery and that particular vascular bed.

The complexities of such differential regulation of contractility may be clearly demonstrated by studies from this laboratory on the *in vivo* and *in situ* effects of the Hoffman-LaRoche ionophore X-537A (RO 2-2985) (Schwartz *et al.*, 1974; Hanley *et al.*, 1975). When this compound is injected at a 1 mg/kg dose in the conscious chronically instrumented dog, there is a large increase in arterial pressure due to a positive ionotropic effect of this material on the heart. However, after the central aortic pressure has returned to normal, renal blood flow as well as coronary artery blood flow increases significantly. Subsequent isolation and *in vitro* study of renal, femoral and coronary artery strips indicate that the ionophore seems to have specific effects upon norepinephrine or K^+ induced contractions of renal arteries as opposed to those of femoral arteries. The nature of the ionophore suggests that the mechanism of regulation of contractility in the renal artery is different from that in other vascular beds. As a result, one theoretically could (after defining mechanisms of contractile regulation in various vascular beds) design vascular site-specific drugs such that increased blood flow could be directed to occur in only one area. Naturally, this type of approach is far in the future and, prior to the development of such therapeutic agents, a specific characteristic of each vascular bed and its regulatory mechanism must be defined.

MITOCHONDRIA

Successful isolation and characterization of smooth muscle mitochondria has been hampered by many difficulties. Because of the large quantity of connective tissue in the large arteries generally used, standard tissue disruption and subsequent isolation of these organelles have not been very successful. Despite these technical problems, some workers have characterized Ca^{2+} binding to fractions which they suggest (on the basis of appropriate enzyme markers) are mitochondria. However, even though Ca^{2+} binding is stimulated by ATP and inhibited by sodium azide, it is very difficult to ascribe these characteristics to functionally intact phosphorylating mitochondria since various oxidative parameters have rarely been measured. Recently, however, a number of investigators (Batra, 1975; Wrogemann and Stevens, 1977; Vallieres *et al.*, 1975; Wikstrom *et al.*, 1975 and this laboratory) have succeeded in isolating smooth muscle mitochondria and characterizing them by virtue of their various oxidative capacities. Some of the groups have studied Ca^{2+} binding as well. Until very recently, most of the mitochondrial preparations isolated from vascular smooth muscle had relatively low oxidation rates and relatively low respiratory control index values (Morrison *et al.*, 1970). Stevens and Wrogemann (1970), however, isolated tracheal smooth muscle mitochondria which had an oxygen uptake rate of close to 100. Neither of these groups studied the Ca^{2+} binding capacities of those organelles. The previous aortic tissue mitochondrial studies lacked data on Ca^{2+} binding or release characteristics as well. Batra and Daniel (1971), however, did study ATP dependent Ca^{2+} binding to uterine mitochondrial preparations without measuring oxidative capacities of the preparation. In addition, Hess and Ford (1977), and Webb and Bhalla (1976a) have reported that same type of study, i.e., ATP dependent Ca^{2+} uptake of mitochondria isolated from aortic tissue. Vallieres *et al*. (1975) studied substrate utilization and Ca^{2+} transport by mitochondria isolated from both the main pulmonary artery and mesenteric vein. They expressed their state 3 oxygen uptake measurements as per mg of mitochondrial protein, which was specifically normalized with respect to cytochrome oxidase activity. These workers showed (with succinate as substrate) that Q_{O_2} was of the order of 117 in the main pulmonary artery and somewhat lower (92) in the mesenteric vein. In addition, they also studied the appropriate oxidative parameters related to Ca^{2+} binding respiratory control index and ADP/O ratios using a dual beam spectrophotometer. Calcium ion uptake by pulmonary artery mitochondria and mesenteric vein mitochondria could be stimulated by the respiratory substrate. This was the first demonstration of a specific substrate dependent Ca^{2+} binding to mitochondria of vascular smooth muscle.

Our laboratory has also studied Ca^{2+} accumulation by mitochondria isolated from canine aorta. Table I shows the substrate utilization for oxidative phosphorylation capacities of the mitochondria. The three substrates used also supported Ca^{2+} binding to the mitochondrial fraction. These were glutamate-malate, pyruvate-malate and succinate. The oxidative details are outlined in Table I.

Of considerable interest in these present experiments was Ca^{2+} binding and release capacity in the presence of 5 mM succinate as compared to 5 mM ATP. The characteristics of Ca^{2+} binding to and release from these preparations are indicated in Figure 2. A specific difference in the nature of the binding/release cycle was dependent on the "energizer" used to induce the binding. For example, ATP dependent binding of Ca^{2+} seemed to occur at a much slower rate than binding dependent on succinate. In addition, the succinate dependent Ca^{2+} binding was released more readily, probably due to oxygen depletion, in the same manner as seen with cardiac muscle (Sordahl, 1975).

Clearly, recent work has demonstrated that coupled mitochondria can be isolated from various sources of smooth muscle, and that these mitochondria are capable of Ca^{2+} sequestration in response to both ATP and appropriate respiratory substrates. The

TABLE I.   RESPIRATORY PARAMETERS OF ISOLATED CANINE AORTIC MITOCHONDRIA[a]

Substrate[b]	State 3	State 4	RCI	ADP/O
		(natoms/0/mg/min)		
Glutamate Malate (11)	73.0 ± 5.5	23.4 ± 1.9	3.3 ± 0.2	2.64 ± 0.2
Pyruvate Malate (4)	65.3 ± 2.5	32.5 ± 1.7	2.2 ± 0.2	2.93 ± 0.3
Succinate (4)	79.9 ± 7.0	39.5 ± 3.3	2.1 ± 0.1	1.61 ± 0.03

[a]*1-2 mg protein were incubated at 30° C for a 5 minute equilibration period in a Gilson oxygraph. The incubation solution contained substrate at 5 mM as indicated, 10 mM K_2HPO_4, 0.25 M sucrose, 10 mM Tris HCl pH 7.4, and in the case of succinate, 2 μg rotenone. 500 nmoles ADP were added to initiate state 3 respiration.*

[b]*Numbers in parentheses represent total number of separate experiments.*

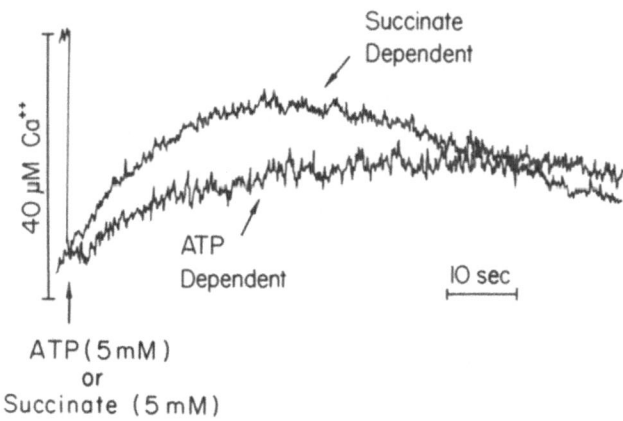

Figure 2.   Dual beam spectrophotometric traces of Ca^{2+} binding to and release from canine aortic mitochondria. The Ca^{2+} sensitive dye, murexide, was used to measure Ca^{2+} binding. In the two curves, Ca^{2+} binding was induced with 5 mM succinate or 5 mM ATP.

characteristics of the Ca^{2+} binding observed also apparently
depend upon the nature of the induction.

The question of whether these organelles play a direct role
in the regulation of $[Ca_i]$ of Figure 1 remains unanswered.   In
cardiac muscle, Scarpa (1976) has suggested that the kinetics
of Ca^{2+} uptake by these organelles are not rapid enough to be
involved in beat to beat regulation of that tissue.   Carafoli
(1976), however, suggests that this is not the case and has
presented extensive data indicating that the Na^+ releasing effect
of Ca^{2+} binding to cardiac mitochondria is of physiologic importance.

The possible direct role of mitochondria in regulation
of cytoplasmic Ca^{2+} of smooth muscle is not yet clear.   Vallieres
et al. (1975) have suggested that the organelles may serve as
reserve sinks of Ca^{2+} as has been suggested for cardiac muscle.
These workers do, however, show that smooth muscle mitochondria
can sequester large amounts of Ca^{2+} without becoming uncoupled.
Because of the relatively slow rate of contraction and relaxation of the smooth muscle, arguments used against mitochondrial
involvement for cardiac and skeletal muscle cannot really be
applied to smooth muscle.   In addition, as discussed earlier, Ca^{2+}
requirements vary among smooth muscle types.   As a result, until
these quantitative differences are worked out, the involvement
of these organelles in Ca^{2+} regulation must still be considered
a possibility.

CONCLUSIONS

In order to establish specific mechanisms of action for
the multitude of drugs affecting smooth muscle contractility,
the inter-relationships between possible regulatory areas must
be determined.   Subcellular studies suggest complex relationships among the various organelles and these are further complicated by the probability that different smooth muscles may well
possess different mechanisms for the regulation of cytoplasmic
Ca^{2+} levels.   As a result, much more fundamental work needs to
be done before the specific mechanisms of various drugs can be
elucidated.   To date, the Ca^{2+} regulatory mechanisms in smooth
muscles are essentially unknown, and we can only begin to define
the inter-relationships between different subcellular organelles.

Acknowledgements

The original data in this paper was supported by HL 16947.
Dr. Allen is an Established Investigator of the American Heart
Association. The author is grateful to Dr. Charles Seidel for
much helpful discussion, and to Ms. Loris Barrett for her assistance in the preparation of this manuscript.

REFERENCES

Allen, J. C., 1977, Ca^{++} binding properties of canine aortic
microsomes. Lack of effect of c-AMP, *Blood Vessels* 14: 91.

Andersson, R. G., and Nilsson, K. B., 1977, Role of cyclic nucleotide metabolism and mechanical activity in smooth muscle, *in*
"The Biochemistry of Smooth Muscle" (N. L. Stephens, ed.),
pp. 263-292, University Park Press, Baltimore.

Batra, S. C., and Daniel, E. E., 1971, ATP dependent Ca^{++} uptake
by subcellular fractions of uterine smooth muscle, *Comp. Biochem.
Physiol.* 38a: 369.

Batra, S. C., 1975, The role of mitochondria in the regulation
of myoplasmic Ca^{++} concentration in smooth muscle, *in* "Calcium
Transport in Contraction and Secretion" (E. Carafoli, F.
Clementi, W. Drabikowski, and A. Margreth, eds.), pp. 87-94,
North-Holland Publishing Company, Amsterdam.

Besch, H. R., Jones, L. R., and Watanabe, A. M., 1976, Intact
vesicles of canine cardiac sarcolemma, Evidence from vectorial
properties of Na^+,K^+-ATPase, *Circ. Res.* 39: 586.

Bremel, R. D., 1974, Myosin linked Ca^{++} regulation in vertebrate
smooth muscle, *Nature* 252: 405.

Carafoli, E., 1976, Mitochondria Ca^{++} transport and Ca^{++} binding
proteins, *in* "Mitochondria: Bioenergetics, Biogenesis and
Membrane Structure" (Lester Packer and A. Gomez-Puyou, eds.),
pp. 47-60, Academic Press, New York.

Carsten, M. E., 1969, Role of Ca^{++} binding by sarcoplasmic reticulum in the contraction and relaxation of uterine smooth muscle,
J. gen. Physiol. 53: 414.

Devine, C. E., Somlyo, A. V., and Somlyo, A. P., 1973, Sarcoplasmic
reticulum and excitation-contraction coupling in mammalian smooth
muscles, *J. Cell Biol.* 52: 690.

Diamond, J., 1977, Evidence for dissociation between cyclic nucleo-
tide levels and tension in smooth muscle, *in* "Biochemistry of
Smooth Muscle" (N. L. Stephens, ed.), pp. 343-362, University
Park Press, Baltimore.

Driska, S., and Hartshorne, D. J., 1975, The contractile proteins
of smooth muscle. Properties in components of a Ca^{++} sensitive
actomyosin from chicken gizzard, *Arch. Biochem. Biophys.* 167:
203.

Ebashi, S., Toyo-oka, T., Nonomura, Y., 1977, Gizzard troponin, *in* "The Biochemistry of Smooth Muscle" (N. L. Stephens, ed.), pp. 551-558, University Park Press, Baltimore.

Ford, G. E., and Hess, M. L., 1975, Ca^{++} accumulating properties of subcellular fractions of bovine vascular smooth muscle, *Circ. Res.* 37: 580.

Fitzpatrick, D. F., Landon, E. J., Debbas, G., Hurwitz, L., 1972, Ca^{++} pump in vascular smooth muscle, *Science* 176: 305.

Hanley, H. G., Lewis, R. M., Hartley, C. J., Franklin, D., and Schwartz, A., 1975, Effects of an inotropic agent, RO 2-2985 (X537A) on regional blood flow and myocardial function in chronically instrumented conscious dogs and anesthetized dogs, *Circ. Res.* 37: 215.

Hess, M. L., and Ford, G. D., 1974, Ca^{++} accumulation by subcellular fractions from vascular smooth muscle, *J. Mol. Cell. Cardiol.* 6: 275.

Hurwitz, L., Fitzpatrick, D. F., Debbas, G., and Landon, E. J., 1973, Localization of Ca^{++} pump activity in smooth muscle, *Science* 179: 384.

Morrison, E. S., Scott, R. F., Kroms, M., and Pastori, S. J., 1970, A method for isolating aortic mitochondria exhibiting high respiratory control, *Biochem. Med.* 4: 47.

Namm, D. H., and Peter, J. P., 1976, Occurrence and function of cyclic nucleotides in blood vessels, *Blood Vessels* 13: 24.

Peters, T. J., Muller, M., and DeDuve, C., 1972, Lysosomes of the arterial wall, Isolation and subcellular fractionation of cells from normal rabbit aorta, *J. Exp. Med.* 136: 1117.

Scarpa, A., 1976, Kinetic and thermodynamic aspects of mitochondrial Ca^{++} transport, *in* "Mitochondria, Bioenergetics, Biogenesis and Membrane Structure" (L. Packer and A. Gomez-Puyou, eds.), pp. 31-45, Academic Press, New York.

Schwartz, A., Lewis, R. M., Hanley, H. G., Munson, R. G., Dial, F. D., Ray, M. V., 1974, Hemodynamic and biochemical effects of a new positive inotropic agent. Antibiotic ionophore RO 2-2985, *Circ. Res.* 34: 102.

Sobieszek, A., and Bremel, R. D., 1975, Preparation and properties of vertebrate smooth muscle myofibril and actomyosin, *Eur. J. Biochem.* 55: 49.

Sordahl, L. A., 1975, Effects of Mg^{++}, ruthenium red and the antibiotic ionophore A-23187 on initial rates of Ca^{++} uptake and release by heart mitochondria, *Arch. Biochem. Biophys.* 167: 104.

Stauber, W. T., and Schottelius, B. A., 1975, An isopycnic zonal centrifugation study of smooth muscle organelles isolated from hog carotid artery, *Proc. Soc. Exp. Biol. Med.* 150: 529.

Stephens, N. L., ed., 1977, "The Biochemistry of Smooth Muscle", University Park Press, Baltimore.

Stephens, N. L., and Wrogemann, K., 1970, Oxidative phosphorylation in smooth muscle, *Amer. J. Physiol.* 219: 1796.

Vallieries, J., Scarpa, A., Somlyo, A. P., 1975, Subcellular
    fractions of smooth muscle, Isolation, substrate utilization
    and Ca^{++} transport by main pulmonary artery and mesenteric vein
    mitochondria, *Arch. Biochem. Biophys.* 170: 659.
Webb, R. C., and Bhalla, R. C., 1976a, Ca^{++} sequestration by sub-
    cellular fractions isolated from vascular smooth muscle, Effect
    of cyclic nucleotides and prostaglandins, *J. Molec. Cell Cardiol.*
    8: 145.
Webb, R. C., and Bhalla, R. C., 1976b, Altered calcium sequestra-
    tion by subcellular fractions of vascular smooth muscle from
    spontaneously hypertensive rats, *J. Mol. Cell. Cardiol.* 8: 651.
Wei, J. W., Janis, R. A., Daniel, E. E., 1976a, Isolation and
    characterization of plasma membrane from rat mesenteric arteries,
    Blood Vessels 13: 279.
Wei, J. W. Janis, R. A., Daniel, E. E., 1976b, Studies on sub-
    cellular fractions from mesenteric arteries of spontaneously
    hypertensive rats, Alterations in both Ca^{++} uptake and enzyme
    activities, *Blood Vessels* 13: 293.
Wei, J. W., Janis, R. A., Daniel, E. E., 1976c, Ca^{++} accumulation
    in enzymatic activities of subcellular fractions from aortas
    and ventricles of genetically hypertensive rats, *Circ. Res.*
    39: 133.
Wei, J. W., Janis, R. A., Daniel, E. E., 1977, Relationship between
    blood pressures of spontaneously hypertensive rats and altera-
    tions in membrane properties of mesenteric arteries, *Circ. Res.*
    40: 299.
Wrogeman, K., and Stephens, N. L., 1977, Oxidative phosphorylation
    in smooth muscle, *in* "The Biochemistry of Smooth Muscle" (N.
    L. Stephens, ed.), pp. 41-50, University Park Press, Baltimore.

CHAPTER 8

ROLE OF CALCIUM IN THE ACTIONS OF AGENTS

AFFECTING MEMBRANE PERMEABILITY

James W. Putney, Jr.

Department of Pharmacology
Wayne State University School of Medicine
Detroit, Michigan 48201

INTRODUCTION

It has been apparent from the earliest electrophysiological measurements that extracellular Ca^{2+} plays a role in maintaining membrane stability and in long-term control of membrane permeability. Endogenous neurotransmitters and hormones, known to affect membrane permeability in a number of tissues, do not affect the level of extracellular Ca^{2+} (though surface binding may be affected), but quite often modulate the intracellular Ca^{2+} concentration. Thus, if Ca^{2+} were to play a role in alteration (rather than maintenance) of membrane permeability, then an action of intracellular Ca^{2+} should be evident. Recent investigations have demonstrated that this is indeed the case. The membranes of diverse cell types have been shown to respond to elevation of intracellular Ca^{2+} usually with an elevation in permeability to K^+. In the red cell, this relationship has been demonstrated by several techniques although no endogenous receptor mechanisms capable of controlling this process under physiological conditions have been identified. Excitable cells behave similarly and (as discussed below) changes in intracellular Ca^{2+} may mediate receptor-dependent as well as voltage-dependent changes in K^+ permeability.

The nature of Ca^{2+} action in exocrine cells has only recently become apparent. Here the magnitude of change is large (and easily quantitated) because of the osmotic gradients necessary to produce bulk flow of water. Also, the cells not only have the same advantage as does the red cell in lacking voltage-dependent parameters, but also afford the investigator the additional flexibility of studying any of several receptors mechanisms

controlling Ca^{2+} flux under physiological conditions. The following discussion is devoted primarily to the development of exocrine
gland preparations as models for study of the role of Ca^{2+} in the
actions of agents affecting membrane permeability.

EXOCRINE GLANDS: A SPECIAL CASE OF STIMULUS-SECRETION COUPLING

     The term stimulus-secretion coupling describes the sequence
of events between the initial stimulation of secretory cells and
the appearance of secretory product in the extracellular milieu
(Rubin, 1974). For neurotransmitter release and many endocrine
organs, the problem of stimulus-secretion coupling involves the
characterization of ionic and macromolecular events leading to
the secretion of prepackaged materials. The process presumably
involves exocytosis: the fusion of the membranes of the storage
organelles and plasmalemma such that secretory products are released without traversing the cytoplasm of the cell (Rubin, 1974;
Butcher, 1978; but see Rothman, 1975). The universal signal
triggering exocytosis is believed to be an increase in the intracellular concentration of Ca^{2+} ions (Rubin, 1974).

     Exocytosis occurs in the exocrine glands. The mechanism,
although different in quantitative and kinetic aspects, is qualitatively similar to that occurring in nerve endings and endocrine
organs. The importance of Ca^{2+} as a mediator of exocytosis of
prepackaged enzymes has been previously affirmed in the exocrine
pancreas (Case, 1974; Williams, 1974), parotid salivary gland
(Leslie et al., 1976; Putney et al., 1977b) and lacrimal gland
(Putney et al., 1977a). In addition, the exocrine glands secrete
or regulate the flow of water and salts, and in this respect are
functionally akin to other epithelial tissues (intestine, kidney,
toad bladder, etc.). Though the term stimulus-secretion coupling
has been applied to the regulation of water flow in exocrine
glands, it is important to note that the regulation of water flow
and the process of membrane fusion are distinctly unique phenomena.
No structural rearrangements are necessary for the bulk transport
of water. Since water transport is believed to be mediated by
changes in ion distribution that create osmotic gradients, research
in the past has been directed toward unmasking receptor-controlled
ion permeability changes that might produce such gradients. There
is no a priori reason why Ca^{2+} need function in such an arrangement; membrane receptors could conceivably be linked directly to
the relevant ion channels that regulate osmotic flow of electrolytes and water. The use of second messengers, however, can
provide for a considerable amplification of response such that
the opening of a few Ca^{2+} channels could result in the activation
of many additional channels owing to the sizable Ca^{2+} gradient
across the plasmalemma of most cells. In fact, as discussed

below, large shifts in electrolytes can be induced through several receptor mechanisms in exocrine glands. These shifts appear to be universally regulated by Ca^{2+}-controlled ion channels.

CALCIUM AS A GENERAL REGULATOR OF MEMBRANE PERMEABILITY

Extracellular Ca^{2+} has been known for some time to be required for general membrane integrity. In the absence of divalent cations, membranes become leaky and depolarized; excitation parameters become inactivated (Putney and Askari, 1978). In many cases such as squid axon, other divalent cations (notably Mg^{2+}) can substitute for Ca^{2+}; (Frankenhaeuser and Hodgkin, 1957). In some tissues, however, Mg^{2+} will not protect cells from the enhancement of membrane permeability due to Ca^{2+} omission. Both excitable and inexcitable cells may demonstrate a specific dependence on extracellular Ca^{2+}. In the parotid gland, tissues incubated in the absence of Ca^{2+} and Mg^{2+} gain significant quantities of Na^+ and lose K^+; 1.0 mM Mg^{2+} can totally block this effect (Putney *et al.*, 1977b). Calcium ion omission elevates K^+ efflux, but 1.0 mM Mg^{2+} prevents the increase (Table I). In rabbit atria, Ca^{2+} omission elevates K^+ efflux significantly even when Mg^{2+} is present; liver appears to behave similarly (Table I). The significance of this observation is not clear. Whether the phenomenon represents a qualitative or quantitative difference in regulation of membrane permeability by extracellular Ca^{2+} (and Mg^{2+}) will require more extensive investigation.

Just as lowering external Ca^{2+} can increase membrane permeability, increasing intracellular Ca^{2+} can produce a similar (though greater) effect. In the extensively studied cellular membrane system of the red cell, Ca^{2+} activation of K^+ efflux has been estimated by preparing resealed ghosts containing EGTA (ethyleneglycol bis(aminoethyl ether)-N,N'-tetraacetic acid)-Ca^{2+} buffers or by stimulating Ca^{2+} entry with the divalent cationophore A23187 (Simons, 1976a, b; Lew and Ferreira, 1976). Curiously, these techniques yield quite disparate values for the K_m for intracellular Ca^{2+}. With EGTA-Ca^{2+} buffers and resealed ghosts, the internal Ca^{2+} concentration of cells can be tightly controlled; the preparation is somewhat leaky, however, and contains no ATP. Under these conditions, K^+ efflux is half maximally stimulated by 4×10^{-7} M Ca^{2+} (Simons, 1976a, b). The use of the ionophore A23187 permits Ca^{2+}-loading of intact cells with normal (?) levels of ATP. Although this preparation is more physiological than resealed ghosts, the estimation of intracellular Ca^{2+} is less certain and depends on a theoretical treatment relating total cell Ca^{2+} to intracellular ionized Ca^{2+} (Ferreira and Lew, 1976). However, errors in estimation of internal Ca^{2+} cannot explain the magnitude of difference

TABLE I.   EFFECT OF Ca OMISSION ON K^+ EFFLUX IN RAT PAROTID GLAND, RABBIT ATRIA AND GUINEA PIG LIVER

Tissue	Mg^{2+}	k_e (%/min)	
		$+ Ca^{2+}$	$- Ca^{2+}$
Rat Parotid[a]	0	$3.78 \pm .07(64)$[e]	$4.95 \pm .22(32)$[f]
Rat Parotid[b]	1.0	$3.56 \pm .12(10)$	$3.55 \pm .06(10)$
Rabbit Atrium (left)[c]	2.5	$1.44 \pm .06(15)$	$1.70 \pm .07(15)$[f]
Guinea Pig Liver[d]	1.2	$1.27 \pm .04(30)$	$2.31 \pm .01(40)$[f]

[a] *Putney, 1976a.*
[b] *Putney, 1977.*
[c] *Putney and R. J. Parod, unpublished.*
[d] *Putney and S. J. Weiss, unpublished.*
[e] *Mean $\pm$ 1 S.E.M., (n) = number of determinations.*
[f] *Significantly greater than in the absence of Ca^+ (P < .05).*

in K_m values obtained. With the latter method, Lew and Ferreira (1976) estimate the K_m for Ca^{2+}-induced K^+ efflux to be of the order of 1.2×10^{-3} M, almost four orders of magnitude greater than that obtained with ghosts. The difference cannot presently be determined as resulting from an alteration in the nature of the Ca^{2+} site due to reversible hemolysis or to the action of intracellular substances (ATP or metabolites) in the intact cells. It is important to note, however, that the maximum increase in K^+ efflux is greater than three orders of magnitude over the resting flux. Thus, changes in internal Ca^{2+} in the micromolar range could still mediate measurable increases in K^+ flux (Lew and Ferreira, 1976).

The functional significance of the control of K^+ permeability by Ca^{2+} in red cells is unknown. In excitable cells, such a system may contribute to the rectifying current responsible for membrane repolarization after an action potential. Depolarization of excitable membranes activates Ca^{2+} influx (Putney and Askari, 1978). Accordingly, the K^+ permeability of a number of excitable tissues can be increased by small increases in intracellular Ca^{2+} (Meech and Standen, 1975; Krnjevic and Lisiewicz, 1972; Isenberg, 1975; Bassingthwaighte *et al.*, 1976).

The rather ubiquitous nature of the Ca^{2+}-K^+ interaction raises the possibility that Ca^{2+} may play a role in the action of neurotransmitters and hormones that affect K^+ permeability through specific receptor mechanisms. In liver, the activation of α-adrenergic receptors stimulates K^+ efflux. Extracellular Ca is not required, but release of tissue Ca^{2+} by the α-adrenergic agonist phenylephrine has been observed (Putney and Weiss, unpublished). In rabbit atria, a rather clear-cut independence of Ca^{2+} and of the muscarinic stimulation of K^+ permeability can be demonstrated. Enhanced K^+ efflux due to carbachol is independent of the extracellular Ca^{2+} concentration and the cholinergic agonist has no demonstrable effect on influx or efflux of Ca^{2+} (Putney and Parod, unpublished).

In the exocrine glands, control of K^+ permeability may be involved in regulation of water flow. Here, the role of Ca^{2+} as intermediate in receptor-stimulated K^+ permeability has been unequivocally demonstrated. Although studies now have been largely restricted to the parotid gland of the rat, recent observations suggest that the basic mechanism of Ca^{2+}-controlled K^+ efflux may apply to the submaxillary salivary gland (Martinez *et al.*, 1976) and to the lacrimal gland as well (see below). Thus, the exocrine glands are proving to be useful alternatives to the red cell as a model for Ca^{2+} control of membrane permeability. Due to the receptor-linked Ca influx mechanisms present, the investigator is afforded the advantage of pharmacological methods for controlling internal Ca^{2+} (see below).

ROLE OF CALCIUM IN AGONIST-INDUCED PERMEABILITY CHANGES IN EXOCRINE GLANDS

That the first few drops of stimulated saliva contain high concentrations of K^+ has puzzled and intrigued exocrine physiologists for two decades (Burgen, 1956; Schneyer *et al.*, 1972). It was apparent from the earliest measurements that much of the K^+ in the "potassium transient" (as it is called) was derived from the glandular cells themselves (Burgen, 1956; Burgen and Emmelin, 1961). A good deal of speculation has been put forth affirming and denying the importance of K^+ transport in both the initiation and maintenance of salivary secretion. The exact locus of the ionic events responsible for water flow in the salivary glands is still a mystery, however, owing largely to our inability to examine transport and permeability phenomena occurring specifically at the apical (luminal) membrane of acinar cells. Nonetheless, the studies of K^+ transport by salivary glands have revealed such

an elaborate regulatory system for this ion, controlled by the
same substances that control the flow of saliva, that the importance of K^+ at some step in the generation of transepithelial
water flow seems assured.

Much of our present understanding of the control of ion
permeabilities in salivary glands is attributable to the work of
Michael Schramm and Zvi Selinger who developed an *in vitro* salivary
gland preparation with slices of the rat parotid gland (Bdolah
et al., 1964; Babad *et al.*, 1967; Schramm and Selinger, 1974,
1975). This preparation is reasonably homogenous, being composed
80 to 85% of a single type of serous acinar cell. Also, for
unknown reasons, the parotid slices survive *in vitro* and maintain
ion gradients better than most epithelial slice systems (Leslie
et al., 1976). Initially, Schramm and Selinger found that the
slices were an ideal tool for the study of amylase release induced
through β-adrenergic receptor mechanisms and cyclic AMP. Subsequent
studies revealed two other receptor mechanisms (α-adrenergic and
cholinergic), both of which mediated loss of K^+ from the slices.
The K^+ release is striking; the slices lose up to 60% of intracellular K^+ in about five minutes. Extracellular Ca^{2+} is abso-
lutely required for K^+ release by these mechanisms (Selinger *et
al.*, 1973). Once K^+ is released, an appropriate blocking agent
(i.e., phentolamine or atropine) or removal of Ca^{2+} with EGTA
permits the reuptake of K^+ by the slices. Finally, a similar
K^+ release can be induced by the divalent cationophore A23187,
again requiring external Ca^{2+} ions (Selinger *et al.*, 1974). These
observations are compatible with a mechanism whereby the activation
of α-adrenergic or cholinergic receptors stimulates Ca^{2+} influx
and the resulting increase in intracellular Ca^{2+} triggers the
release of cellular K^+. Recent studies by Rudich and Butcher
(1976) suggest that a third receptor, for certain peptides, can
stimulate K^+ release by a similar mechanism.

Electrophysiological studies with the mouse parotid also
show that cholinergic or α-adrenergic receptor activation increases membrane permeability to K^+. The membrane potential of
mouse parotid acinar cells is about -70 mV and appears to be
largely a K^+ diffusion potential (Pedersen and Petersen, 1973).
Muscarinic or α-adrenergic receptor activation produces a hyperpolarization of 12-13 mV; β-receptor activation causes slight
(7 mV) depolarization. The hyperpolarization response to drugs
is unaffected by 10^{-3} M ouabain, a concentration sufficient to
block electrogenic Na^+ pumping in the parotid. Further, the
response can be potentiated by decreasing, and inhibited by increasing, the external K^+ concentration. Assuming that the drugs
enhance membrane permeability to K^+, these effects are predictable
from the known relationship between membrane potential and K^+
equilibrium potential as a function of extracellular K^+.

However, the electrical measurements in the parotid differed from the chemical determinations in two respects: First, the loss of K^+ measured by atomic absorption suggested that cholinergic and α-adrenergic agonists produced a sustained increase in K^+ permeability, while the electrical responses were transient. Second (and most important), in contrast to the release of K^+, the hyperpolarization was unaffected by omission of Ca^{2+} from the bathing medium, even in the presence of EGTA (Petersen and Pedersen, 1974). Measurements of K^+ flux with isotope techniques have served to reconcile these discrepancies (Putney, 1976a). The distributions and fluxes of ^{42}K and ^{86}Rb in parotid slices are virtually indistinguishable, and the latter may thus be employed as a marker for K^+ flux. With this technique, unidirectional efflux of K^+ can be monitored under nearly steady-state conditions. Such measurements revealed that both a transient phase and a sustained phase of efflux occur in response to carbachol, phenylephrine (Putney, 1976a) or substance P (unpublished). Only the later, sustained phase of release is dependent on the presence of Ca^{2+} in the bathing medium and is blocked by La^{3+}, a cation known to act by interfering with Ca^{2+} movement and binding at superficial sites (Weiss, 1974). Thus it appears that the observations of Schramm and Selinger and those of Petersen and Pedersen are not in conflict. The electrical measurement of a transient Ca^{2+}-independent increase in K^+ conductance corresponds to the transient K^+ efflux measured with ^{86}Rb, and the Ca^{2+}-dependent net loss of K^+ (measured by atomic absorption) is probably represented in the ^{86}Rb experiments by the sustained, Ca^{2+}-dependent increase in K^+ efflux. Since the flow of saliva is similarly Ca^{2+}-dependent and sustained (Douglas and Poisner, 1964; Petersen *et al.*, 1967), it has been argued that the sustained phase of release is of greater functional significance than the electrically measurable transient (Putney, 1976a). More recent experiments (discussed below) suggest that the transient and sustained phases of release are probably manifestations of the same molecular events. A comparison of the results obtained when K^+ efflux is studied by the three different approaches is schematically presented in Figure 1.

Because of the various physiological functions associated with Ca^{2+}, the demonstration that a process has a requirement for Ca^{2+} does not necessarily mean that Ca^{2+} mediates that process by entering the cell. Such a mechanism (Ca^{2+} influx) generally requires documentation from three independent lines of evidence: (1) requirement of Ca^{2+} for activity, (2) measurable Ca^{2+} flux that can be related to activity, and (3) the ability of an ionophore for Ca^{2+} (preferably A23187) to mimic the effect of the agonist that is believed to act through stimulating Ca^{2+} influx (Putney and Askari, 1978). Criterion (1) is easily demonstrated, and, as mentioned earlier, A23187 can stimulate net K^+ release and can also stimulate efflux of ^{86}Rb (Putney, 1976a). A study

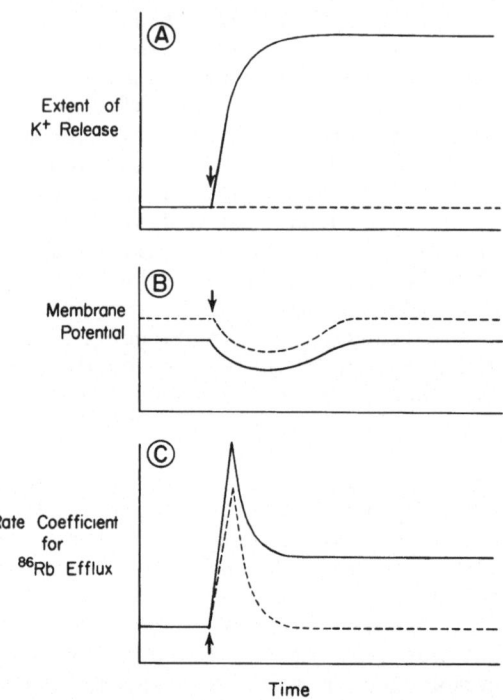

Figure 1. Schematic representation of various approaches to the
study of Ca^{2+} and K^+ permeability in the parotid gland. The
arrows indicate the points of addition of muscarinic or α-adrenergic
agonist. Solid lines indicate results obtained in the presence
of Ca^{2+}; dashed lines, results obtained in the absence of Ca^{2+}.
(A) Extent of K^+ release measured according to Schramm and Selinger
(1974). Parotid slices are incubated in a small volume of Ringer's
and the net loss of cellular K^+ is assayed by measuring an increase
in medium K^+ by atomic absorption (or with K^+ electrode). The
effect is sustained, and omission of external Ca^{2+} qualitatively
blocks the response. (B) Effect of agonists on membrane potential
(after Petersen and Pedersen, 1974). Cholinergic and α-adrenergic
stimuli produce hyperpolarization due to increased membrane conductance to K^+. The response is transient and unaltered by Ca^{2+}
omission. (C) Unidirectional efflux of K^+ measured with ^{86}Rb
(Putney, 1976a). Slices are loaded with ^{86}Rb and then the rate
of efflux of the isotope followed as an index of K^+ efflux. A
transient efflux occurs that is Ca^{2+}-independent (as in [B]) and
a sustained phase follows that requires Ca^{2+} (as in [A]).

of ^{45}Ca fluxes in the parotid has demonstrated that carbachol significantly increases Ca^{2+} influx into a slowly exchanging (presumably cellular) compartment (Putney, 1976b). The extra Ca^{2+}
influx can be blocked by atropine or La^{3+} and can be potentiated
by lowering extracellular Na^{+}. Phenylephrine (an α-agonist) also
stimulates Ca^{2+} influx, but isoproterenol does not (Putney *et al.*,
1977b, but see Miller and Nelson, 1977). Thus, the three criteria
mentioned above can all be met, and it is reasonable to conclude
that agents enhancing K^{+} permeability in the parotid do so by
first increasing membrane permeability to Ca^{2+}. The resulting
elevation in intracellular Ca^{2+} produces the enhanced membrane
permeability to K^{+}, presumably by interacting at some specific
site on the inner aspect of the plasmalemma.

In a number of tissues, stimulation of muscarinic receptors
produces an increase in cellular content of cyclic 3',5'-guanosine
monophosphate (cGMP) leading some to propose that this cyclic
nucleotide might be involved in the coupling of receptor activation to tissue response (Goldberg *et al.*, 1975). In the parotid,
cholinergic and α-adrenergic agonists both increase tissue cGMP
levels (Butcher *et al.*, 1976a, b) but substance P does not (Rudich
and Butcher, 1976). This latter observation discourages schemes
implicating cGMP as an obligatory intermediate since the quality
of the three receptor mechanisms in effecting K^{+} efflux appears
identical (Putney, 1977 and see below). In addition, the increase
in cGMP due to submaximal concentrations of carbachol or phenylephrine can be potentiated by the phosphodiesterase inhibitor
1-methyl-3-isobutylxanthine without potentiating K^{+} efflux (Butcher
et al., 1976a, b). These observations render doubtful any role
for cGMP in the regulation of K^{+} permeability in the parotid gland.

What, then, is the mechanism underlying the transient increase
in K^{+} efflux? Two possibilities are apparent: (1) there could
exist two populations of receptors for each agonist, one mediating
transient and the other sustained responses; or (2) the same
receptors could mediate both phases of the response. When scaled
to the same maximum, agonist-dose-response curves for the transient
and sustained responses are practically superimposable (Putney,
1976a). This relationship obtains for both carbachol and phenylephrine (similar data for substance P are not available) even though
the ratio of transient to sustained release is greater for carbachol
than for phenylephrine. Such reasoning suggests (but does not
prove) that the same receptors mediate both phases of release.
Other observations (below) serve to shore up this supposition and
to add the conclusion that the transient and sustained responses
are probably both consequences of the same molecular phenomenon.

The transient response to an agonist is, by definition, a
self-limiting process. Even though the agonist is still present

the response has undergone a process of inactivation. Surprisingly, it was observed that this inactivation phenomenon is not receptor-specific; when one agonist produces a transient release of K^+, another agonist, known to act on different receptors, can no longer produce a response. The term "cross-receptor inactivation" has been used to describe this phenomenon (Putney, 1977).

Figure 2 shows the results of experiments that reveal the mechanism of cross-receptor inactivation and of the transient response as well. So that the transient response could be studied in isolation, the Ringer's solutions for these experiments contained no added Ca^{2+} and 10^{-4} M EGTA. In panel A, prevention of the transient due to carbachol (added at [1]) by atropine (experiment with dashed line) prevents cross-receptor inactivation, since a normal response to substance P can be obtained at [3]. If, however, carbachol is displaced from muscarinic receptors by atropine after the fact (at [2], experiment with solid line), then the response to substance P (at [3]) fails. This is not due to the failure of atropine to displace carbachol from the receptors, as evidenced by Panel B. Here the occupation by carbachol (added at [1]) of muscarinic receptors is revealed by reintroducing Ca^{2+} (1.0 mM, at [3]) and thus unmasking the activated sustained phase of the response (solid line). The reintroduction of Ca^{2+} fails to stimulate K^+ release, however, if, as in Panel A, atropine is added 4 min prior to the addition of Ca^{2+}. This suggests that atropine has effectively displaced carbachol from the muscarinic receptors but could not reactivate the mechanism necessary to permit a transient response to substance P.

Panels C and D (Fig. 2) show that while Ca^{2+} is not required initially for the transient response, its presence is required for reversal of cross-receptor inactivation. In Panel C, carbachol was added at (1), followed by atropine at (2), and substance P and Ca^{2+} at (3). The combination of substance P and Ca^{2+} produced an increase in K^+ efflux where neither agent was capable of acting alone. In Panel D, a more complicated sequence shows that Ca^{2+} can restore the ability of substance P to produce a transient in the absence of Ca^{2+}. Carbachol was added at (1), and while the muscarinic receptors were occupied, Ca^{2+} (1.0 mM) was added (at [2]). Then, while Ca^{2+} was present, the muscarinic receptors were cleared (atropine at [3]), then Ca^{2+} removed (by 3 mM EGTA at [4]) and finally substance P was added (at [5]). Under these conditions, and in the absence of ionized calcium, substance P produced a transient response similar to that obtained when cross-receptor inactivation had been prevented by atropine (as in Panel A).

These experiments provide information, not only about cross-receptor inactivation and the nature of the transient, but about

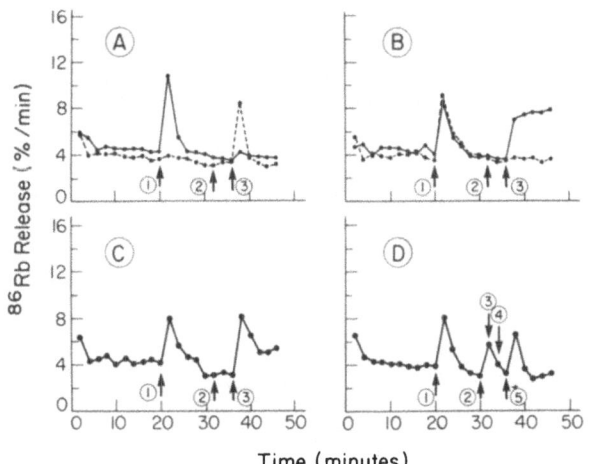

Time (minutes)

Figure 2. Release of ^{86}*Rb and cross-receptor inactivation in parotid slices. Slices were loaded with* ^{86}*Rb and efflux then monitored in a Ringer's solution containing no added Ca*$^{2+}$ *and* 10^{-4} *M EGTA, so that the Ca*$^{2+}$*-independent transient response could be studied. For details and preliminary experiments, see Putney (1977). The following concentrations were employed: carbachol,* 10^{-5} *M; substance P,* 10^{-7} *M; atropine,* 10^{-4} *M; Ca*$^{2+}$*, 1.1 x* 10^{-3} *M; excess EGTA, 3 x* 10^{-3} *M. Agents were added at the times indicated by the arrows and were always present until the end of the experiment. All experiments: (1) = carbachol.*

A: (●————●), (2) = atropine, (3) = substance P;
(●— — — —●), 0-46 min = atropine, (2) = no addition,
*   (3) = substance P.*
B: (●————●), (2) = no addition, (3) = Ca^{2+}*;*
(●— — — —●), (2) = atropine, (3) = Ca^{2+}*.*
C: (2) = atropine, (3) = substance P + Ca^{2+}*.*
D: (2) = Ca^{2+}*, (3) = atropine, (4) excess EGTA,*
*   (5) = substance P.*
Taken from Putney (1977) with kind permission of the Journal of Physiology and the Cambridge University Press.

receptor regulation of Ca^{2+} transport in general. The interpretation is that the receptors activate inward Ca^{2+} transport systems which, in the inactive state, bind (a) calcium ion(s) at a locus inaccessible to EGTA. Upon activation, the bound Ca^{2+} is released and initiates the transient K$^+$ efflux. If the system is turned off while transporting Ca^{2+} inward, membrane-associated Ca^{2+} is retained; if no Ca^{2+} is available, the system is inactivated and incapable of producing a second transient. The most

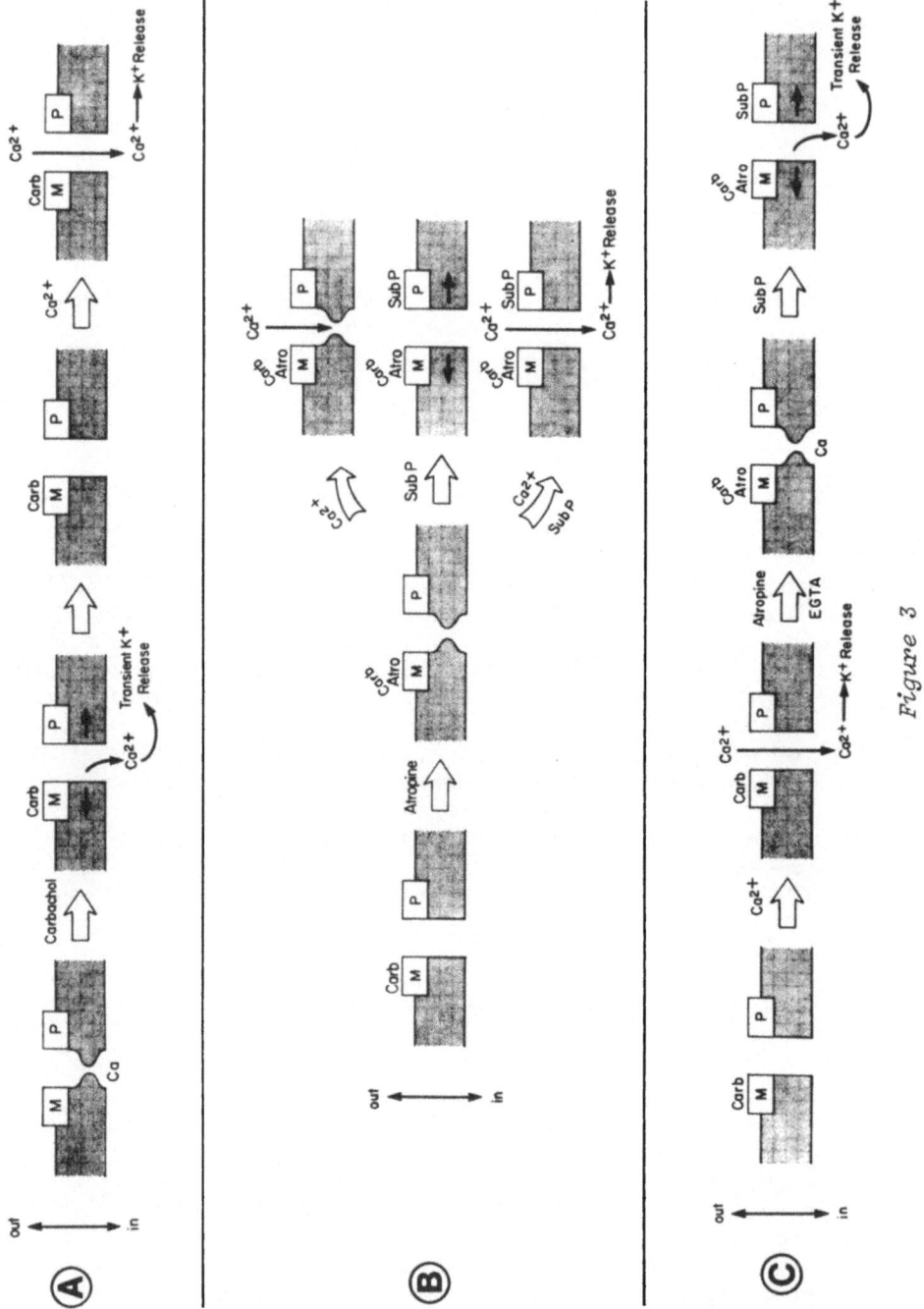

Figure 3

Figure 3. Model depicting co-regulation of a single Ca^{2+} influx site by a muscarinic receptor (M) and peptide receptor (P). In all cases, the outer aspect of the plasmalemma is toward the top of the page. Calcium ion is assumed absent extracellularly except where specified. Panel A: This illustration depicts the basic features of the model. The binding of Carbochol (carb) to the muscarinic receptor activates the Ca^{2+} influx site which dissociates (a) bound calcium ion(s) and triggers a transient release of K^{+} (^{86}Rb). The addition of other agonists can produce no further response. Since the Ca^{2+} channels (or sites) are still activated, readdition of extracellular Ca^{2+} will produce K^{+} release (Figure 2b). Panel B: This diagram serves to illustrate other key experiments for Figure 2. Here, carbachol can be easily removed from its receptor by atropine (atro). Addition of either Ca^{2+} or substance P alone fails to produce K^{+} release (Figures 2a, b), Ca^{2+}, because the channels are closed, and substance P because Ca^{2+} bound to the influx site has been depleted by prior exposure to carbachol. Substance P and Ca^{2+} in combination produce effective K^{+} release as Ca^{2+} may move inward via the transport system activated by substance P. Panel C: Finally the experiment demonstrating that Ca^{2+} is the missing factor necessary for transient release (Figure 2d) is schematically represented here. Calcium ion is reintroduced into the medium, is permitted entry, and mediates K^{+} release. If, under these conditions, the channels are inactivated by atropine and Ca^{2+} subsequently removed with EGTA, then bound Ca^{2+} is restored to the binding site. Reactivation by substance P, in the absence of external Ca^{2+}, produces transient K^{+} release. Taken from Putney (1977) with kind permission of the Journal of Physiology and the Cambridge University Press.

striking consequence of this scheme is that if activation of one receptor mechanism inactivates the others, all three receptors must regulate the same Ca^{2+} influx sites (Putney, 1977). Conversely, each Ca^{2+} influx site is presumably controlled by at least three distinct receptors. A schematic illustration of this interpretation is presented in Figure 3.

The physiological significance of such an arrangement is not clear. A precedence does exist in the control of another second messenger, cyclic AMP, by separate receptors. The evidence suggests that several different receptors can regulate the same adenylate cyclase molecules in a number of tissues (Putney and Askari, 1978). Such multivalent coupling mechanisms may provide protection from a deleterious "overload" in case several receptor systems are activated simultaneously.

Apparently, muscarinic receptors can stimulate Ca^{2+} influx in the rat lacrimal gland as well. The stimulation of exocytosis by carbachol requires Ca^{2+} in the bathing medium (Putney et al., 1977a), and the ability of carbachol to enhance uptake of ^{45}Ca is correlated with the stimulation of exocytosis (Keryer and Rossignol, 1976). Recent experiments suggest that this Ca^{2+} influx may also affect K^+ permeability in a manner similar to the parotid. Thus, carbachol induces a biphasic increase in release of ^{86}Rb from rat exorbital lacrimal gland slices and this response is blocked by atropine (Figure 4). When Ca^{2+} is omitted from the Ringer's solution, the later phase fails, while the transient persists. This effect is reversible since efflux returns if Ca is reintroduced to the Ringer's. The resemblance of this phenomenon to K^+ efflux in the parotid suggests that similar mechanisms may underly both processes.

Recent studies have shown that other ionic events are associated with the response of the parotid to secretagogues (Putney and Parod, 1978). Carbachol significantly increases the uptake of ^{22}Na by parotid slices (Figure 5, Top) without affecting the size of the extracellular space (Putney and Parod, 1978). This effect requires the presence of Ca^{2+} ions in the Ringer's solution. Carbachol also appears to activate the Na^+, K^+-pump in the parotid, as measured by ouabain-sensitive uptake of ^{86}Rb (Figure 5, Bottom). This effect requires not only extracellular Ca^{2+} but also extracellular Na^+. In fact, the Na^+ reduction from 125 mM to 5 mM which causes a reversal of the carbachol effect suggests an inhibition of the pump. These results can be explained by assuming that the trigger for pump activation is the increase in cell Na^+. When the Na^+ gradient is reversed (by lowering Na^+ in the Ringers to 5 mM), carbachol may cause a net outward movement of Na^+ and the decrease in cell Na^+ leads to an inhibition of the pump. In support of this, increasing cell Na^+ by removal of external K^+ can also stimulate ^{86}Rb uptake (measured in Ringer's containing normal K^+; Putney and Parod, 1978). These effects on Na^+ distribution have been far less extensively characterized than on the Ca^{2+}-K^+ system. The relative importance of Na^+ and K^+ and their interactions will require continued investigation.

The discussion to this point has dealt with describing a control system whereby Ca^{2+} influx modulates other ion permeabilities. Little is known, however, about the mechanisms by which intracellular Ca^{2+} affects other ion channels or about the mechanisms by which receptor activation mediates Ca^{2+} influx. Some speculation has appeared recently concerning the latter phenomenon.

It has been known for some time that muscarinic receptor activation causes an increase in phospholipid turnover (Hokin, 1974). Virtually all cells that respond to muscarinic stimuli are believed to show this effect, and it is possible that other Ca^{2+}-mediated receptor activities behave similarly (Michell

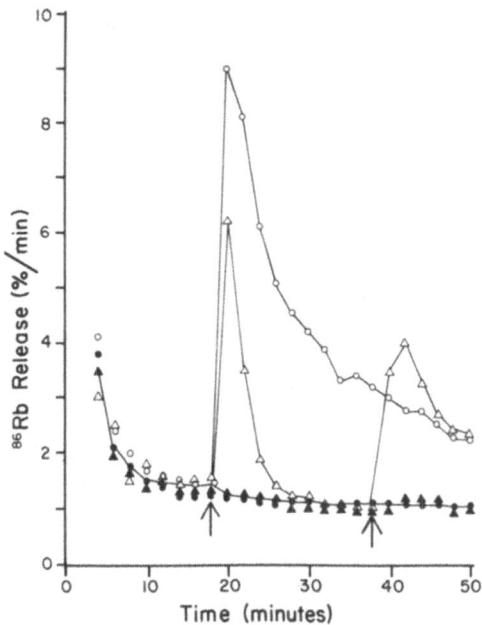

*Figure 4. Release of ^{86}Rb from lacrimal slices by carbachol.
The protocol was similar to that employed for figure 2.●━━━━━●,
control; ○━━━━━○, 10^{-5} M carbachol 18-50 min; ▲━━━━━▲, 10^{-4}
M atropine 12-50 min, 10^{-5} M carbachol 18-50 min; △━━━━△, no
added Ca^{2+} + 10^{-4} M EGTA 0-50 min, 10^{-5} M carbachol 18-50 min,
3.1 mM Ca^{2+} 38-50 min. Each point is the mean from four separate
experiments. The standard errors were generally less than 10% of
the means. Taken from Putney et al. (1977) with kind permission
of Life Sciences and Pergammon Press.*

et al., 1976). In the parotid, both muscarinic and α-adrenergic
agonists, but not β-adrenergic agonists, increase the incorporation
of ^{32}P into phosphatidylinositol (Oron et al., 1975) and decrease
the fraction of total phospholipid present as phosphatidylinositol
(Jones and Michell, 1976). When ^{32}P incorporation is measured,
most of the label is found in microsomes derived from rough endoplasmic reticulum, an observation that has led some to doubt the
relevance of this phenomenon to surface membrane and receptor
mediated phenomena (Hokin, 1974; Oron et al., 1975). R. H. Michell,
however, realized that the incorporation of ^{32}P into phospholipid
was secondary to the breakdown of phosphatidylinositol. This
breakdown, he reasoned, could represent an initial membrane event,
perhaps even the opening or activation of Ca^{2+} channels (Michell
et al., 1976). Inspection of the time course of incorporation of

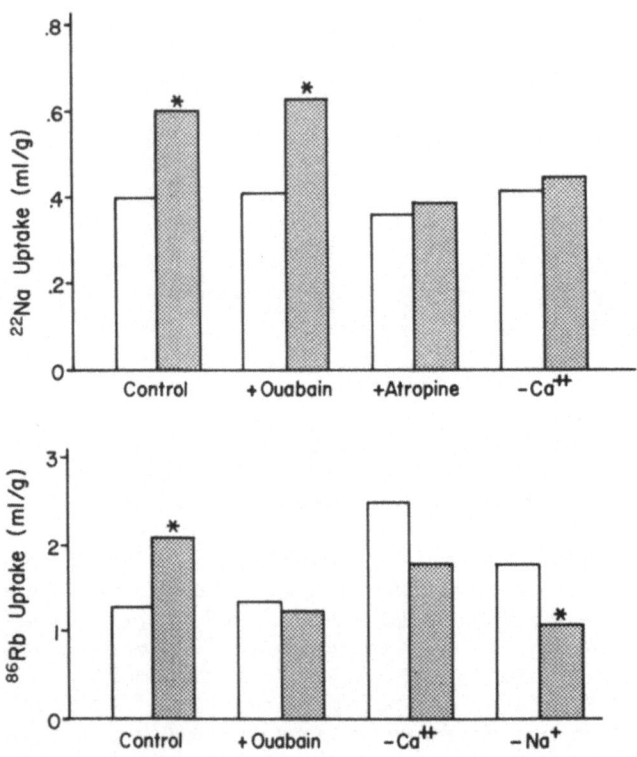

*Figure 5. Stimulation of Na^+ uptake and Na^+-K^+-pumping by carbachol
in parotid gland. Open bars indicate control values, and stipled
bars values obtained in the presence of carbachol. * indicates
statistically significant values. For standard errors and experimental procedures, see Putney and Parod (1978). (A) Carbachol
significantly increases ^{22}Na uptake. This response is blocked
by atropine but not ouabain and requires external Ca^{2+}. (B)
Carbachol also significantly stimulates ^{86}Rb influx; the response
is blocked by ouabain indicating that Na^+, K^+-pumping is increased.
Calcium ion is required for the effect. When all but 5 mM of
Na^+ is substituted with Li^+, carbachol decreases ^{86}Rb uptake. The
figure summarizes data originally reported in different format by
Putney and Parod (1978).*

[32]P due to epinephrine in the parotid reveals a considerable lag time (Oron *et al.*, 1976) which is consistent with such a view. The strongest points of evidence relating the phospholipid effect to the early events in receptor action concern the relationship of Ca^{2+} to the effect. First, the phospholipid effect does not require Ca^{2+} in the bathing medium, while virtually all other consequences of muscarinic activation have such a requirement (including synthesis of cGMP). Second, when endogenous receptors and Ca^{2+} channels are bypassed by using the ionophore A23187, no phospholipid effect is obtained (Oron *et al.*, 1975), while K^+ release, exocytosis and cGMP synthesis, all occur (Butcher, 1975). These observations are consistent with a mechanism by which autonomic receptor activation stimulates dephosphorylation of some membrane constituent resulting in activation of a Ca^{2+} channel or carrier. These same observations suggest that activation of the K^+ channel by Ca^{2+} does not involve phosphate transfer since the ionophore does not appear to affect the phosphate distribution. Further investigations in this area may reveal the exact molecular events associated with receptor control of ion channels in general.

SUMMARY AND GENERAL CONCLUSIONS

Stimulus-secretion coupling, as it applies to water flow in epithelial tissues, involves the elucidation of mechanisms by which hormones and neurotransmitters regulate membrane permeability to, and transport of, osmotically active ions. As Ca^{2+} appears to be a universal intermediate for exocrine function, proposed coupling schemes could embody Ca^{2+} as a regulator of membrane permeability.

External calcium ions play an important role in regulating membrane permeability. In many cases, Mg^{2+} can substitute in this role, but this may not be universally true. The stimulation of membrane permeability to K^+ by intracellular Ca^{2+} has been extensively studied in the red cell, although the physiological significance of the phenomenon in these cells is not clear. In the case of excitable tissues, the slow inward Ca^{2+} current may feed back and contribute to the delayed K^+ current that provides for repolarization following an action potential.

Another system where K^+ permeability is controlled by internal Ca^{2+} is the salivary glands (and perhaps other exocrine glands). Here, the stimulation of water flow by neurotransmitters and peptides probably involves (at least in part) an increase in membrane permeability to K^+. However, measurements of K^+ efflux made with different techniques were in conflict as to the Ca^{2+}-dependence of the response. The use of ^{86}Rb as a marker for unidirectional K^+ flux has resolved the discrepancy and has revealed that secretagogues cause both transient and sustained phases of K^+ efflux. The sustained phase of efflux requires ionized calcium in the bathing medium while the transient does not. The sustained phase is probably triggered by a sustained influx of Ca^{2+} since (1) Ca^{2+} is required for the effect, (2) the effect can be mimicked by the divalent cationophore A23187, and (3) agents that stimulate K^+ efflux also stimulate Ca^{2+} influx. The transient response is believed due to a pulse of Ca^{2+} released from membrane binding sites associated with the same Ca^{2+} channels (or carriers) that mediate the Ca^{2+} influx. The phenomenon of cross-receptor inactivation was observed whereby the production of a transient response through one receptor negated additional responses due to other receptors. This demonstrates that these same Ca^{2+} channels are each controlled by at least three different receptors; muscarinic, α-adrenergic and peptide (substance P).

Preliminary studies suggest that the lacrimal glands are under similar control. Carbachol will increase K^+ efflux in a biphasic manner; the sustained efflux requires Ca^{2+} while the transient efflux does not.

Muscarinic receptor activation has also been shown to increase Na^+ uptake in the parotid and the resulting elevation in internal Na^+ serves to stimulate the Na^+, K^+-pump. This effect is also Ca^{2+}-dependent but will require more extensive investigation to establish its role in the overall process of stimulus-secretion coupling.

A re-examination of the phospholipid effect whereby phospholipid turnover is stimulated by neurotransmitters and hormones suggests that phosphotidylinositol breakdown may be one of the steps involved in the activation of Ca^{2+} channels by these agents. The evidence suggests, however, that a different mechanism is involved in the opening of K^+ channels by intracellular Ca^{2+}.

The studies described here underscore the importance of Ca^{2+} in the actions of secretagogues on exocrine glands. Beyond this, they illustrate the utility of the exocrine glands as a model for Ca^{2+} controlled ion permeabilities in general. In the parotid, Ca^{2+} can be introduced into the cells through physiologic pathways by activating the receptor-linked Ca^{2+} channels, or by the use of ionophores (thus by-passing membrane receptor mechanisms). This system is uncomplicated by the field-dependent parameters of excitable tissues while offering greater experimental flexibility than the erythrocyte. Additionally, since the responses produced are passive permeability changes, the measurements are less vulnerable to artifacts produced by fatigue or substrate depletion than such processes as exocytosis or muscle contraction. These considerations make the exocrine glands ideal tools for studying the cellular pharmacology and physiology of early events in drug-receptor mechanisms that utilize Ca^{2+}.

Acknowledgements

Work from the authors laboratory described in this review was supported by grants from the NIH, #DE-04067 and EY-01978.

REFERENCES

Babad, H., Ben-Zvi, R., Bdolah, A., and Schramm, M., 1967, The mechanism of enzyme secretion by the cell. 4. Effects of inducers, substrates and inhibitors on amylase secretion by rat parotid slices, *Eur. J. Biochem.* 1: 96.

Bassingthwaite, J. B., Fry, C. H., and McGuigan, J. A. S., 1976, Relationship between internal calcium and outward current in mammalian ventricular muscle; a mechanism for the control of the action potential duration? *J. Physiol. (London)* 262: 15.

Bdolah, A., Ben-Zvi, R., and Schramm, M., 1964, The mechanism of enzyme secretion by the cell. II. Secretion of amylase and other proteins by slices of rat parotid gland, *Arch. Biochem. Biophys.* 104: 58.

Burgen, A. S. V., 1956, The secretion of potassium in saliva, *J. Physiol. (London)* 132: 20.

Burgen, A. S. V., and Emmelin, N. G., 1961, "Physiology of the Salivary Glands," Edward Arnold Ltd., London.

Butcher, F. R., 1975, The role of calcium and cyclic nucleotides in α-amylase release from slices of rat parotid: Studies with the divalent cation ionophore A-23187, *Metabolism* 24: 409.

Butcher, F. R., 1978, Regulation of exocytosis, *in* "Biochemical Action of Hormones, Vol. 5" (G. Litwack, ed.), Academic Press, in press.

Butcher, F. R., McBride, P. A., and Rudich, L., 1976a, Cholinergic regulation of cyclic nucleotide levels, amylase release and K^+ efflux from rat parotid glands, *Mol. Cell. Endocrin.* 5: 243.

Butcher, F. R., Rudich, L., Emler, C., and Nemerovski, M., 1976b, Adrenergic regulation of cyclic nucleotide levels, amylase release and potassium efflux in rat parotid gland, *Mol. Pharmacol.* 12: 862.

Case, R. M., 1974, The role of calcium and of cyclic AMP in pancreatic secretory processes, *in* "Secretory Mechanisms of Exocrine Glands" (N. A. Thorn and O. H. Petersen, eds.), pp. 344-354, Munksgaard, Copenhagen.

Douglas, W. W., and Poisner, A. M., 1963, The influence of calcium on the secretory response of the submaxillary gland to acetylcholine or to noradrenaline, *J. Physiol. (London)* 165: 528.

Ferreira, H. G., and Lew, V. L., 1976, Use of ionophore A23187 to measure cytoplasmic Ca buffering and activation of the Ca pump by internal Ca, *Nature* 259: 47.

Frankenhaeuser, B., and Hodgkin, A. L., 1957, The action of calcium on the electrical properties of squid axons, *J. Physiol. (London)* 137: 218.

Goldberg, N. D., Haddox, M. K., Nicol, S. E., Glass, D. B., Sanford, C. H., Kuehl, F. A., Jr., and Estensen, R., 1975, Biological regulation through opposing influences of cyclic GMP and cyclic AMP: The Yin Yang hypothesis, *in* "Advances in Cyclic Nucleotide Research, Vol. 5." (G. I. Drummond, P. Greengard and G. A. Robison, eds.), pp. 307-330, Raven Press, New York.

Hokin, M. R., 1974, Breakdown of phosphatidylinositol in the pancreas in response to pancreozymin and acetylcholine, *in* "Secretory Mechanisms of Exocrine Glands" (N. A. Thorn and O. H. Petersen, eds.), pp. 101-112, Munksgaard, Copenhagen.

Isenberg, G., 1975, Is potassium conductance of cardiac Purkinje fibres controlled by $[Ca^{2+}]_i$?, *Nature* 253: 273.

Jones, L. M., and Michell, R. H., 1976, Cholinergically stimulated phosphatidylinositol breakdown in parotid-gland fragments is independent of the ionic environment, *Biochem. J.* 158: 505.

Keryer, G., and Rossignol, B., 1976, Effect of carbachol on [45]Ca uptake and protein secretion in rat lacrimal glands, *Amer. J. Physiol.* 230: 99.

Krnjevic, K., and Lisiewicz, A., 1972, Injections of calcium ions into spinal motoneurones, *J. Physiol. (London)* 225: 363.

Leslie, B. A., Putney, J. W., Jr., and Sherman, J. M., 1976, α-adrenergic, β-adrenergic and cholinergic mechanisms for amylase secretion by rat parotid gland *in vitro, J. Physiol. (London)* 260: 351.

Lew, V. L., and Ferreira, H. G., 1976, Variable Ca sensitivity of a K-selective channel in intact red-cell membranes, *Nature* 263: 336.

Meech, R. W., and Standen, N. B., 1975, Potassium activation in *Helix aspera* neurones under voltage clamp: A component mediated by calcium influx, *J. Physiol. (London)* 249: 211.

Michell, R. H., Jafferji, S., and Jones, L. M., 1976, Receptor occupancy dose-response curve suggests that phosphatidylinositol breakdown may be intrinsic to the mechanism of the muscarinic cholinergic receptor, *FEBS Lett.* 69: 1.

Miller, B. E., and Nelson, D. L., 1977, Calcium fluxes in isolated acinar cells from rat parotid: The effect of adrenergic and cholinergic stimulation, *J. Biol. Chem.* 252: 3629.

Oron, Y., Lowe, M., and Selinger, Z., 1975, Incorporation of inorganic [32P] phosphate into rat parotid phosphatidylinositol. Induction through activation of *alpha* adrenergic and cholinergic receptors and relation to K^+ release, *Mol. Pharmacol.* 11: 79.

Pedersen, G. L., and Petersen, O. H., 1973, Membrane potential measurement in parotid acinar cells, *J. Physiol. (London)* 234: 217.

Petersen, O. H., and Pedersen, G. L., 1974, Membrane effects mediated by alpha- and beta-adrenoceptors in mouse parotid acinar cells, *J. Memb. Biol.* 16: 353.

Petersen, O. H., Poulsen, J. H., and Thorn, N. A., 1967, Secretory potentials, secretory rate, and water permeability of the duct system in the cat submandibular gland during perfusion with calcium-free Locke's solution, *Acta Physiol. Scand.* 71: 203.

Putney, J. W., Jr., 1976a, Biphasic modulation of potassium release in rat parotid gland by carbachol and phenylephrine, *J. Pharmacol. Exp. Ther.* 198: 375.

Putney, J. W., Jr., 1976b, Stimulation of ^{45}Ca influx in rat parotid gland by carbachol, *J. Pharmacol. Exp. Ther.* 199: 526.

Putney, J. W., Jr., 1977, Muscarinic, α-adrenergic and peptide receptors regulate the same calcium influx sites in the parotid gland, *J. Physiol. (London)* 268: 139.

Putney, J. W., Jr., and Askari, A., 1978, Modification of membrane function by drugs, *in* "The Physiological Basis for Disorders of Biomembranes" (T. E. Andreoli, J. F. Hoffman and D. D. Fanestil, eds.), in press, Plenum Press, New York.

Putney, J. W., Jr., and Parod, R. J., 1978, Calcium-mediated effects of carbachol on cation pumping and Na uptake in rat parotid gland slices, *J. Pharmacol. Exp. Ther.*, in press.

Putney, J. W., Jr., Parod, R. J., and Marier, S. H., 1977a, Control by calcium of protein discharge and membrane permeability to potassium in the rat lacrimal gland, *Life Sci.* 20: 1905.

Putney, J. W., Jr., Weiss, S. J., Leslie, B. A., and Marier, S. H., 1977b, Is calcium the final mediator of exocytosis in the rat parotid gland?, *J. Pharmacol. Exp. Ther.* 203: 144.

Rothman, S. S., 1975, Protein transport by the pancreas, *Science* 190: 747.

Rubin, R. P., 1974, "Calcium and the Secretory Process", Plenum Press, New York.

Rudich, L., and Butcher, F. R., 1976, Effect of substance P and eledoisin on K$^+$ efflux, amylase release and cyclic nucleotide levels in slices of rat parotid gland, *Biochim. Biophys. Acta* 444: 704.

Schneyer, L. H., Young, J. A., and Schneyer, C. A., 1972, Salivary secretion of electrolytes, *Physiol. Rev.* 52: 720.

Schramm, M., and Selinger, Z., 1974, The function of α- and β-adrenergic receptors and a cholinergic receptor in the secretory cell of rat parotid gland, *in* "Advances in Cytopharmacology, Vol. 2", (B. Ceccarelli, F. Clementi and J. Meldolesi, eds.), pp. 29-32, Raven Press, New York.

Schramm, M., and Selinger, Z., 1975, The functions of cyclic AMP and calcium as alternative second messengers in parotid gland and pancreas, *J. Cyclic Nucleotide Res.* 1: 181.

Selinger, Z., Batzri, S., Eimerl, S., and Schramm, M., 1973, Calcium and energy requirements for K^+ release mediated by the epinephrine α-receptor in rat parotid slices, *J. Biol. Chem.* 248: 369.

Selinger, Z., Eimerl, S., and Schramm, M., 1974, A calcium ionophore simulating the action of epinephrine on the α-adrenergic receptors, *Proc. Nat. Acad. Sci. U. S. A.* 71: 128.

Simons, T. J. B., 1976a, The preparation of human red cell ghosts containing calcium buffers, *J. Physiol. (London)* 256: 209.

Simons, T. J. B., 1976b, Calcium-dependent potassium exchange in human red cell ghosts, *J. Physiol. (London)* 256: 227.

Weiss, G. B., 1974, Cellular pharmacology of lanthanum, *Annu. Rev. Pharmacol.* 14: 343.

Williams, J. A., 1974, Intracellular control mechanisms regulating secretion by exocrine and endocrine glands, *in* "Secretory Mechanisms of Exocrine Glands", (N. A. Thorn and O. H. Petersen, eds.), pp. 389-399, Munksgaard, Copenhagen.

SECTION III

CALCIUM IN DRUG ACTION:

SOME SPECIFIC BIOLOGICAL SYSTEMS

   In the preceding two sections, emphasis was placed on approaches and techniques employed to analyze cellular and subcellular Ca^{2+} distribution and binding and to determine how alterations (including drug-induced actions) in Ca^{2+}-mediated events can influence responsiveness and reactivity of an impressive range of biological processes. In this third and final section, similar considerations are still present, but overall emphasis shifts to presentation of a sequence of system-oriented chapters. In each of these chapters, the Ca^{2+}-related actions of relevant pharmacological agents are examined in terms of a specific type of biological preparation.

   For example, in the first chapter of this section, the central role of release of intracellular Ca^{2+} in a varied set of responses in platelets is documented. Even in this relatively uncomplicated biological system, the effects of Ca^{2+} appear to be both ubiquitous and of considerable importance. In the next chapter (Chapter 10) attention is focused on specific components of a very complex system, membrane receptors and synaptic vesicles of the central nervous system. It has become increasingly clear in recent years that alterations in synaptic Ca^{2+} are an integral component of the mechanism of action of such important agents as the opiate drugs, and our current understanding of these relationships is presented. In contrast to the recent and tentative nature of our concepts concerning opiate-Ca^{2+} interactions, the subject matter of the next chapter (Chapter 11) concerns a system (the neuromuscular junction) for which some extremely sophisticated methodology and views of the roles of Ca^{2+} have evolved. However, underlying the precise but descriptive hypothesis for Ca^{2+} as the initiator of

neurohumoral agent release at the neuromuscular junction is a much
less established picture of events at the molecular or ionic level.
A somewhat similar situation exists for Ca^{2+} roles in drug-induced
desensitization at the skeletal muscle motor end-plate (Chapter
12). Both electrophysiological and ionic analysis have clearly
established a central role for Ca^{2+} in the pharmacologically
important process. However, the molecular events underlying these
Ca^{2+}-related events remain to be elaborated. In striated muscle
fibers (Chapter 13), the essential role of Ca^{2+} in excitation-
contraction coupling is firmly established. The focal point for
current investigative efforts concerns the relationships between
cellular Ca^{2+} release (and rebinding) and associated metabolic
events (respiration, cyclic nucleotide levels). Use of agents
such as ryanodine which act directly in some manner at intracellular sites to alter the release-rebinding Ca^{2+} cycle promises to
clarify some remaining mechanism-related questions concerning
control and regulation of intracellular Ca^{2+} levels. Finally, in
the last chapter (Chapter 14), some drug-related effects on Ca^{2+}
binding and distribution in vascular smooth muscle are presented
within the context of a Ca^{2+}-dependent relationship between the
manner in which Ca^{2+} is bound and utilized by the smooth muscle
cell and the type or degree of response elicited by each particular
drug.

In all of the chapters in this section, an increasing emphasis
is placed upon subcellular and molecular approaches. The general
and cellular models employed for the roles of Ca^{2+} in drug action
provide a satisfactory framework for description of physiological
events and pharmacological actions. However, in all of the biological systems discussed, the critical questions being asked are
increasingly molecular in nature and the techniques being employed
are designed to provide useful information at this level. Thus,
the chapters in this section may well provide good experimental
models of differing types of investigations of the varied roles of
Ca^{2+} in drug action in specific biological systems. In view of
the diversity of such relationships, the applicability of these
rationales and approaches to investigation of interactions of
drugs with other biological systems should be both appropriate and
beneficial.

CHAPTER 9

THE ROLE OF CALCIUM IN BLOOD PLATELET

FUNCTION

Maurice B. Feinstein

Department of Pharmacology
University of Connecticut Health Center
Farmington, Connecticut 06032

PHYSIOLOGICAL FUNCTIONS OF PLATELETS

The platelet occupies a central position in the hemostatic
reactions which protect the integrity of the vascular system in
the case of injury. The arrest of bleeding occurs as the result
of a complex series of responses involving contractile activity
of the blood vessel wall, the formation of a platelet plug at the
site of injury, the coagulation of plasma due to the conversion
of fibrinogen to fibrin, and the contraction or retraction of the
clot. One of the most significant properties of the platelet is
its ability to adhere avidly to subendothelial tissue exposed by
damage to the endothelium (Baumgartner, 1972). This interaction
with connective tissue sets in motion a remarkable series of
physical and biochemical transformations of the platelet resulting
in a rapid formation of the platelet plug and consolidation of the
clot. The clotting process is activated in parallel to platelet
activation and is in fact facilitated substantially by properties
of the platelets themselves (Walsh, 1974).

The responses of the platelet to stimulation involve several
fundamental types of responses: (a) changes in cell shape and
membrane surface properties leading to cellular adhesion, (b) the
release of preformed substances stored within secretory granules
which facilitate platelet aggregation, promote clot formation,
and influence vasomotor activity, (c) the stimulus-induced synthesis of potent platelet aggregating and vasoactive factors from
endogenous phospholipid arachidonic acid stores, and (d) cellular
contractile activity.

Failure of platelets to function normally due to one type of defect or another in these responses leads to bleeding tendencies of varying degrees of severity (Weiss, 1975; Stuart, 1975). On the other hand, the formation of platelet-fibrin thrombi and the release of vasoconstrictor substances under pathological conditions can result in the occlusion of blood vessels leading to a wide variety of acute clinical syndromes which are a leading cause of morbidity and mortality. Besides their obvious hemostatic functions platelets may also play a role in inflammatory and immunological processes (Smith *et al.*, 1976; Nachman and Weksler, 1972; DesPrez and Marney, 1971).

This chapter is concerned specifically with a consideration of the role of calcium ion in platelet function. The involvement of Ca^{2+} in platelet responses to stimulation is widespread, encompassing nearly all aspects of the cellular responses to stimuli. A full understanding of platelet physiology demands the elucidation of the various functions of Ca^{2+} and the mechanisms by which the platelet regulates Ca^{2+} disposition. Although the following discussion will attempt to point out important areas of Ca^{2+} involvement, it will become apparent that in many cases the subject is only in the early stages of development.

THE ROLE OF CALCIUM IN PLATELET SHAPE CHANGE, AGGREGATION AND THE RELEASE REACTION

The platelet normally circulates in the blood as a smooth-surfaced disc. Upon stimulation it rapidly alters its shape to that of a sphere with many pseudopodia. The change in shape is normally followed by the adhesion of platelets to one another forming large masses, or aggregates, and the secretion of storage granules by a process termed the "release reaction." A wide variety of substances can produce this remarkable effect, *i.e.* adenosine diphosphate (ADP), thrombin, collagen, epinephrine, serotonin, arachidonic acid, the Ca^{2+} ionophore A23187 and many others (Mustard and Packham, 1970). Platelet secretory granules contain a wide variety of substances, many of which play an important role in facilitating platelet aggregation or the clotting process; *e.g.* ADP, ATP, serotonin, Ca^{2+}, fibrinogen, and platelet factor 4 (anti-heparin factor) (Figure 1). In some cases lysosomal-like granules (alpha-granules) containing acid hydrolases are also released to a limited degree. Concurrently with these events important procoagulant activities, including platelet factor 3, appear at the membrane surface (Walsh, 1974; Seegers, 1971; Marcus, 1969) to catalyze formation of the clotting enzyme thrombin. Calcium ion is importantly involved in these reactions as it catalyzes necessary protein transitions of factor X and prothrombin, and is required for their binding to phospholipid (Nelsestuen *et al.*, 1976).

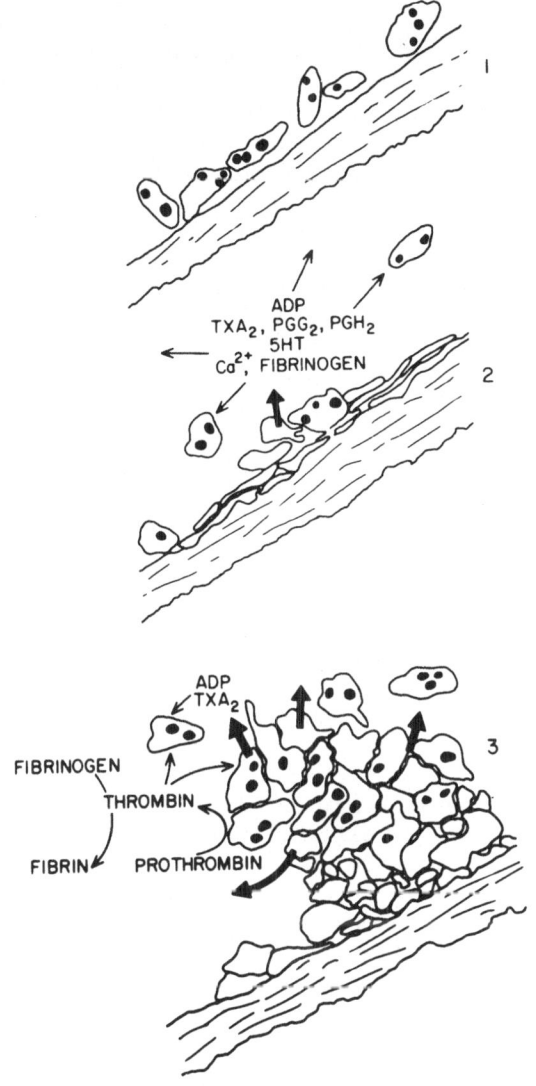

Figure 1. Diagrammatic representation of platelet interactions with subendothelium of a damaged blood vessel. (1) Circulating platelets begin to contact subendothelial constituents. (2) Platelets adherent to subendothelium change shape and adhere to other platelets. Platelets release ADP, along with other contents of the secretory granules, and newly synthesized PG endoperoxides and thromboxane A$_2$ which diffuse into the immediate area to stimulate other platelets. (3) Platelet plug grows rapidly facilitated by platelet-derived aggregating factors. Thrombin formation may be promoted as a result of platelet factor 3 activity appearing in the surface membrane. Thrombin stimulates platelet aggregation, release reaction and TXA$_2$ synthesis, and also catalyzes the formation of a fibrin clot.

Platelet shape change does not require the presence of external Ca^{2+} since it occurs in the presence of high external concentrations of EDTA. However, prolonged exposure to EDTA prevents shape change induced by ADP, which may result from a depletion of membrane-bound divalent cations (Born, 1972). Shape change is induced by the calcium ionophore A23187 (Gerrard et al., 1974) indicating that the morphological transformations are induced by an internal translocation of Ca^{2+}. LeBreton et al. (1976) employing low concentrations of chlortetracycline as a flourescent probe for membrane-bound Ca^{2+} demonstrated what appeared to be a redistribution of Ca^{2+} away from membrane sites during ADP and A23187-induced shape change. High concentrations of chlortetracycline inhibited shape change presumably by chelating intracellular Ca^{2+}.

External Ca^{2+} is essential for platelet aggregation and is probably involved in cell surface adhesion reactions, but the mechanisms involved have not been elucidated. The dependency of the release reaction on external Ca^{2+} is variable. In some species (e.g. pig), and especially at low temperatures, the addition of Ca^{2+} to the medium enhanced secretion (Grette, 1962). External Ca^{2+} is necessary for collagen-induced release (Feinstein et al., 1976; Hovig, 1963) and it enhances secretion induced by low concentrations of thrombin (Mürer, 1972). However, secretion induced by high concentrations of thrombin is unimpaired by the absence of external Ca^{2+} (Miller et al., 1975; Mürer, 1972; Sneddon, 1972; Wolfe and Shulman, 1970; Morse et al., 1965). Some experiments indicate that the release reaction elicited by A23187 may be facilitated by the presence of extracellular Ca^{2+} (Feinstein and Fraser, 1975; Worner and Brossmer, 1975; Massini and Lüscher, 1974). Feinman and Detwiler (1975) believe that the apparent partial requirement for external Ca^{2+} was due to its necessity for aggregation, and that platelet aggregation facilitates the release reaction (Massini and Lüscher, 1972) especially at low concentrations of stimulating agent. Regardless of the role of external Ca^{2+} it is clear that the platelet must contain internal stores of Ca^{2+} which can be mobilized by suitable stimuli to activate secretion of storage granules and other platelet responses. Furthermore, for reasons to be discussed later, it is not likely that a direct Ca^{2+} influx from the extracellular space into the cell is responsible for inducing secretion.

The release reaction is similar to comparable processes in endocrine glands and other secretory cells in its requirement for energy, which can be supplied by either oxidative phosphorylation or anaerobic glycolysis. A fall in a metabolic pool of ATP occurs during the release reaction (Holmsen et al., 1969) along with the accumulation of endproducts of adenine nucleotide metabolism, notably hypoxanthine. It is considered likely that this energy is

expended in an internal contraction wave, and that secretion is
dependent upon a contractile process involving Ca^{2+}-activated
platelet actomyosin (Day and Holmsen, 1971b; White, 1971; Grette,
1962). Yet another role for Ca^{2+} may involve its ability to
facilitate membrane fusion (Papahadjopoulos et al., 1977), an
essential step in exocytosis.

Since ADP is a powerful aggregating agent and is released
along with other contents of the secretory granules it was long
assumed to be the agent ultimately mainly responsible for initiating shape change and aggregation due to collagen, epinephrine,
serotonin and thrombin (Izrael et al., 1974). Besides having a
direct aggregating effect of its own, low concentrations of ADP
(ineffective alone) synergistically promote aggregation by low
concentrations of other aggregating agents (Packham et al., 1973;
Silver et al., 1973; Baumgartner and Born, 1968). Other recently
discovered mediators of platelet aggregation are produced by
oxidative metabolism of arachidonic acid to form prostaglandin
endoperoxides (PGG_2 and PGH_2) and thromboxane A_2 (TXA_2). These
potent substances are not stored, but are rapidly synthesized at
the time when platelets are stimulated. Both types of mediators
play a significant role in platelet aggregation and secretion.
Released ADP can be destroyed enzymatically by the addition of
creatine phosphate plus creatine phosphokinase to the medium in
which platelets are suspended (Izrael et al., 1974), and prostaglandin endoperoxide synthesis can be blocked by non-steroidal
antiinflammatory drugs. Aggregation due to low concentrations of
ADP is inhibited by indomethacin, but at concentrations above
10 μM aggregation is unaffected, although the release reaction
is blocked (Claesson and Mahlmsten, 1977). Collagen-induced
aggregation was completely blocked only when the appearance of
both mediators was blocked simultaneously (Packham et al., 1977).
Previously degranulated platelets (depleted of releasable ADP)
can be aggregated by arachidonic acid (Kinlough-Rathbone et al.,
1975 and A23187 (Feinstein et al., 1976; Kinlough-Rathbone et al.,
1976, 1975). Thus, ADP release is not essential for aggregation
when internal Ca^{2+} can be mobilized directly by the ionophore,
or when sufficient TXA_2 is synthesized. Aggregation and secretion
produced by high concentrations of thrombin or A23187 are independent of both ADP and prostaglandin endoperoxide synthesis (Packham
et al., 1977).

Mechanisms must therefore exist for initiating platelet aggregation and the release reaction independently of the formation
of PG endoperoxides and TXA_2, or the release of ADP (Packham et al.,
1977). The factors responsible are not known, but the result most
likely depends upon mobilization of cellular Ca^{2+} stores. This
pathway is most apparent at high levels of stimulation, especially
by thrombin and A23187. At low levels of stimulation by these

agents, as well as by collagen, the contribution of PG endoperoxides, TXA_2 and released ADP is of great significance, and in some
circumstances essential for maximal platelet activation. ADP,
PG endoperoxides and TXA_2 can therefore be viewed as intermediary
amplifiers of the fundamental cellular reactions leading to aggregation and the release reaction. Stimulation can be brought about
by multiple or redundant pathways leading to the same basic platelet response. Addition of PG endoperoxides and TXA_2 to platelets
normally elicits release of ADP (Claesson and Mahlmsten, 1977),
and under some conditions exogenous ADP can induce PG endoperoxide
formation (Mustard *et al.*, 1975). Platelets defective in one pathway may be activated by other mechanisms. For example, platelets
whose ability to aggregate was compromised by blocking PG endoperoxide synthesis could be induced to aggregate normally if
storage pool deficient platelets (which could not release ADP,
but could make PG endoperoxides) were present (Gerrard *et al.*,
1975).

Holmsen (1974) proposed an important conceptual framework for
understanding platelet responses to stimulation. The principle
points of this hypothesis are: (1) The normal platelet function
sequence (*i.e.* shape change, aggregation, release reaction) is
not a chain reaction in the sense that an initial step is a necessary trigger for the following step. Thus, each of the characteristic platelet responses occurs in *parallel* with others, not in
series, and therefore any step may be bypassed without necessarily
affecting the other responses. This is evident from many examples
in the literature of conditions in which one or more steps of the
sequence is absent or grossly deficient, while others are normal.
(2) Each of the platelet responses is considered to be brought
about by the triggering of a "basic cellular reaction," the intensity of which varies as a function of the stimulus strength. The
basic cellular reaction is proposed to be *cellular contraction*,
requiring ATP as its energy source and Ca^{2+} for activation of
the contractile machinery. All inducers of energy-dependent primary aggregation will act by causing mobilization of cellular
Ca^{2+} so as to activate one or more of the contractile systems of
the cell specifically concerned with the particular functional
responses. Calcium ion is therefore proposed as the primary intracellular messenger or transmitter of information from the surface
membrane, where stimulating agents react with their receptors, to
the internal contractile machinery. (3) Each of the specific
platelet responses has a different requirement for energy expenditure and contractile activity. ATP utilization increases as the
platelet response spreads in intensity from shape change to
aggregation and release reaction (Holmsen, 1974).

The responses to the Ca^{2+} ionophore A23187 increase as a
function of concentration implying that the magnitude and nature

of the response to the ionophore is a function of the amount of internal Ca^{2+} that is mobilized. One can add a further condition to Holmsen's hypothesis, namely that sites of Ca^{2+} mobilization and action may be highly localized within the cell. Shape change, for example, may specifically involve Ca^{2+} interactions with the surface membrane and associated microfibrils and microtubules without involving other organelles or contractile elements deeper within the cell interior. Upon this system proposed by Holmsen it is also necessary to add additional controls which make the regulation of platelet function more complex, but also add elements for finer control. Although the various platelet responses are essentially independent of each other there is no doubt that under physiological conditions they significantly influence each other. As previously noted, although ADP may not be essential for aggregation its secretion by release of granules, or from damaged vascular tissue, certainly acts as a positive amplifier of response to other stimuli. Similarly, as will be discussed later, the production of PG endoperoxides and TXA_2 serves as a positive feedback amplification system (Mürer et al., 1976). We may conclude that there are several mechanisms for the mobilization of cellular Ca^{2+} and various types of stimuli can act synergistically to recruit Ca^{2+}. In addition other mechanisms exist for negative feedback and the limitation of platelet responses. Some of these involve antagonism of either the mobilization of activator Ca^{2+} or the Ca^{2+}-dependent reactions.

CALCIUM IN PLATELETS: INTRACELLULAR LOCALIZATION, TRANSPORT, AND MOBILIZATION BY STIMULI

The hypothesis that increased intracellular free Ca^{2+} is essential for stimulus-secretion coupling (Rubin, 1974; Douglas, 1968) has been strongly supported by experiments with Ca^{2+}-ionophores. These ionophores (e.g. A23187) which render membranes highly permeable to Ca^{2+} (and Mg^{2+}) have been found to release secretory granules from mast cells (Cochrane and Douglas, 1974; Foreman et al., 1973), adrenal medulla (Cochrane et al., 1975), β-cells of the pancreas (Charles et al., 1975), neurohypophysis (Russel et al., 1974) and the platelet (Mürer et al., 1976; Feinstein and Fraser, 1975; Feinman and Detwiler, 1974; Massini and Lüscher, 1974; White et al., 1974; Yuen and Macey, 1974). Although in some cases the secretory response of the platelet to A23187 is facilitated by the presence of extracellular Ca^{2+} the release reaction occurs in the presence of Ca^{2+} chelators. It is clear that in the platelet, as in some other cells (Ridgeway et al., 1977; Babcock et al., 1976; Schroeder and Strickland, 1974; Steinhardt and Epel, 1974), the ionophore can release internal stores of Ca^{2+} into the cytoplasm. The lipophilic ionophore would be expected to easily gain access to internal organelles of the platelet which may sequester Ca^{2+}. A23187 causes Ca^{2+} release from mitochondria in intact sperm (Babcock $et\ al.$, 1976), the isolated sarcoplasmic reticulum from skeletal or cardiac muscle (Scarpa $et\ al.$, 1972) and from the microsomal fraction of sonicated platelets (Käser-Glanzmann $et\ al.$, 1977).

Thrombin and collagen, however, must be assumed to be unable to gain direct access to internal organelles. Therefore, if Ca^{2+} is released by thrombin or collagen from sites other than in the surface membrane there must be mechanisms which convey the effect of protein-receptor interaction to the internal organelles.

The ability of platelet stimulating agents to mobilize intracellular Ca^{2+} must be assumed on the basis of indirect evidence since direct measurement of free intracellular Ca^{2+} has not yet been possible. Secretion and cellular contractile activity presumably reflect Ca^{2+}-mediated events, but the actual reactions involved in the secretory process remain unknown or uncertain. However, Ca^{2+} mobilization by stimuli can also be deduced from the activation of several enzymatic processes which occur concurrently. These Ca^{2+}-dependent activities include: (1) activation of phosphorylase, measured as a rise in glucose-1-phosphate within seconds of stimulation (Detwiler, 1972), (2) activation of phosphorylase b kinase (Gear and Schneider, 1975), and (3) activation of phospholipase A_2 (Pickett $et\ al.$, 1977; Pickett and Cohen, 1976; Bills $et\ al.$, 1976; Hamberg $et\ al.$, 1975; Hamberg and Samuelsson, 1974; Schoene and Iacono, 1973; Smith $et\ al.$, 1973).

Among the principal unresolved problems regarding the role of Ca^{2+} in platelet function are: (1) the localization of internal Ca^{2+} stores, (2) the localization and mechanism of Ca^{2+}-transport or binding systems which can maintain a low resting level of free Ca^{2+} in the cytoplasm, (3) the mechanisms by which Ca^{2+} is mobilized by various kinds of stimuli to activate different aspects of platelet function, (4) the precise molecular nature of Ca^{2+} regulation of contractile protein activity and the release of storage granules, and (5) the nature of the interactions between Ca^{2+}, cyclic nucleotides and protein kinases which modulate platelet function.

Platelets have very large stores of Ca^{2+} which, if uniformly distributed in cell water, would give a concentration of about 15 mM. The precise distribution of Ca^{2+} in the platelet is poorly understood. Such information is important because specific platelet responses may be governed by localized molecular events, and therefore by regional variations in free and bound Ca^{2+} levels. A large proportion of platelet Ca^{2+} is released along with ADP and serotonin (Mürer, 1969), suggesting that it is contained in the secretory granules. X-ray microprobe analysis shows that dense bodies (Takaya, 1975; Martin $et\ al.$, 1974; Skaer $et\ al.$,

1974) and alpha-granules (Sato *et al.*, 1975) are major sites of concentration of Ca^{2+}. Calcium ion localized in the nucleoids of alpha-granules disappeared rapidly after stimulation by thrombin (Sato *et al.*, 1975) and might be involved in activation of platelet responses. Other definitive sites for Ca^{2+} were not found, but in some cases fixation and post-fixation with osmium probably resulted in the loss of Ca^{2+} (Oschman *et al.*, 1974). Unfortunately total platelet Ca^{2+} was not measured chemically prior to, and after, preparation of samples to assess the magnitude of any Ca^{2+} loss.

Steiner and Tateishi (1974) reported that in intact platelets various aggregating agents which released about the same amount of ^{14}C-serotonin (*e.g.* 72-88%) released widely varying amounts of Ca^{2+}; *e.g.* ADP 2.4%, epinephrine 3.2%, collagen 40.2%, and thrombin 79.8%. It is evident that these results are incompatible with those studies which indicated that most of the platelet Ca^{2+} is contained in the secretory granules and is released along with ADP and serotonin. Salganicoff *et al.* (1975) suggested that Ca^{2+} released by thrombin and other aggregating agents comes not only from the dense granules which contain serotonin and adenine nucleotides, but also from another type of granule. Detwiler and Feinman (1973) demonstrated different kinetics for the release of Ca^{2+} and ATP and also concluded that the source of Ca^{2+} released by thrombin was not the secretory granules but rather some other organelle, such as the dense tubular system (DTS), involved in excitation-secretion coupling. Release of Ca^{2+} from the platelet would presumably reflect net efflux from the cytoplasm. If this view is correct the net loss of Ca^{2+}, but not serotonin or ADP, should be a function of the concentration of extracellular Ca^{2+}. Such experiments have not been reported. Lages *et al.* (1975) found that the Ca^{2+} content of platelets with storage pool disease was reduced by about 60%. This finding is consistent with a granule location for most of the cell Ca^{2+}.

In disrupted platelets the most extensive studies on the distribution of Ca^{2+} have been conducted by Steiner and Tateishi (1974) and Salganicoff *et al.* (1975). Steiner and Tateishi found 98% of platelet Ca^{2+} was bound to protein. About 21% of membrane Ca^{2+} was linked to lipids, primarily sphingomyelin and phosphatidylcholine. Although the granule fraction obtained from platelets disrupted by the glycerol lysis technique contained the highest specific activity (nm/mg protein) of Ca^{2+} it represented only 13% of total Ca^{2+}. At least 60% of platelet Ca^{2+} was present in the soluble fraction. Salganicoff *et al.* (1975) disrupted platelets with a French press. In their experiments preservation of organelles appeared superior since 80% of total Ca^{2+} was associated with particulate fractions. The highest specific activity of Ca^{2+} was in a fraction containing mitochondria, α-granules and

dense bodies.   Further subfractionation of the mitochondrial-granule
fraction resulted in significant separation of serotonin and Ca^{2+}.
Most (70%) of the Ca^{2+} was associated with membrane fractions different than those which contained 80% of the serotonin, although
the principle serotonin fraction had the highest specific activity
for Ca^{2+}.   The possible loss of Ca^{2+} from certain fractions and
the redistribution of diffusible Ca^{2+} during the gradient separation procedure was not assessed.   In neither of these studies
were marker enzymes for smooth endoplasmic reticulum measured.

        Calcium ion is associated with microsomal membrane fractions,
obtained from platelet homogenates, since these membrane vesicles
can accumulate Ca^{2+} in the presence of ATP (Käser-Glanzmann et al.,
1977; Robblee et al., 1973; Statland et al., 1969; Grette, 1963).
It has been suggested that this activity may be derived from the
dense tubule system (smooth endoplasmic reticulum) of the platelet
which could function in a manner similar to the sarcoplasmic reticulum of muscle (White, 1972a), i.e. it would sequester Ca^{2+} to
maintain low free Ca^{2+} activity in the cytosol, and would also be
capable of releasing the stored Ca^{2+} under the influence of suitable
stimuli.   Compared to a surface membrane fraction prepared by the
glycerol-lysis method of Barber and Jamieson (1970) the microsomal
fraction was enriched in cytochromes P450 and b_5, NADH-cytochrome
C reductase, NADPH-cytochrome C reductase, and glucose-6-phosphatase
(Cinti and Feinstein, 1976; Feinstein and Fraser, unpublished data).
These activities are usually markers for the endoplasmic reticulum
in other cells. Ca^{2+}-ATPase activity can be detected cytochemically
in the plasma membrane (White and Krivit, 1965), the open canalicular system (OCS) (Cutler et al., 1978) which represents extensive
invaginations of the surface membrane into the cell interior, and
the dense tubular system (Figures 2, 3).   These results suggest
that Ca^{2+} transport ATPases may reside in the membranes of the
dense tubules as well as in regions of the surface membrane, especially the open canalicular system.   However, more definitive biochemical evidence is required to conclusively establish the precise
localization and properties of Ca^{2+} transport enzymes.   In assess-
ing the overall cellular regulation of platelet Ca^{2+} it will also
be necessary in the future to more fully explore the potentialities
of mitochondria and secretory granules as organelles for Ca^{2+}-
transport.   It must be concluded that the studies performed up to
the present time provide no clear definitive picture of either the
quantitative subcellular localization of calcium in platelets or
the sources of activator Ca^{2+}.

        The mechanisms by which platelet aggregating agents induce a
rise in cytoplasmic Ca^{2+} is unknown, but several possibilities can
be considered (Figure 4).   (1) Increased membrane permeability to
Ca^{2+} through a membrane channel or endogenous ionophore coupled
to the receptor protein.   Although some effects of collagen are

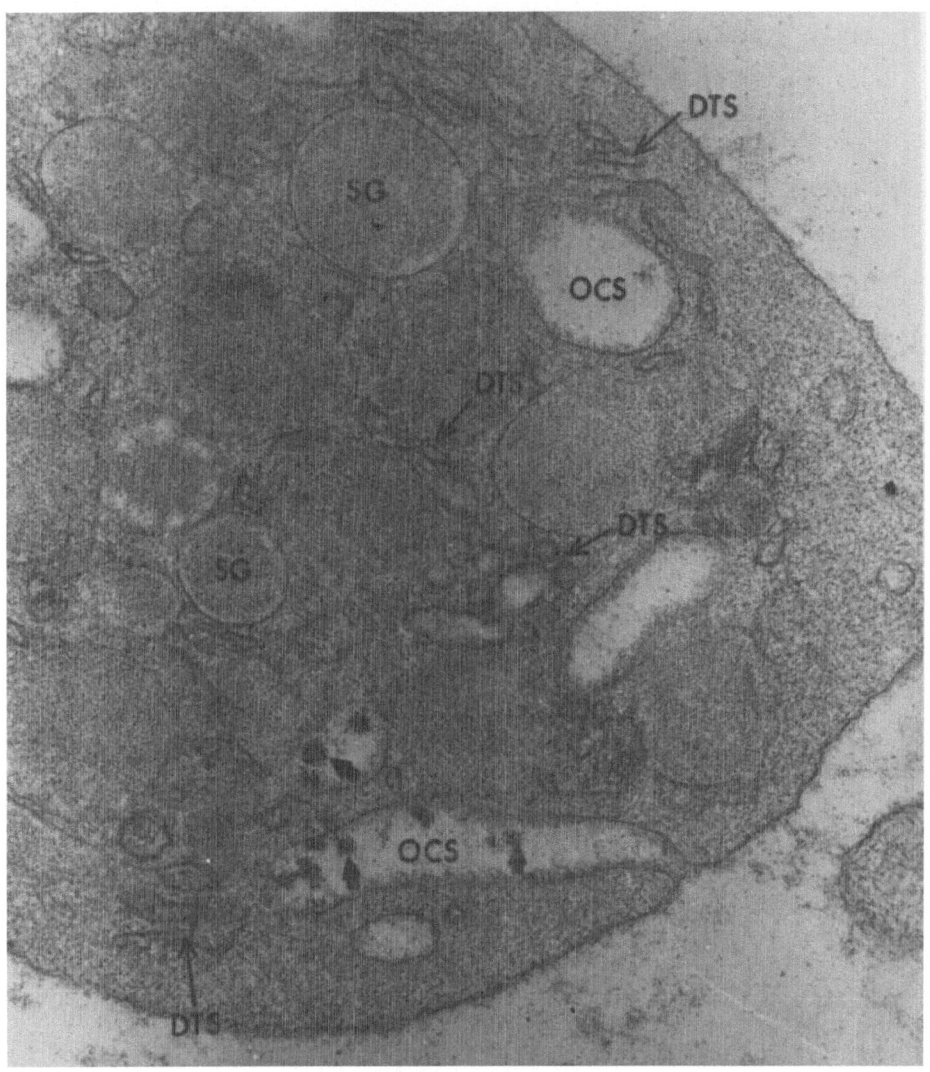

Figure 2. Ca²⁺-activated ATPase activity in platelets. Electron micrograph of a platelet incubated in cytochemical media to demonstrate Ca²⁺-ATPase activity prior to fixation in 1.25% glutaraldehyde for 30 minutes. Reaction product is seen only in portions of the open canalicular system (arrows). The dense tubular system (DTS), the cell surface, secretory granules (SG) and the rest of the cell is free of reaction product. The section is unstained.

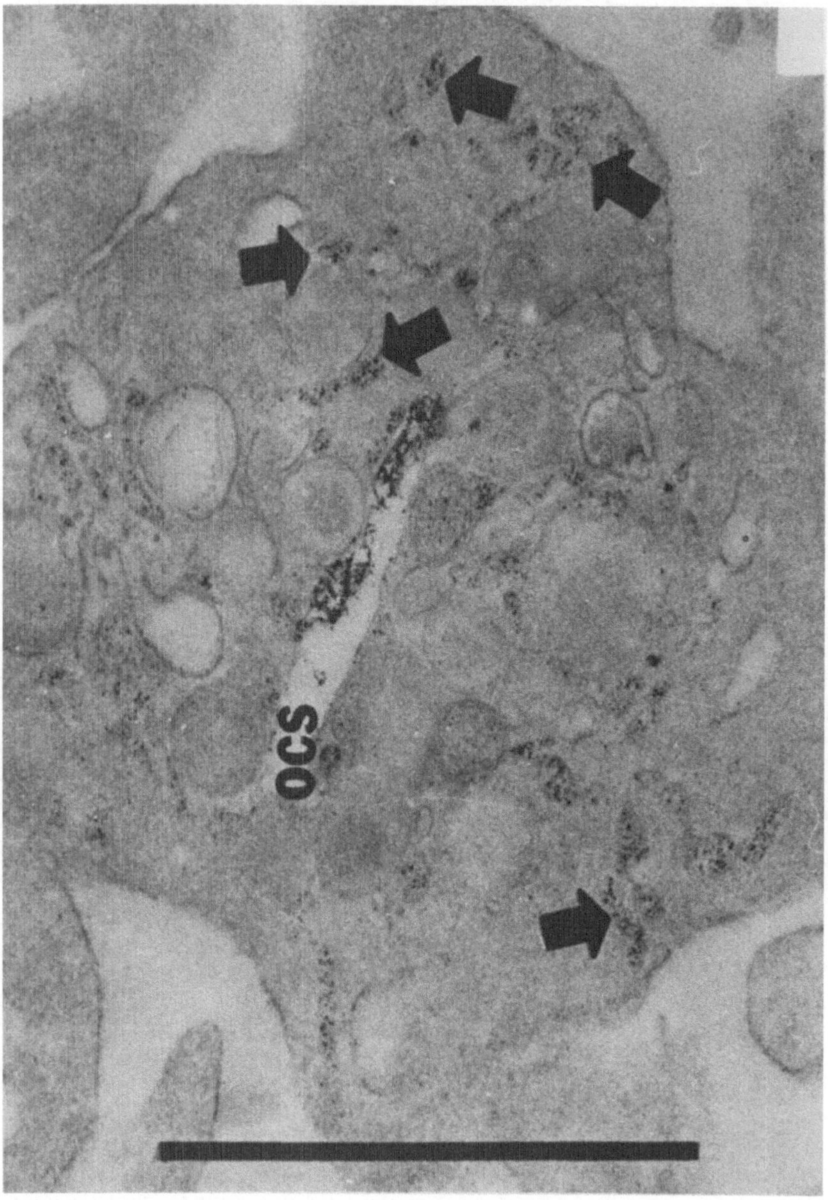

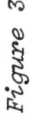

Figure 3

Figure 3. Ca^{2+}-activated ATPase activity in platelets. Electron micrograph of a platelet fixed for 15 minutes in 1.25% glutaraldehyde and then incubated in cytochemical media to demonstrate Ca^{2+}-ATPase activity. Reaction product is seen in the dense tubular system (arrows) and a portion of the open canalicular system (OCS). The cell surface is free of reaction product. The section is unstained. Bar represents 1μ.

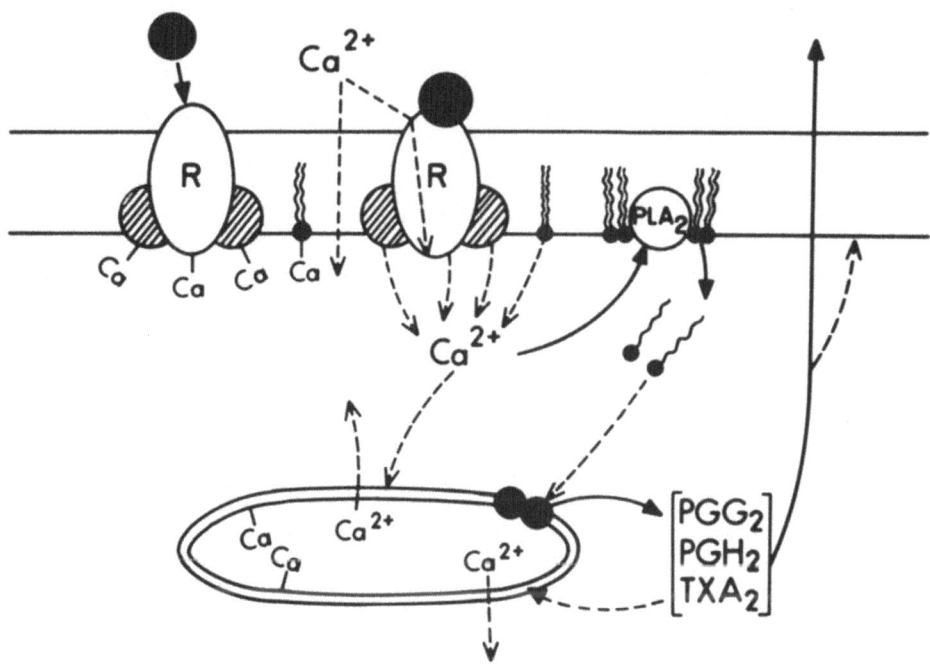

Figure 4. Possible mechanisms for the mobilization of Ca^{2+} during platelet activation. Platelet stimulating agents (●) interact with membrane receptors (R). This might cause an influx of Ca^{2+} through the lipid domain of the membrane or through a protein channel. Alternatively Ca^{2+} bound to the receptor, or to proteins or lipids closely associated with the receptor, is released into the cytoplasm. A rising cytoplasmic Ca^{2+} concentration may induce additional Ca^{2+} release from internal organelles such as the dense tubular system. Ca^{2+} also activates phospholipase A_2 (PLA_2) to form free arachidonic acid which serves as substrate for synthesis of prostaglandin endoperoxides (PGG_2, PGH_2) and thromboxane A_2 (TXA_2). The latter may release Ca^{2+} from intracellular organelles or from the surface membrane.

partially inhibited by verapamil (Haslam and Lynham, 1976) a blocking agent for Ca^{2+} channels in some tissues, it is unlikely that Ca^{2+} influx is the immediate trigger for excitation since no studies show that it occurs early enough. (2) Ca^{2+} bound to the inner surface of the membrane may be released as a result of conformational changes induced in receptor proteins by aggregating agents, or alteration of a transmembrane electrical potential. (3) Additional internal stores of Ca^{2+} may be released by: (a) Ca^{2+}-induced Ca^{2+} release, such as occurs in muscle cells under certain conditions (Fabiato and Fabiato, 1977), with released surface membrane Ca^{2+} serving as the trigger, (b) an intracellular transmitter substance (*e.g.* PG endoperoxides, thromboxane A_2, cyclic nucleotides) formed in response to the stimulus which would release Ca^{2+} from an internal organelle, (c) a surface membrane depolarization which might be conveyed internally along the DTS initiated at sites of close apposition of the OCS-DTS membranes (White, 1972a,b).

No studies have conclusively demonstrated the existence of any of these mechanisms for recruiting Ca^{2+}. With regard to membrane potential-linked events Horne and Singer (1976) reported that thrombin and collagen produced a hyperpolarization, measured with a fluorescent cyanine dye. This may be due to a sudden increase in K^+ permeability since K^+ efflux increases as a result of stimulation. K^+ efflux has been attributed to release by the secretory process, but studies with electron-probe microanalysis revealed no K^+ emission from platelet dense bodies (Skaer *et al.*, 1974). Increased ^{42}K efflux in response to thrombin reached a maximum in less than 30 sec and was blocked by the local anesthetic tetracaine (Feinstein and Sha'afi, unpublished experiments). This suggests that K^+ loss from the cytoplasm may occur as a result of a stimulus-induced increase of free Ca^{2+}, *i.e.* the so-called Gardos effect (Gardos, 1958). A23187 has been shown to depolarize pancreatic acinar cells in conjunction with its stimulation of amylase secretion (Poulsen and Williams, 1977). The depolarization seemed due to a Ca^{2+} mediated increase in Na^+ permeability. The effects of A23187 on platelet Na^+ and K^+ have not yet been reported, but thrombin does increase Na^+ uptake concurrently with loss of K^+ (Feinstein and Fraser, unpublished data). Platelets treated with the monovalent cation ionophores monensin and nigericin very rapidly lose nearly all their K^+ and take up Na^+ (Feinstein *et al.*, 1977a). This would also be expected to produce depolarization of a K^+-dominated membrane potential. No secretion or platelet aggregation occurred under these conditions and furthermore these K^+-depleted platelets aggregated maximally when stimulated by thrombin, A23187 or collagen. Therefore, there is no convincing evidence at present that would link platelet excitation to membrane potential changes. The small size of platelets obviously severely limits the kinds of experiments which can be performed to answer the pertinent questions.

LeBreton *et al.* (1976) utilizing chlortetracycline as a fluorescent probe for membrane-bound calcium reported that Ca^{2+} was
apparently released from the surface membrane by ADP and that this
response persisted, along with shape change, despite the presence
of TMB-6, a local anesthetic-like drug which blocked secretion
(LeBreton and Dinerstein, 1977). This implies that another and
larger internal pool of Ca^{2+} must be mobilized to elicit secretion.
A similar conclusion with respect to platelet activation by thrombin and A23187 was reached by Charo *et al.* (1976b) and Feinstein
et al. (1976) employing TMB-8 and local anesthetics which are
antagonists of intracellular Ca^{2+}. Mobilization of this additional
source of Ca^{2+} might take place by Ca^{2+}-induced Ca^{2+} release, a
process which in muscle is very susceptible to blockade by local
anesthetics (Thorens and Endo, 1975; Ford and Podolsky, 1972).
Another possibility is that the membrane pool of Ca^{2+} stimulates
production of another intracellular transmitter which can mobilize
additional Ca^{2+}. Likely candidates are thromboxane A_2 and/or the
PG endoperoxides whose synthesis is initiated by Ca^{2+}-dependent
activation of phospholipase A_2. One of the presumed sources of
activator Ca^{2+} is the dense tubular system (Robblee *et al.*, 1973;
1972a,b; Statland *et al.*, 1969; White and Krivit, 1967). It is
therefore quite significant that thromboxane synthetase activity
has been reported (Gerrard *et al.*, 1976) to be localized to the
DTS. PG endoperoxides and TXA_2 could act as ionophores to release
Ca^{2+} from the DTS (Gerrard *et al.*, 1976) but direct evidence concerning such a mechanism of action is not conclusive (Reed, 1977).
The fact that certain smooth muscles are stimulated to contract
by TXA_2 indicates that this agent can bring about the mobilization
of cellular Ca^{2+}. Verapamil, which affects influx of external Ca^{2+}
in smooth muscle (Haeusler, 1972) had no effect on contractions
due to TXA_2. Local anesthetics which can inhibit smooth muscle
contraction due to the mobilization of intracellular Ca^{2+} stores
(Feinstein and Paimre, 1969) were also able to inhibit TXA_2 induced contraction of the rabbit aorta and platelet aggregation
Feinstein *et al.*, 1977b).

The extent of Ca^{2+} exchangeability in platelets has been the
subject of controversy (Mürer and Holme, 1970; Wallach *et al.*,
1958; Odell and Upton, 1955). The most detailed analysis (Steiner
and Tateishi, 1974) indicated that Ca^{2+} uptake was markedly temperature and pH dependent. ^{45}Ca uptake was increased by extracellular K^+ and was reduced by Na^+. Attainment of a steady-state of
^{45}Ca between platelets and the medium required more than two hours.
The ^{45}Ca uptake curves suggested the existence of three compartments for cellular Ca^{2+}; a surface compartment representing 13%
of the total space, an intracellular compartment of 57%, and the
remainder non-exchangeable. However, conclusions about the number
of compartments and their capacity appears premature since, at

physiological concentrations of extracellular Ca^{2+}, not more than 5% of total cellular calcium was exchangeable (Steiner and Tateishi, 1974).

   Platelet stimulation by thrombin (Massini and Lüscher, 1974; Robblee et al., 1973) collagen (Feinstein et al., 1976) and A23187 (Feinstein et al., 1976; Feinstein and Fraser, 1975; Mürer et al., 1975; Massini and Lüscher, 1974; White et al., 1974) is accompanied by an enhanced uptake of ^{45}Ca from the incubation medium. However, except for an experiment of Massini and Lüscher (1974) with A23187, none of the available evidence indicates that the uptake of Ca^{2+} occurs early enough to be considered a causal event. Local anesthetics block ^{45}Ca uptake elicited by collagen (Feinstein et al., 1976). Thrombin-induced uptake of ^{45}Ca is greatest when the platelets have been exposed to the isotope only briefly prior to stimulation (Feinstein and Fraser, unpublished results). When pre-equilibration of unstimulated platelets with ^{45}Ca is allowed to occur for 45-60 min thrombin-induced uptake becomes progressively reduced. This result indicates that ^{45}Ca uptake in thrombin-stimulated platelets is probably due to an increased rate of exchange with a Ca^{2+} pool that can completely, but slowly, equilibrate with extracellular ^{45}Ca in unstimulated cells. PGE_1 plus theophylline strongly inhibits thrombin-induced ^{45}Ca uptake (Feinstein et al., 1977b). This effect will be considered more thoroughly when the role of cAMP in platelet function is discussed.

   Uptake of ^{45}Ca due to A23187 is increased by local anesthetics (Feinstein et al., 1976), PGE_1 and dibutyryl cyclic AMP (Feinstein and Fraser, unpublished data). Uptake of ^{45}Ca due to A23187 probably occurs by two processes facilitated by the ionophore, i.e. (1) net uptake of Ca^{2+} and (2) exchange with free intracellular Ca^{2+}. Local anesthetics and increased platelet cyclic AMP must potentiate one or the other of these mechanisms for ^{45}Ca uptake. Pretreatment of platelets with thrombin greatly reduces ^{45}Ca uptake when the isotope and ionophore are added subsequently. A possible explanation for this effect is that thrombin causes the release of a Ca^{2+} pool with which ^{45}Ca can exchange in the presence of A23187, such as in the DTS or the secretory granules.

   It is apparent that a number of complex mechanisms are at work which can affect ^{45}Ca fluxes during stimulation and that much additional work will be required to unravel all the complexities of platelet calcium metabolism. Note also that effects of a drug on ^{45}Ca fluxes need not correlate with its ultimate influence on platelet function. Thus, the enhancement of ionophore-induced ^{45}Ca uptake by local anesthetics and PGE_1 occurs concurrently with their inhibition of ionophore-induced secretion and aggregation.

CALCIUM REGULATION OF PLATELET CONTRACTILE PROTEINS

It is well established that platelet actomyosin ATPase activity is sensitive to Ca^{2+} (Harris *et al.*, 1974; Abramowitz *et al.*, 1975; Bettex-Galland and Lüscher, 1965) but the molecular details are far from being worked out. ATPase activity of platelet actomyosin is similar to that of smooth muscle in that Ca^{2+} ATPase activity greatly exceeds that of Mg^{2+} ATPase activity (Harris *et al.*, 1974; Abramowitz *et al.*, 1975). Calcium ion has also been reported to be a positive allosteric effector of myosin ATPase activity (Malik *et al.*, 1974). Calcium sensitivity of platelet actomyosin varies with ionic strength, pH and Mg^{2+} concentrations as well as the presence of additional protein factors. Calcium ion control is actin-linked (Cohen *et al.*, 1973) and protein fractions with troponin-like activity have been described (Puszkin *et al.*, 1975; Cohen *et al.*, 1973; Thorens *et al.*, 1973). However, pure troponin components have not been isolated.

In cardiac muscle the phosphorylation of troponin subunits, notably Tn-I (Bailin, 1977; Ray and England, 1976; Reddy and Wyborny, 1976; Solaro *et al.*, 1976) and Tn-T by a cyclic AMP-dependent protein kinase decreases the Ca^{2+} sensitivity of actomyosin ATPase activity. Dephosphorylation by a phosphatase increases Ca^{2+} sensitivity. Whether platelet troponin-like proteins are affected similarly is unknown, but this is a potential area for regulation of Ca^{2+} actions by cyclic AMP.

Several neurosecretory tissues (*e.g.* brain, ganglia, adrenal medulla and cortex) contain a modulator protein which closely resembles muscle troponin C (Vanaman *et al.*, 1976). This modulator protein can serve as a Ca^{2+}-dependent activator of actomyosin ATPase, 3':5'-cyclic nucleotide phosphodiesterase and adenylate cyclase. The protein seems to be distributed in both cytoplasm and membranes. Binding to the latter is increased by Ca^{2+}. The troponin-like activity in platelets could be related to this modulator protein which in the presence of Ca^{2+} could serve to activate actomyosin, and perhaps to stimulate the breakdown of cyclic AMP as well, so as to facilitate the release reaction.

Platelet myosin-actin interaction appears to depend upon the phosphorylation of the 20,000 dalton light chain of myosin (Adelstein and Conti, 1975). Phosphorylation is catalyzed by an endogenous cyclic nucleotide-independent protein kinase which, unlike the analogous smooth muscle kinase, does not require Ca^{2+}. Dephosphorylation by a platelet phosphatase reduces ATPase activity Adelstein and Conti, 1975).

Weber (1976) has proposed several criteria for a contractile system responsible for intracellular movements, *i.e.*: close

apposition of actin and myosin at some time so as to allow molecular interactions and reversible anchoring of the contractile system
to the plasma membrane and to those organelles that have to be
moved, perhaps by an assembly-disassembly process. Microfilaments
in the platelet can be decorated with heavy meromyosin and therefore contain actin (Behnke, 1971). Behnke proposed that the
cytoplasm contained G-actin monomers in equilibrium with F-actin
filaments. In the resting platelet much of the actin may be in
a non-polymerized form. Stimulation of platelets causes microfilaments to appear more abundantly in the cytoplasm. Abramowitz
et al. (1975) reported the presence of two forms of platelet actin,
one which polymerizes similarly to muscle actin. The other in
contrast polymerizes in the absence of Ca^{2+} and ATP, and depoly-
merizes in their presence. It was postulated that the latter form
of actin served a structural function but its real role is not
known. Myosin filaments are not identifiable in the electron
microscope, but the presence of myosin in the microfilaments of
a number of cells has been revealed utilizing fluorescent-labelled
myosin antibodies (Pollard, 1976; Weber and Groeschel-Stewart, 1975).
The presence of both actin and myosin in microfilaments, at some
time, would provide the basis for contractile activity. But
mechanochemical coupling need not require filaments formed from
polymerized myosin (Oplatka et al., 1974). Tropomyosin is present
in microfilaments (Lazarides, 1976) and may provide sites for binding of troponin-like proteins that may confer Ca^{2+} sensitivity.

Cytochalasin B can inhibit clot retraction, aggregation and
the release reaction, but its effects are quite complex and concentration dependent (Haslam et al., 1975). Cytochalasin B is
presumed to affect the integrity of microfilaments, but other
studies show that this compound may act by binding to platelet
myosin and inhibiting its ATPase activity (Puszkin et al., 1971).

Platelets also contain microtubules which are believed to
play a role in the formation of the cytoskeleton. The role of
microtubules in platelet functions is not clear. Although microtubule disrupting agents (colchicine, vinblastine) affect platelet
shape and may inhibit secretion at unusually high concentrations
(Friedman and Detwiler, 1975), platelet aggregation and clot retraction are unaffected by disruption of microtubules (Boyle-Kay
and Fudenberg, 1973). Some high molecular weight polypeptides
(200,000 mol. wt.) may be associated with tubulin preparations
(55,000 mol. wt.). They have associated Mg^{2+} or Ca^{2+} stimulated
ATPase activity (Crawford, 1976), but it is not known whether
these polypeptides correspond to the dyneins of cilia and flagella
which are involved in sliding movements of microtubules. Platelet
microtubules are disassembled in the presence of Ca^{2+}. A Ca^{2+}
flux from the membrane surface may affect microtubule structure
and thus lead to shape changes.

The complex interrelationships and interactions between micro-tubules and microfilaments, their involvement in platelet responses to stimuli, and the role of Ca^{2+} in regulating their functions remain to be fully worked out.

PROSTAGLANDINS, PROSTAGLANDIN ENDOPEROXIDES, AND THROMBOXANES

Arachidonic acid induces shape change, aggregation and the release reaction in platelets (Silver et al., 1973; Vargaftig and Zirinis, 1973). This fatty acid is metabolized by two main pathways in the platelet (Figure 5); one route is catalyzed by a cytoplasmic lipoxygenase (Nugteren, 1975) and the other pathway is initiated by a membrane-bound enzyme system, prostaglandin endoperoxide synthetase (Hamberg and Samuelsson, 1973; Nugteren and Hazelhoff, 1973) which converts the fatty acid to the labile endoperoxide PGG_2. PGG_2 can be reduced to PGH_2 by a reductase. These endoperoxides serve as precursors for the synthesis of prostaglandins PGD_2, PGE_2 and $PGF_{2\alpha}$ which is a minor pathway for endoperoxide metabolism (Hamberg et al., 1974a). The endoperoxides are mainly converted to a highly unstable intermediate, thromboxane A_2 (TXA_2) which spontaneously breaks down to a stable endproduct, thromboxane B_2 (TXB_2) (Hamberg et al., 1975). Additional metabolic products of the endoperoxides, which may be formed non-enzymatically, include 12-hydroxy-8,10-heptadecadienoic acid (HHT) and malondial-dehyde (MDA). The latter is readily detected by a colorimetric assay and is a convenient indicator of PG endoperoxide formation (Smith et al., 1976). The prostaglandin endoperoxides and TXA_2 are highly potent inducers of platelet aggregation and secretion (Hamberg et al., 1974b; Willis et al., 1974). TXA_2 is also a powerful stimulant of vascular smooth muscle (Needleman et al., 1976a; Svensson et al., 1975) and is the major component of rabbit aorta contracting substance (RCS) from guinea pig lung and platelets. TXA_2 is formed by a microsomal enzyme (Needleman et al., 1976b) termed thromboxane synthetase. Prostaglandin endoperoxides, TXA_2, TB_2 and other stable endproducts of arachidonate metabolism are produced when platelets are stimulated by collagen, thrombin and A23187 (Pickett et al., 1977; Feinstein et al., 1977; Mahlmsten et al., 1975; Hamberg et al., 1974; Smith et al., 1974). Non-steroidal antiinflammatory agents such as aspirin and indomethacin inhibit the prostaglandin endoperoxide synthetase (Smith and Willis, 1971; Vane, 1971) preventing the formation of PGG_2, PGH_2 and TXA_2 and thereby completely blocking arachidonate-induced aggregation. Recently a number of relatively selective inhibitors of thromboxane synthetase have been described, such as imidazole (Moncada et al., 1977; Needleman et al., 1977) and 9,11-azoprosta-5,13 dienoic acid (Gorman et al., 1977), which has led to controversy about whether or not PG endoperoxides can initiate platelet aggregation without being converted to TXA_2. Furthermore, initial conclusions that

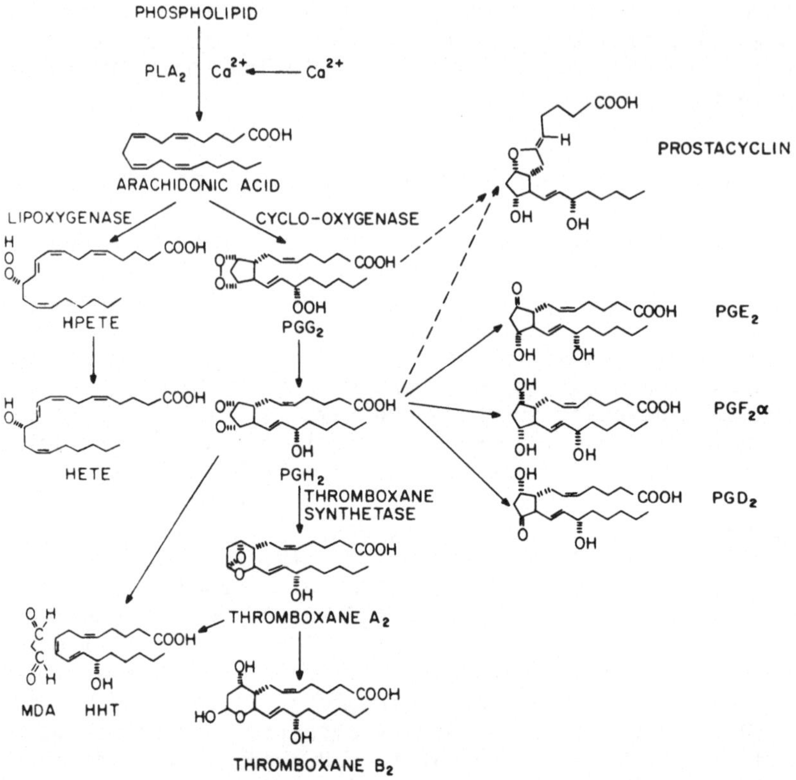

Figure 5. Metabolic pathways of arachidonic acid in platelets. Formation of arachidonate is initiated by translocation of intra- cellular Ca^{2+} to activate PLA_2. Prostacyclin formation (dashed arrows) occurs in blood vessel walls.

the formation of PGG_2 is essential for normal aggregation due to various stimulating agents because of its role in initiating the release reaction (Mahlmsten *et al.*, 1975) have been contested and it has also been concluded that TXA_2 formation is not essential for platelet aggregation (Needleman *et al.*, 1976). Minkes *et al.* (1977) concluded that the formation of PG endoperoxides or TXA_2 is not required for the initiation of release reaction since the concentration of thrombin required to induce maximum serotonin release from platelets was significantly less than that required to stimulate maximum formation of MDA. However, their data shows that at the concentration of thrombin which produced maximal re- lease of serotonin and ADP the amount of MDA formed was about 700 pmol/ml platelet suspension, a concentration of 0.7 μM. At least an equivalent amount of PG endoperoxides must therefore have been

formed. The amount of RCS produced was equivalent to that formed
by adding 400-800 ng/ml (about 1-2 μM) PGH_2 to the platelet suspensions. PGG_2 added exogenously at 0.6 μM was found to release
45-60% of platelet ADP (Mahlmsten et $al.$, 1975). From this data
it is evident that concentrations of thrombin which cause a maximal release reaction produce significant amounts of PG endoperoxides and TXA_2, sufficient in fact to have elicited substantial
release by themselves when added exogenously.

     Aggregation due to collagen can occur despite a block of PG
synthetase depending upon the concentration (Gordon and MacIntyre,
1974; Zucker and Peterson, 1970; O'Brien, 1968) and the type of
collagen used (Nyman, 1977). Collagen-induced aggregation resistant to aspirin and indomethacin has been attributed to the action
of released ADP (Packham et $al.$, 1977). It has further been
suggested (Nyman, 1977) that the aspirin-resistant effect of
collagen does not involve the specific platelet collagen receptor,
but rather possibly a proteolytic step involving membrane-bound
complement (Chater, 1976). Aggregation due to low concentrations
of thrombin and A23187 is also partially depressed by PG synthetase inhibitors, whereas at higher concentrations aggregation and
the release reaction are unaffected (Fukami et $al.$, 1976; Feinstein
and Fraser, 1975; White et $al.$, 1974; Smith and Willis, 1971; Evans
et $al.$, 1968). Recently Vargaftig (1976) has reported that inhibition of thrombin and carrageenan-induced platelet aggregation by
aspirin and indomethacin was reversible by washing the platelets,
whereas the inhibition of PG synthetase persisted. Thus, the non-
steroidal antiinflammatory agents may have an additional pharmacological action on platelets, unrelated to the effects on PG
endoperoxide synthesis, and which may involve antagonism of Ca^{2+}
(Northover, 1977; Whittle, 1976).

     The role of PGE_2 and $PGF_{2\alpha}$ in platelet function is not well
understood. Low concentrations of PGE_2 decrease cyclic AMP and
enhance ADP-induced aggregation. Higher concentrations have the
direct opposite effect. Another prostaglandin PGD_2, which is
produced during platelet stimulation, is an even more potent inhibitor of aggregation than PGE_1. Its formation may represent an
important internal negative feedback pathway to limit platelet
aggregation (Oelz et $al.$, 1977).

     Blood vessel walls contain an enzyme which can convert PG
endoperoxides to a prostaglandin termed, prostacyclin (PGI_2, PGX)
which is a vasodilator and a potent inhibitor of platelet aggregation (Grygleswski et $al.$, 1976). PGI_2 strongly stimulates platelet
adenylate cyclase activity (Best et $al.$, 1977) and thereby inhibits
PLA_2 activation as well (Lapetina et $al.$, 1977). The formation in
blood vessel walls of PGI_2 from PG endoperoxides originating from
stimulated platelets represents yet another important negative

feedback pathway limiting the growth of platelet thrombi (Gryglewski *et al.*, 1976). It has been suggested (Gorman *et al.*, 1977) that *in vivo* the thromboxane synthetase inhibitor azo analog I could divert platelet PGH_2 toward prostacyclin synthesis and thereby be of value in the treatment of vascular problems associated with platelet aggregation and vascular spasm.

The enzyme phospholipase A2 (PLA_2) occupies a strategic position in the pathway for generation of PG endoperoxides, prostaglandins and TXA_2 since little free arachidonate is present intracellularly and neither the PG endoperoxides nor their byproducts are stored in cells (Kunze and Vogt, 1971). Activation of PLA_2 results in the release of free arachidonate from certain membrane phospholipids (Blackwell *et al.*, Bills *et al.*, 1976; Derksen and Cohen, 1975) and a non-mitochondrial burst of O_2 consumption due to oxidation of the fatty acid (Fukami *et al.*, 1976; Pickett and Cohen, 1976). PLA_2 specifically requires Ca^{2+} for activity (Wells, 1974, 1972) and is, therefore, essentially inactive in unstimulated platelets. Release of intracellular Ca^{2+} by platelet stimulating agents activates PLA_2 with the resultant formation of PG endoperoxides and TXA_2. The Ca^{2+} ionophore A23187 activates PLA_2 producing a fall in phospholipid arachidonate (Pickett *et al.*, 1977), an O_2 burst (Feinstein *et al.*, 1977b; Pickett *et al.*, 1977) and the formation of RCS (Feinstein *et al.*, 1977b). The effects of A23187 are greater than thrombin (Pickett *et al.*, 1977) and occur in the absence of extracellular Ca^{2+}.

Activation of PLA_2 can be blocked by several types of inhibitors. Antimalarials, such as mepacrine prevent the formation of RCS elicited by bradykinin in guinea pig lung (Vargaftig and Hai, 1975). Mepacrine inhibits aggregation of platelets produced by collagen and thrombin and blocks the release of arachidonate from phospholipids (Blackwell *et al.*, 1977). PLA_2 from several sources can be inhibited by drugs with local anesthetic activity (Kunze *et al.*, 1976) by competitive inhibition of Ca^{2+} binding to the enzyme or interaction with the substrate. Local anesthetics (*e.g.* dibucaine, tetracaine) inhibit malondialdehyde and RCS formation in platelets exposed to collagen, thrombin and A23187, but not when exogenous arachidonate is added (Feinstein *et al.*, 1977b). Furthermore, these drugs do not affect the formation of platelet aggregating factors (PG endoperoxides and TXA_2) from arachidonate by platelet microsomes (Feinstein and Fraser, unpublished results). Although the local anesthetics clearly can block PLA_2 activation in platelets it should be borne in mind that they also have additional actions since they inhibit aggregation and the release reaction induced by arachidonic acid, or by PG endoperoxides and TXA_2 generated from arachidonate by platelet microsomes (Feinstein *et al.*, 1977b).

In common with mast cells, neutrophils, and basophils the secretory activity of rabbit platelets was found to be inhibited by irreversible organophosphorous inhibitors of serine esterases (Henson *et al.*, 1976). These inhibitors are much more effective if present during the period of platelet stimulation than if they are preincubated with platelets and then washed out prior to stimulation. Thus, their target sites are made much more available in a stimulated platelet. It was proposed that the platelet enzymes which are inactivated by the organophosphorus compounds exist in a proenzyme (zymogen) form which is activated by the stimulus (Henson *et al.*, 1976).

The serine-esterase inhibitor, phenylmethanesulfonyl fluoride (PMSF) has been found (Feinstein *et al.*, 1977b) to block malonaldehyde formation and arachidonate oxidation induced in human platelets by collagen and thrombin, but not by A23187 or arachidonic acid. Inactivation of thrombin directly by PMSF, measured by blood clotting and platelet aggregation assays, was too slow to account for this result (see also, Seegers *et al.*, 1965). Furthermore, thrombin-induced aggregation was normal in the same platelets in which malonaldehyde formation was blocked by PMSF. PMSF was much more effective when it was present during the period of exposure of platelets to collagen or thrombin. Preincubation of PMSF with unstimulated platelets followed by washing out prior to addition of the stimulus had little effect. These experiments indicate that a stimulus-activated serine-esterase (protease) is involved in the activation of platelet phospholipase A_2 by collagen and thrombin and may account for the inhibition of the release reaction by serine-esterase inhibitors.

Cyclic 3',5'-AMP also inhibits PLA_2 activation (Feinstein *et al.*, 1977b; Lapetina *et al.*, 1977; Minkes *et al.*, 1977), not by a direct effect on the enzyme but rather by preventing the mobilization of Ca^{2+} necessary for PLA_2 activity (Feinstein *et al.*, 1977b).

INTERRELATIONSHIPS BETWEEN CALCIUM AND CYCLIC NUCLEOTIDES

The various functions of platelets are regulated to a significant degree by cyclic AMP (Salzman, 1972). Platelet aggregation and the release reaction are inhibited by agents which increase the level of cellular cyclic AMP. Prostaglandin E_1 (PGE_1) for example is a powerful inhibitor of many types of stimulating agents, *i.e.* ADP, epinephrine, collagen, thrombin, A23187 and TXA_2. PGE_1 is believed to act by stimulation of platelet adenylate cyclase (Smith and Macfarlane, 1974). The actions of PGE_1 are markedly potentiated by phosphodiesterase inhibitors, and are duplicated for the most part by dibutyryl cyclic AMP. Other more physiologically significant prostaglandins, such as PGD_2 and PGI_2

(prostacyclin) are also more potent stimulators of adenylate cyclase (Best *et al.*, 1977; Gorman *et al.*, 1977b; Tateson *et al.*, 1977) and inhibitors of platelet aggregation (Gryglewski *et al.*, 1976; Smith *et al.*, 1974). PGI_2 induces much greater accumulation of cyclic AMP than either PGD_2 or PGE_1. PGI_2 is made in arterial walls from PG endoperoxides (Best *et al.*, 1977; Gryglewski *et al.*, 1976) and may represent a negative feedback pathway by which PG endoperoxides released from aggregating platelets are converted to an agent which can inhibit or reverse platelet aggregation. PGD_2 on the other hand can be formed within stimulated platelets (Oelz *et al.*, 1977) non-enzymatically or by an endoperoxide - PGD_2 isomerase (Nugteren and Hazelhof, 1973). Collagen, thrombin, epinephrine and arachidonate (but not ADP) stimulated PGD_2 synthesis (Oelz *et al.*, 1977) which was blocked by indomethacin. PGD_2, like PGE_1, can inhibit platelet responses to collagen, epinephrine, ADP, PG endoperoxides and TXA_2.

Since a rise in cyclic AMP inhibits platelet responses, many investigators have attempted to determine if the resting state is maintained by cyclic AMP and if the concentration of this nucleotide must be reduced for aggregation and the release reaction to occur. Experiments along these lines have produced conflicting conclusions (Haslam and Taylor, 1971; Salzman, 1972). A problem with studies concerning cyclic nucleotide levels during aggregation is that cyclic variations may occur. Legarde and Dechavanne (1977) showed that thrombin produced a very early (5 sec) decrease in cyclic AMP which returned to normal, or even above normal over a period from 15 sec - 3 min after stimulation. The rebound in cyclic AMP was blocked by indomethacin suggesting that prostaglandin synthesis (*e.g.* PGE_2, PGD_2) was responsible for a secondary stimulation of cyclase activity. The rise in cyclic AMP after thrombin was accompanied by an increase in platelet prostaglandin synthesis (Droller, 1976). Other work has shown that platelet stimulation *in vitro* can occur without a measurably significant fall in basal levels of total cyclic AMP (Macfarlane and Mills, 1975; Haslam and Taylor, 1971) probably because the basal rate of cyclic AMP synthesis *in vitro* is quite low.

When adenylate cyclase is initially stimulated by PGE_1 so as to raise the concentration of cyclic AMP then a fall in cyclic AMP often occurs upon the addition of an aggregating agent (Claesson and Mahlmsten, 1977; Mills and Smith, 1971). This could be due to a direct effect of the aggregating agent on the cyclase as is the case with epinephrine (Zieve and Greenough, 1969), but the effect is often not observed in broken cell preparations. Since both basal and PGE_1-stimulated adenylate cyclase activity is inhibited by Ca^{2+} (Rodan and Feinstein, 1976; Vigdahl *et al.*, 1969) it is possible that Ca^{2+} mobilized by aggregating agents may contribute to the fall in cyclic AMP that has been observed. The

Ca^{2+}-ionophore A23187 has no effect on the cyclase in platelet homogenates but it strongly prevents the synthesis of cyclic AMP in intact platelets induced by PGE_1 (Rodan and Feinstein, 1976). In this case it seems clear that enough Ca^{2+} was mobilized in the cell by the ionophore to inhibit cyclase activity. Whether suffi- cient Ca^{2+} is mobilized by other aggregating agents to effectively inhibit adenylate cyclase remains to be determined. Thromboxane A_2 and PGH_2 also inhibit PGE_1 and PGI_2 stimulated formation of cyclic AMP in intact cells (Claesson and Mahlmsten, 1977; Miller *et al.*, 1977) perhaps indirectly by release of intracellular Ca^{2+}. The inhibition of adenylate cyclase by Ca^{2+} may represent an im- portant mechanism for positive feedback since cyclic AMP antagonizes Ca^{2+} in the platelet.

PGE_1 and dibutyryl cyclic AMP inhibit secretion and aggrega- tion due to A23187 (Feinstein and Fraser, 1975; White *et al.*, 1974). Cyclic AMP may affect the amount of Ca^{2+} that can be mobilized by aggregating agents, or inhibit reactions which are stimulated by Ca^{2+}. The spontaneous reversibility of platelet aggregation under some conditions, including stimulation by low concentrations of A23187, indicates that cellular mechanisms must exist to bind or re-accumulate released Ca^{2+}. Other recent experiments show that cyclic AMP regulates free Ca^{2+} levels in the platelet. As previous- ly mentioned, the activation of phospholipase A_2 by thrombin and collagen in intact platelets is antagonized by conditions which increase cyclic AMP levels. MDA and RCS formation and the O_2 burst induced by stimulation is blocked by PGE_1, dibutyryl cyclic AMP and prostacyclin (Feinstein *et al.*, 1977b; Lapetina *et al.*, 1977; Minkes *et al.*, 1977). The addition of A23187 overcomes the inhibition of PLA_2 activation, thereby demonstrating that cyclic AMP inhibits PLA_2 activity, not by a direct effect on the enzyme but rather by restricting the availability of Ca^{2+} to the enzyme (Feinstein *et al.*, 1977b). Furthermore, the increased uptake of ^{45}Ca by thrombin-treated platelets, which is likely due to exchange with free intracellular Ca^{2+}, is also inhibited by elevated plate- let cyclic AMP (Feinstein *et al.*, 1977b).

Grette (1963) isolated a factor which inhibited superprecipi- tation of platelet actomyosin and whose action could be reversed by addition of Ca^{2+}. This "relaxing factor" was later shown to consist of membranous vesicles which accumulate Ca^{2+} in the pre- sence of ATP (Robblee *et al.*, 1973; Statland *et al.*, 1969). The first direct evidence linking this transport system controlling cytoplasmic free Ca^{2+} levels to regulation by cyclic AMP comes from recent experiments of Käser-Glanzmann *et al.* (1977). They found that isolated platelet membrane vesicles (sedimenting be- tween 19,000 x g and 40,000 x g) which could actively accumulate Ca^{2+} in the presence of ATP and oxalate lost much of their transport efficacy when they were washed in the absence of ATP. Their ability

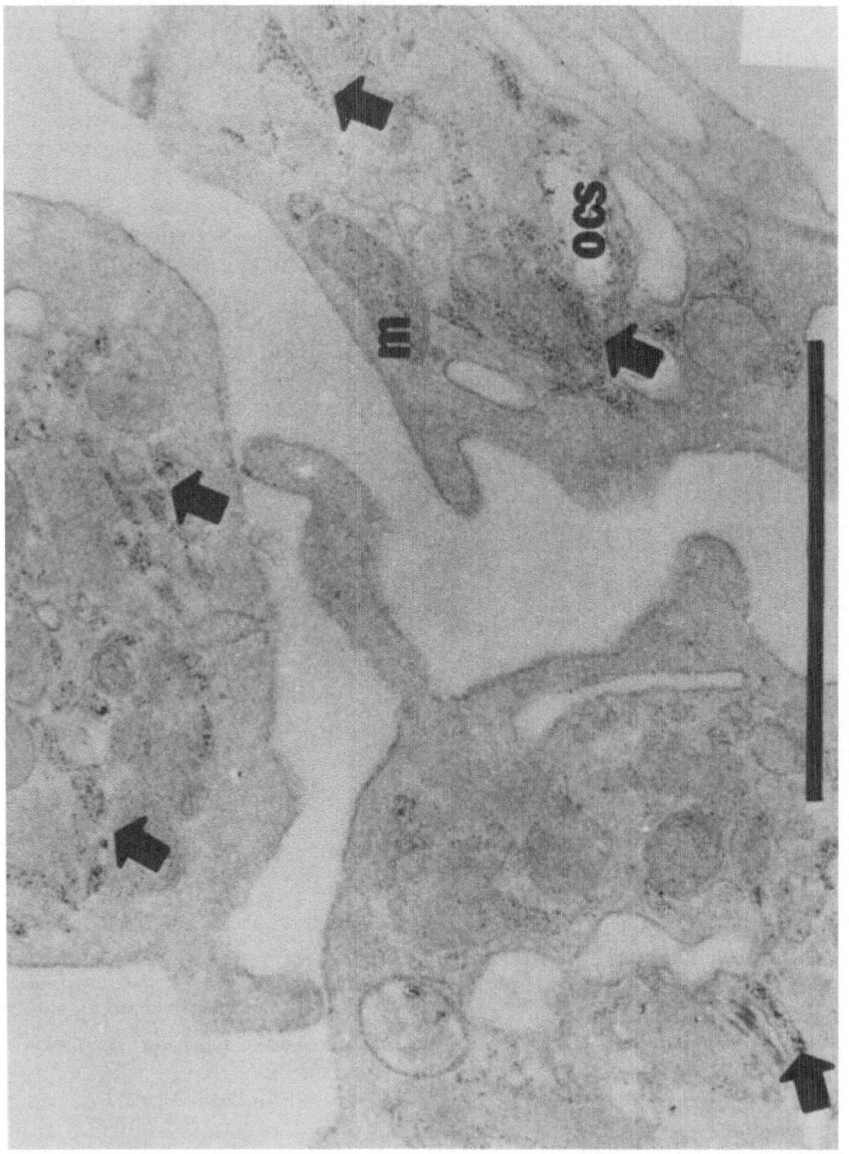

Figure 6

Figure 6. Cytochemical localization of adenylate cyclase activity in platelets. Electron micrograph of 3 platelets which were fixed in 1.25% glutaraldehyde for 15 minutes and then incubated in cytochemical media containing PGE₁, theophylline and adenylyl imidodiphosphate [APP(NH)P] to demonstrate adenylate cyclase activity. Reaction product is seen almost exclusively in the dense tubular system (arrows). A portion of the open canalicular system (OCS) in one of the cells shows a small amount of reaction product. Bar represents 1μ.

to accumulate Ca^{2+} was stimulated up to 3-fold by the addition of cyclic AMP and a platelet protein kinase preparation. It is uncertain whether the effect was to increase Ca^{2+} binding to the membranes, or to facilitate the translocation of Ca^{2+} to the vesicle interior.

Platelet membrane fractions which accumulate Ca^{2+} are also rich in adenylate cyclase activity (Rodan and Feinstein, 1976, and unpublished observations). However, there is no conclusive biochemical evidence that both enzymatic activities are present in the same organelle. Cyclic AMP-protein kinase stimulated accumulation of Ca^{2+} has been demonstrated previously in various types of muscle (Kirchberger *et al.*, 1972; Tada *et al.*, 1974; Andersson and Nilsson, 1972) and it was reported that adenylate cyclase activity was present in the sarcoplasmic reticulum. The presence of adenylate cyclase activity in the SR of cardiac muscle has recently been disputed (Engelhard *et al.*, 1976). In chicken skeletal muscle adenylate cyclase and Ca^{2+}-transport activities are in different subfractions of the SR (unpublished data). Cytochemically adenylate cyclase was found predominantly in the terminal cisternae of the SR.

Calcium-stimulated ATPase activity can be demonstrated cyto chemically in the DTS of intact platelets (Cutler *et al.*, 1978). The open canalicular system (OCS) also displayed similar ATPase activity. Most interestingly, in view of the effect of cyclic AMP on Ca^{2+} transport, the DTS also strongly reacts cytochemically for adenylate cyclase activity (Cutler *et al.*, 1978) (Figure 6). These experiments support the view that the DTS is an intracellular Ca^{2+}-"sink", but they do not yet prove it conclusively. Furthermore, the potentiality of the OCS and the rest of the surface membrane to transport Ca^{2+} remains unknown. Soluble cytoplasmic proteins could also play a role in the buffering of Ca^{2+} levels similar to that of parvalbumins in certain types of muscle (Gerday and Gillis, 1977). It is not known whether such proteins exist in the platelet, or whether their ability to bind Ca^{2+} could be influenced by cyclic AMP.

Since A23187 can "short circuit" a Ca^{2+}-pump and release accumulated Ca^{2+} (Käser-Glanzmann *et al.*, 1977) it is difficult to completely account for the ability of cyclic AMP to antagonize the ionophore's effects on aggregation and secretion. If Ca^{2+} binding were increased by cyclic AMP then the pool of free Ca^{2+} available to be released would be reduced. On the other hand, cyclic AMP may have effects besides that on Ca^{2+} transport which affect platelet aggregation and secretion. Regulation of the phosphorylation of membrane proteins could affect both the ability of cells to adhere together and the intracellular membrane fusion necessary for exocytosis. Several proteins in platelet homogenates, membranes or intact cells have been shown to be phosphorylated by endogenous protein kinases. Membrane polypeptide chains of 52K, 31K and 20K daltons were found to be phosphorylated by Steiner (1975). Phosphorylation was inhibited by Ca^{2+} and only the 52K peptide phosphorylation was cyclic AMP dependent. Booyse *et al.* (1973) found one major membrane protein of 44K daltons to be phosphorylated by cyclic AMP-dependent protein kinase. A minor phosphorylated component of 18-20K daltons was also detected. In intact platelets loaded with $^{32}PO_4$ proteins of 40-42K and 20K daltons showed increased labelling in cells stimulated with thrombin (Lyons *et al.*, 1975), collagen and A23187 (Haslam and Lynham, 1976). Phosphorylation of these proteins was decreased by PGE_1 and dibutyryl cyclic AMP in one study (Lyons *et al.*, 1975). Haslam and Lynham reported that phosphorylation of the 42K dalton protein, induced by collagen, was blocked substantially by a number of agents which inhibited serotonin release (*e.g.* indomethacin, tetracaine, verapamil, dibutyryl cyclic AMP, PGE_1, cytochalasin B and N-ethylmaleimide). It was suggested that the 42K protein was involved in the release reaction and that Ca^{2+} directly or indirectly stimulated protein kinase activity. Platelet protein kinases described up to this time have all been reported to be inhibited by Ca^{2+} (Lyons *et al.*, 1975; Steiner, 1975). However, Assaf (1977) recently reported that a cyclic nucleotide-independent protein kinase from human platelets phosphorylated platelet actomyosin best in the presence of Mg^{2+} plus low concentrations ($5 \times 10^{-5}M$) of Ca^{2+}.

Cyclic GMP levels in platelets are increased by a number of platelet stimulating agents including ADP, collagen and arachidonic acid (Davies *et al.*, 1976; Glass *et al.*, 1975). This points to a mechanism perhaps common to all stimuli as the causative factor affecting the concentration of this cyclic nucleotide. A rise in cytoplasmic Ca^{2+} levels could be responsible since guanylate cyclase is stimulated by Ca^{2+} (Rodan and Feinstein, 1976). It is not clear however whether the enzyme can be regulated by the range of free Ca^{2+} attained physiologically. Increased cyclic GMP has been linked to secretion, cellular motility, and contractile activity in various types of cells. However, no definitive biochemical function for cyclic GMP in these processes has been elucidated.

SUMMARY

Platelet activation by various stimuli appears to be initiated by the stimulus-induced translocation of intracellular Ca^{2+} stores (Figure 7). The release of internal Ca^{2+} sets in motion an integrated set of responses involving; (1) energy-producing reactions, (2) contraction of actomyosin-containing filaments, (3) alterations in microtubule assembly and distribution, (4) release of granules containing stored products which facilitate aggregation and clotting, (5) change in membrane surface properties leading to cellular adhesion, (6) activation of the synthesis of prostaglandins, PG endoperoxides and thromboxane A_2, and (7) the appearance of procoagulant platelet factor 3 in the surface membrane.

The sources of activator calcium and the mechanisms for its mobilization are not known with certainty. The platelet maintains a low level of free Ca^{2+} by active transport, binding and sequestration within certain organelles. The dense tubular system which contains Ca^{2+}-ATPase, adenylate cyclase and thromboxane synthetase activities is likely to be an important organelle for regulating intracellular Ca^{2+}. The significance of the surface membrane and mitochondria in Ca^{2+} regulation is less well understood.

Mobilization of Ca^{2+} apparently occurs through several mechanisms and platelet stimulating agents can act synergistically with each other. The pharmacological blockade of one route of activation will not prevent platelet aggregation if the stimulus can act through additional pathways. Therefore, blockade of prostaglandin synthetase activity by non-steroidal antiinflammatory agents, or destruction of ADP, by themselves, cannot completely prevent platelet aggregation under certain conditions if other mechanisms for releasing internal Ca^{2+} can be activated. Platelet stimulation is more effectively inhibited when more than a single mechanism for activation is blocked.

One of the most important physiological systems to inhibit platelet activation seems to be the generation of prostaglandins which stimulate adenylate cyclase activity. Cyclic AMP can block platelet activation by preventing a rise in free Ca^{2+}, probably by stimulating Ca^{2+}-transport out of the cytosol. The cyclic nucleotide may also affect phosphorylation of proteins which are involved in Ca^{2+} binding or which play a vital role in cellular aggregation and exocytosis. Two mechanisms for prostaglandin-modulated negative feedback exist; (1) the production of PGE_2 and especially PGD_2 during platelet stimulation, and (2) the synthesis of prostacyclin, by blood vessel walls, from PG

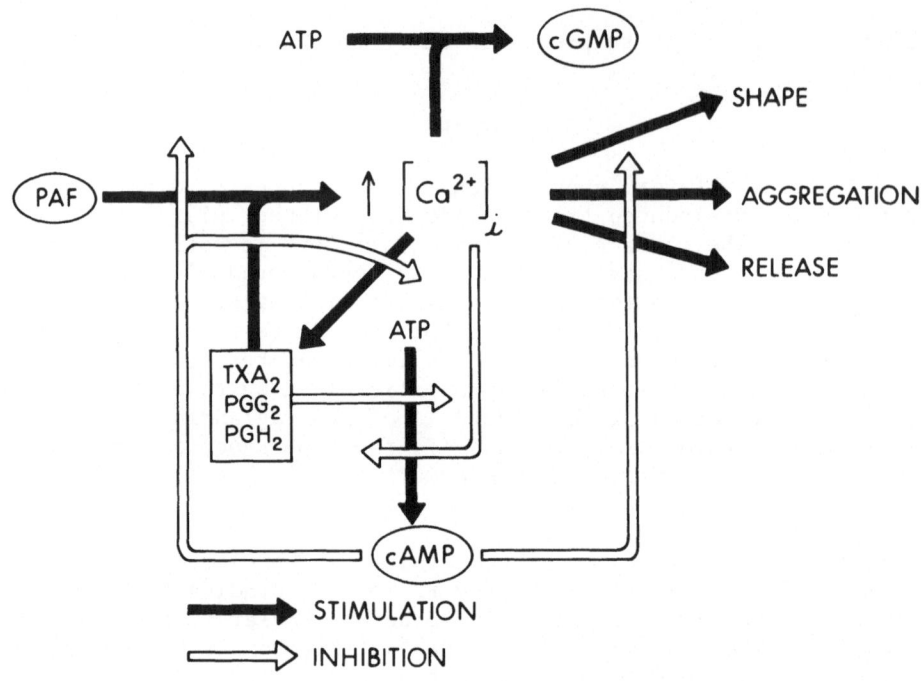

Figure 7. *Interrelationships between Ca^{2+}, cyclic nucleotides and arachidonic acid metabolites. Platelet aggregating factors (PAF) induce a rise in free intracellular calcium activity, $[Ca^{2+}]_i$, thereby initiating reactions leading to shape change, aggregation and the release reaction. Released ADP is itself an aggregating factor. Ca^{2+} initiates synthesis of PGG_2, PGH_2 and TXA_2 which also activate platelets and inhibit adenylate cyclase probably by causing a release of internal Ca^{2+}. Synthesis of cyclic AMP is inhibited directly by Ca^{2+} while that of cyclic GMP is probably stimulated. The role of cyclic GMP is not known but cyclic AMP inhibits platelet activation, in part at least, by antagonizing the rise in free Ca^{2+} and the formation of PG endoperoxides and TXA_2.*

endoperoxides diffusing out of stimulated platelets. Thromboxane synthetase inhibitors could become important pharmacological agents for the treatment of arterial thromboembolism since they could potentially shift synthesis away from TXA_2 formation towards formation of prostacyclin.

REFERENCES

Abramowitz, J. W., Stracher, A., and Detwiler, T. C., 1975, A second form of actin: platelet microfilaments depolymerized by ATP and divalent cations, *Arch. Biochem. Biophys.* 167: 230.

Adelstein, R. S., and Conti, M. A., 1975, Phosphorylation of platelet myosin increases actin-activated myosin ATPase activity, *Nature* 256: 597.

Andersson, R., and Nilsson, K., 1972, Cyclic AMP and calcium in relaxation in intestinal smooth muscle, *Nature (New Biol.)* 238: 119.

Assaf, S. A., 1977, Human platelet protein kinase phosphorylation reaction with platelet membrane and cytoplasmic enzymes and crystallization of a cyclic AMP-independent protein kinase, *Ann. N.Y. Acad. Sci.* 283: 159.

Babcock, D. F., First, N. L., and Lardy, H. A., 1976, Action of the ionophore A23187 at the cellular level. Separation of effects at the plasma and mitochondrial membranes, *J. Biol. Chem.* 251: 3881.

Bailin, G., 1977, Adenosine 3':5'-monophosphate-dependent protein kinase phosphorylation of a bovine cardiac actin complex, *Biophys. J.* 17: 159a.

Barber, A. J., and Jamieson, G. A., 1970, Isolation and characterization of plasma membranes from human blood platelets, *J. Biol. Chem.* 245: 6357.

Baumgartner, H. R., 1972, Platelet interaction with vascular structures, *Thromb. Diath. Haemorrh. Suppl.* 51: 161.

Baumgartner, H. R., and Born, G. V. R., 1968, Effects of 5-hydroxytryptamine on platelet aggregation, *Nature* 218: 137.

Behnke, O., Kristenson, B., and Nielson, L. E., 1971, Electron microscopical identification of platelet contractile proteins, *in* "Platelet Aggregation" (J. Caen, ed.), pp. 3-13, Masson et Cie, Paris.

Best, L. C., Martin, T. J., Russell, R. G. G., and Preston, F. E., 1977, Prostacyclin increases cyclic AMP levels and adenylate cyclase activity in platelets, *Nature* 267: 850.

Bettex-Galland, M., and Lüscher, E. F., 1965, Thrombosthenin, the contractile protein from blood platelets and its relation to other contractile proteins, *Adv. Protein Chem.* 20: 1.

Bills, T. K., Smith, J. B., and Silver, M. T., 1976, Metabolism of [^{14}C] arachidonic acid by human platelets, *Biochim. Biophys. Acta* 424: 303.

Blackwell, G. J., Duncombe, W. G., Flower, R. J., Parsons, M. F., and Vane, J. R., 1977, The distribution and metabolism of arachidonic acid in rabbit platelets during aggregation and its modification by drugs, *Brit. J. Pharmacol.* 59: 353.

Booyse, F. M., Guliani, D., Marr, J. J., and Rafelson, M. E. Jr., 1973, Cyclic adenosine 3',5'-monophosphate dependent protein kinase of human platelets: membrane phosphorylation and regulation of platelet function, *Ser. Haemat.* 6: 351.

Born, G. V. R., 1972, Current ideas on the mechanism of platelet aggregation, *Ann. N.Y. Acad. Sci.* 201: 4.

Boyle-Kay, M., and Fudenberg, H. H., 1973, Inhibition and reversal of platelet activation by cytochalasin B or colcemid, *Nature* 244: 288.

Charles, M. A., Lawecki, J., Pictet, R., Grodsky, G. M., 1975, Interrelationships of glucose, cyclic adenosine 3':5'-monophosphate and calcium, *J. Biol. Chem.* 250: 6134.

Charo, I., Detwiler, T. C., Feinman, R. D., Lubowsky, J., and Zabinski, M. P., 1976a, A new intracellular calcium antagonist has been used to investigate platelet secretion, aggregation, and malondialdehyde formation, *Circ.* 54: 0762.

Charo, I., Feinman, R. D., and Detwiler, T. C., 1976b, Inhibition of platelet secretion by an antagonist of intracellular calcium, *Biochem. Biophys. Res. Commun.* 72: 1462.

Chater, B. V., 1976, The role of membrane bound complement in the aggregation of mammalian platelet by collagen, *Brit. J. Haematol.* 32: 515.

Cinti, D. L., and Feinstein, M. B., 1976, Platelet cytochrome P-450: A possible role in arachidonate-induced aggregation, *Biochim. Biophys. Res. Commun.* 73: 171.

Claesson, H.-E., and Mahlmsten, C., 1977, On the relationship of prostaglandin endoperoxide G_2 and cyclic nucleotides in platelet function, *Eur. J. Biochem.* 76: 277.

Cochrane, D. E., and Douglas, W. W., 1974, Calcium induced extrusion of secretory granules (exocytosis) in mast cells exposed to 48/80 or ionophores A23187 and X-537A, *Proc. Nat. Acad. Sci. U.S.A.* 74: 408.

Cochrane, D. E., Douglas, W. W., Mouri, T., and Nakarato, Y., 1975, Calcium and stimulus-secretion coupling in the adrenal medulla: contrasting stimulating effects of the ionophores X-537A and A23187 on catecholamine output, *J. Physiol. (London)* 252: 363.

Cohen, I., Kaminski, E., and deVries, A., 1973, Actin-linked regulation of the human platelet contractile system, *FEBS Lett.* 34: 315.

Crawford, N., 1976, Platelet microfilaments and microtubules, *in* "Platelets in Biology and Pathology" (J. L. Gordon, ed.), pp. 121-133, North Holland Publishing Co., Amsterdam.

Cutler, L. S., Rodan, G. A., and Feinstein, M. B., 1978, Cytochemical localization of adenylate cyclase and ATPase activity in the dense tubular system of human platelets, submitted for publication.

Davies, T., Davidson, M. M. L., McClenaghan, M. D., Say, A., and Haslam, R. J., 1976, Factors affecting platelet cyclic GMP levels during aggregation induced by collagen and by arachidonic acid, *Thrombosis Res.* 9: 387.

Day, H. J., and Holmsen, H., 1971a, Adenine nucleotides and platelet function, *Ser. Haematol.* 4: 28.

Day, H. J., and Holmsen, H., 1971b, Concepts of the blood platelet release reaction, *Ser. Haemat.* 4: 3.

Derksen, A., and Cohen, P., 1975, Patterns of fatty acid release from endogenous substrates by human platelet homogenates and membranes, *J. Biol. Chem.* 250: 9342.

Des Prez, R. M., and Marney, S. R., Jr., 1971, Immunological reactions involving platelets, *in* "The Circulating Platelet" (S. A. Johnson, ed.), pp. 415-471, Academic Press, New York.

Detwiler, T. C., 1972, Control of energy metabolism in platelets. The effect of thrombin and cyanide on glycolysis, *Biochim. Biophys. Acta* 256: 163.

Detwiler, T. C., and Feinman, R. D., 1973, Kinetics of the thrombin-induced release of calcium (II) by platelets, *Biochemistry* 12: 282.

Douglas, W. W., 1968, Stimulus-secretion coupling: the concept and clues from chromaffin and other cells, *Brit. J. Pharmacol.* 34: 451.

Droller, M. J., 1976, Thrombin-induced platelet prostaglandin and cyclic AMP production and a possible intrinsic modulation of platelet function, *Scand. J. Haematol.* 17: 167.

Engelhard, V. H., Plut, D. A., and Storm, D. R., 1976, Subcellular location of adenylate cyclase in rat cardiac muscle, *Biochim. Biophys. Acta* 451: 48.

Evans, G., Packham, M. A., Nishizawa, E. E., Mustard, J. F., and Murphy, E. A., 1968, The effect of acetylsalicylic acid on platelet function, *J. Exp. Med.* 128: 877.

Fabiato, A., and Fabiato, F., 1977, Calcium release from the sarcoplasmic reticulum, *Circ. Res.* 40: 119.

Feinman, R. D., and Detwiler, T. C., 1974, Platelet secretion induced by divalent cation ionophores, *Nature* 249: 172.

Feinman, R. D., and Detwiler, T. C., 1975, Absence of a requirement for extracellular calcium for secretion from platelets, *Thrombosis Res.* 7: 677.

Feinstein, M. B., and Paimre, M., 1969, Pharmacological action of local anesthetics on excitation-contraction coupling in striated and smooth muscle, *Fed. Proc.* 28: 1643.

Feinstein, M. B., and Fraser, C., 1975, Human platelet secretion and aggregation induced by calcium ionophores. Inhibition by PGE1 and dibutyryl cyclic AMP, *J. gen. Physiol.* 66: 561.

Feinstein, M. B., Fiekers, J., and Fraser, C., 1976, An analysis of the mechanism of local anesthetic inhibition of platelet aggregation and secretion, *J. Pharmacol. Exp. Ther.* 197: 215.

Feinstein, M. B., Henderson, E., and Sha'afi, R. I., 1977a, The effects of alterations of transmembrane Na^+ and K^+ gradients by ionophores (nigericin, monensin) on serotonin transport in human blood platelets, *Biochim. Biophys. Acta* 468: 284.

Feinstein, M. B., Becker, E. L., and Fraser, C., 1977b, Thrombin, collagen and A23187 stimulated endogenous platelet arachidonate metabolism: Differential inhibition by PGE, local anesthetics and a serine-protease inhibitor, *Prostaglandins*, in press.

Ford, L. E., and Podolsky, R. J., 1972, Calcium uptake and force development by skinned muscle fibers in EGTA buffered solutions, *J. Physiol. (London)* 223: 1.

Foreman, J. C., Mongar, J. L., and Gomperts, B. D., 1973, Calcium ionophores and movement of calcium ions following the physiological stimulus to a secretory process, *Nature* 245: 249.

Friedman, F., and Detwiler, T. C., 1975, Stimulus-secretion coupling in platelets. Effects of drugs on secretion of adenosine 5'-triphosphate, *Biochemistry* 14: 1315.

Fukami, M. H., Holmsen, H., and Bauer, J., 1976, Thrombin-induced oxygen consumption, malonyldialdehyde formation and serotonin in human platelets, *Biochim. Biophys. Acta* 428: 253.

Gardos, G., 1958, The function of calcium in the potassium permeability of human erythrocytes, *Biochim. Biophys. Acta* 30: 653.

Gear, A. R. L., and Schneider, W., 1975, Control of platelet glycogenolysis activation of phosphorylase kinase by calcium, *Biochim. Biophys. Acta* 392: 111.

Gerday, C., and Gillis, J. M., 1977, The possible role of parvalbumins in the control of contraction, *J. Physiol.* 258: 96P.

Gerrard, J. M., White, J. G., and Rao, G. H. R., 1974, Effects of the ionophore A23187 on blood platelets. II. Influence on ultrastructure, *Amer. J. Path.* 77: 151.

Gerrard, J. M., White, J. G., Rao, G. H. R., Krivit, W., and Witkop, C. J., 1975, Labile aggregation stimulating substance (LASS): The factor from storage pool deficient platelets correcting defective aggregation and release of aspirin treated normal platelets, *Brit. J. Haematol.* 29: 657.

Gerrard, J. M., White, J. G., and Rao, G. H. R., 1976, Localization of prostaglandin production in the platelet dense tubular system, *Amer. J. Path.* 83: 283.

Glass, D. B., Gerrard, J. M., White, J. G., and Goldberg, N. D., 1975, Cyclic GMP formation in human platelets aggregated by arachidonic acid, *Blood* 46: 1033.

Gordon, J. L., and MacIntrye, D. E., 1974, Inhibition of collagen induced platelet aggregation by aspirin, *Brit. J. Pharmacol.* 50: 469P.

Gorman, R. R., Bundy, G. L., Peterson, D. C., Sun, F. F., Miller, O. V., and Fitzpatrick, F. A., 1977a, Inhibition of human platelet thromboxane synthetase by 9,11-azoprosta-5,13-dienoic acid, *Proc. Nat. Acad. Sci. U. S. A.* 74: 4007.

Gorman, R. R., Bunting, S., and Miller, O. V., 1977b, Modulation of human platelet adenylate cyclase by prostacyclin (PGX), *Prostaglandins* 13: 377.

Grette, K., 1962, Studies on the mechanism of thrombin-catalyzed hemostatic reactions in blood platelets, *Acta Physiol. Scand.* 56 (Suppl. 195): 1.

Grette, K., 1963, Relaxing factor in extracts of blood platelets and its function in the cells, *Nature* 198: 488.

Gryglewski, R. J., Bunting, S., Moncada, S., Flower, R. J., and
  Vane, J. R., 1976, Arterial walls are protected against deposi-
  tion of platelet thrombi by a substance (prostaglandin X) which
  they make from prostaglandin endoperoxides, *Prostaglandins*
  12: 685.
Haeusler, G., 1972, Differential effect of verapamil on excitation-
  contraction coupling in adrenergic nerve terminals, *J. Pharmacol.
  Exp. Ther.* 180: 672.
Hamberg, M., and Samuelsson, B., 1973, Detection and isolation of
  an endoperoxide intermediate in prostaglandin biosynthesis,
  Proc. Nat. Acad. Sci. U. S. A. 70: 899.
Hamberg, M., and Samuelsson, B., 1974, Prostaglandin endoperoxides,
  novel transformations of arachidonic acid in human platelets,
  Proc. Nat. Acad. Sci. U. S. A. 71: 3400.
Hamberg, M., Svensson, J., Wakabayashi, T., and Samuelsson, B.,
  1974a, Isolation and structure of two prostaglandin endoperoxides
  that cause platelet aggregation, *Proc. Nat. Acad. Sci. U. S. A.*
  71: 345.
Hamberg, M., Svensson, J., and Samuelsson, B., 1974b, Prostaglandin
  endoperoxides. A new concept concerning the mode of action and
  release of prostaglandins, *Proc. Nat. Acad. Sci. U. S. A.* 71:
  3824.
Hamberg, M., Svensson, J., and Samuelsson, B., 1975, Thromboxanes:
  a new group of biologically active compounds derived from prostaglandin endoperoxides, *Proc. Nat. Acad. Sci. U. S. A.* 72: 2994.
Harris, G. L., Cone, D. H., and Crawford, N., 1974, Effect of divalent cations and chelating agents on the ATPase activity of
  platelet contractile protein, thrombosthenin, *Biochem. Med.*
  11: 10.
Haslam, R., and Lynham, J. A., 1976, Increased phosphorylation of
  . specific blood platelet proteins in association with the release
  reaction, *Biochem. Soc. Transactions* 4: 694.
Haslam, R. J., and Taylor, A., 1971, Role of cyclic 3',5'-adenosine
  monophosphate in platelet aggregation, *in* "Platelet Aggregation"
  (J. Caen, ed.), pp. 85-93, Masson et Cie, Paris.
Haslam, R. J., Davidson, M. M. L., and McClenaghan, M. D., 1975,
  Cytochalasin B, the blood platelet release reaction and cyclic
  GMP, *Nature* 253: 455.
Henson, P. M., Gould, D., and Becker, E. L., 1976, Activation of
  stimulus-specific serine esterases (proteases) in the initiation
  of platelet secretion. I. Demonstration with organophosphorus
  inhibitors, *J. Exper. Med.* 144: 1657.
Holmsen, H., Day, H. J., and Stormorken, H., 1969, The blood platelet release reaction, *Scand. J. Haematol. (Suppl.)* 8: 1.
Holmsen, H., 1974, Are platelet shape change, aggregation and release reaction tangible manifestations of one basic platelet
  function, *in* "Platelets, Production, Function, Transfusion and
  Storage" (M. Baldini and S. Ellie, eds.), pp. 207-220, Grune
  and Stratton, New York.

Horne, W. C., and Singer, E. R., 1976, The effect of aggregating agents and drugs on the membrane potential of washed human platelets, *Fed. Proc.* 35: 1451.

Hovig, T., 1963, Release of platelet aggregating substance (adenosine diphosphate) from rabbit platelets induced by saline "extract" of tendons, *Thromb. Diath. Haemorrh.* 9: 264.

Izrael, V., Zawilska, K., Jaisson, F., Levy-Toledano, S., and Caen, J., 1974, Effect of a fast removal of plasmatic ADP by the creatine phosphate and creatine phosphokinase system on human platelet function in vitro, *in* "Platelets: Production, Function, Transfusion and Storage" (M. G. Baldini and S. Ebbe, eds.), pp. 187-196, Grune and Stratton, Inc., New York.

Käser-Glanzmann, R., Jakábová, M., George, J. N., and Lüscher, E. F., 1977, Stimulation of calcium uptake in platelet membrane vesicles by adenosine 3',5'-cyclic monophosphate and protein kinase, *Biochim. Biophys. Acta* 466: 429.

Kinlough-Rathbone, R. L., Chahil, A., Packham, M. A., Riemers, H.-J., and Mustard, J. F., 1975, Effects of ionophore A23187 on thrombin-degranulated washed rabbit platelets, *Thromb. Res.* 7: 435.

Kinlough-Rathbone, R. L., Riemers, H.-J., Mustard, J. F., and Packham, M. A., 1976, Sodium arachidonate can induce platelet shape change and aggregation which are independent of the release reaction, *Science* 192: 1011.

Kirchberger, M. A., Tada, M., and Katz, A. M., 1972, Adenosine 3':5'-monophosphate-dependent protein kinase-catalyzed phosphorylation reaction and its relationship to calcium transport in cardiac sarcoplasmic reticulum, *J. Biol. Chem.* 249: 6166.

Kunze, H., and Vogt, W., 1971, Significance of phospholipase A for prostaglandin formation, *Ann. N. Y. Acad. Sci.* 180: 123.

Kunze, H., Nahas, N., Traynor, J. R., and Wurl, M., 1976, Effects of local anesthetics on phospholipases, *Biochim. Biophys. Acta* 441: 93.

Lagarde, M., and Dechavanne, M., 1977, Thrombin decreases platelet cyclic AMP in the absence of prostaglandin synthesis, *Biomedicine* 27: 110.

Lages, B., Scrutton, M. C., Holmsen, H., Day, H. J., and Weiss, H. J., 1975, Metal ion content of gel-filtered platelets from patients with storage pool disease, *Blood* 46: 119.

Lapetina, E. G., Schmitges, C. J., Chandrabose, K., and Cuatrecasas, P., 1977, Cyclic adenosine 3',5'-monophosphate and prostacyclin inhibit membrane phospholipase activity in platelets, *Biochem. Biophys. Res. Commun.* 76: 828.

Lazarides, E., 1976, Actin, α-actinin and tropomyosin interaction in the structural organization of actin filaments in nonmuscle cells, *J. Cell Biol.* 68: 202.

Le Breton, G. C., Dinerstein, R. J., Roth, L. J., and Feinberg, H., 1976, Direct evidence for intracellular divalent cation redistribution associated with platelet shape change, *Biochem.*

Biophys. Res. Commun. 71: 362.

Le Breton, G. C., and Dinerstein, R. J., 1977, Effect of the calcium antagonist TMB-6 on intracellular calcium distribution associated with platelet shape change, *Thrombosis Res.* 10: 521.

Lyons, R. M., Stanford, N., and Majerus, P. W., 1975, Thrombin-induced protein phosphorylation in human platelets, *J. Clin. Invest.* 56: 924.

Macfarlane, D. E., and Mills, D. C. B., 1975, The effects of ATP on platelets: evidence against the central role of released ADP in primary aggregation, *Blood* 46: 309.

Malik, M. N., Rosenberg, S., Detwiler, T. C., and Stracher, A., 1974, Role of Ca^{2+} in the allosteric regulation of platelet actomyosin, *Biochem. Biophys. Res. Commun.* 61: 1071.

Mahlmsten, C., Hamberg, M., Svensson, J., and Samuelsson, B., 1975, Physiological role of an endoperoxide in human platelets: hemostatic defect due to platelet cyclo-oxygenase deficiency, *Proc. Nat. Acad. Sci. U. S. A.* 72: 1446.

Marcus, A. J., 1969, Platelet function, *N. Eng. J. Med.* 280: 1213.

Martin, J. H., Carson, F. L., and Race, G. J., 1974, Calcium-containing platelet granules, *J. Cell. Biol.* 60: 775.

Massini, P., and Lüscher, E. F., 1972, On the mechanism by which cell contact induces the release reaction of blood platelets: the effect of cationic polymers, *Thromb. Diath. Haemorrh.* 27: 121.

Massini, P., and Lüscher, E. F., 1974, Some effects of ionophores for divalent cations on blood platelets. Comparison with the effects of thrombin, *Biochim. Biophys. Acta* 372: 109.

Miller, J. L., Katz, A. J., and Feinstein, M. B., 1975, Plasmin inhibition of thrombin-induced platelet aggregation, *Thromb. Diath. Haemorrh.* 33: 286.

Miller, O. V., Johnson, R. A., and Gorman, R. R., 1977, Inhibition of PGE_1-stimulated cAMP accumulation in human platelets by thromboxane A_2, *Prostaglandins* 13: 599.

Mills, D. C. B., and Smith, J. B., 1971, The control of platelet responsiveness by agents that influence cyclic AMP metabolism, *Ann. N. Y. Acad. Sci.* 201: 391.

Minkes, M., Stanford, N., Shi, M. M. Y., Roth, G. J., Raz, A., Needleman, P., and Majerus, P. N., 1977, Cyclic adenosine 3',5'-monophosphate inhibits the availability of arachidonate to prostaglandin synthetase in human platelet suspensions, *J. Clin. Invest.* 59: 449.

Moncada, S., Bunting, S., Mullane, K., Thorogood, P., Vane, J. R., Raz, A., and Needleman, P., 1977, Imidazole: a selective inhibitor of thromboxane synthetase, *Prostaglandins* 13: 611.

Morse, E. E., Jackson, D. P., and Conley, C. L., 1965, Role of platelet fibrinogen in the reactions of platelets to thrombin, *J. Clin. Invest.* 44: 809.

Mürer, E. H., 1969, Thrombin induced release of calcium from blood platelets, *Science* 166: 623.

Mürer, E. H., 1972, Factors influencing the initiation and the extrusion phase of the platelet release reaction, *Biochim. Biophys. Acta* 261: 435.

Mürer, E. H., and Holme, R., 1970, A study of the release of calcium from human blood platelets and its inhibition by metabolic inhibitors N-ethylmaleimide and aspirin, *Biochim. Biophys. Acta* 222: 197.

Mürer, E. H., Davenport, K., Rausch, M. A., Day, H. J., 1975, Metabolic aspects of the secretions of stored compounds from blood platelets. V. Effect of ionophore A23187 on washed platelets, *Biochim. Biophys. Acta* 451: 1.

Mürer, E. H., Stewart, G. J., Rausch, M. A., and Day, H. J., 1976, Calcium ionophore A23187 (Eli Lilly) effect on platelet function, structure and metabolism, *Thromb. Diath. Haemorrh.* 34: 72.

Mustard, J. F., and Packham, M. A., 1970, Factors influencing platelet function: adhesion, release, and aggregation, *Pharmacol. Rev.* 22: 97.

Mustard, J. F., Perry, D. W., Kinlough-Rathbone, R. L., and Packham, M. A., 1975, Factors responsible for ADP-induced release reaction of human platelets, *Amer. J. Physiol.* 228: 1757.

Nachman, R. L., and Weksler, B., 1972, The platelet as an inflammatory cell, *Ann. N. Y. Acad. Sci.* 201: 131.

Needleman, P., Minkes, M., and Raz, A., 1976a, Thromboxanes: selective bio-synthesis and distinct biological properties, *Science* 193: 163.

Needleman, P., Moncada, S., Bunting, S., Vane, J. R., Hamberg, M., and Samuelsson, B., 1976b, Identification of an enzyme in platelet microsomes which generates thromboxane A_2 from prostaglandin endoperoxides, *Nature* 261: 558.

Needleman, P., Raz, A., Ferendelli, J. A., and Minkes, M., 1977, Application of imidazole as a selective inhibitor of thromboxane synthetase in human platelets, *Proc. Nat. Acad. Sci. U. S. A.* 74: 1716.

Nelsestuen, G. L., Broderius, M., and Martin, G., 1976, Role of γ-carboxyglutamic acid. Cation specificity of prothrombin and factor X-phospholipid binding, *J. Biol. Chem.* 251: 6886.

Northover, B. J., 1977, Effect of indomethacin and related drugs on the calcium ion-dependent secretion of lysosomal and other enzymes by neutrophil polymorphonuclear leukocytes *in vitro*, *Brit. J. Pharmacol.* 59: 253.

Nugteren, D. H., 1975, Arachidonate lipoxygenase in blood platelets, *Biochim. Biophys. Acta* 326: 448.

Nugteren, D. H., and Hazelhof, E., 1973, Isolation and properties of intermediates in prostaglandin biosynthesis, *Biochim. Biophys. Acta* 326: 448.

Nyman, D., 1977, Collagen-induced platelet aggregation: evidence of several mechanisms for the induction of platelet release by collagen, *Thromb. Res.* 10: 743.

O'Brien, J. R., 1968, Effect of salicylates on human platelets, *Lancet* 1968i: 779.

Odell, T. T., and Upton, A. C., 1955, Distribution of Calcium[45] in platelets and bone marrow of rats, *Acta Haematol*. 14: 291.

Oelz, O., Oelz, R., Knapp, H. R., Sweetman, B. J., and Oates, J. A., 1977, Biosynthesis of prostaglandin D_2. I. Formation of prostaglandin D_2 by human platelets, *Prostaglandins* 13: 225.

Oplatka, A., Gadasi, H., Tirosh, R., Laiyed, Y., Muhlrad, A., and Liron, N., 1974, Demonstration of mechanochemical coupling in systems containing actin, ATP and non-aggregating active myosin derivatives, *J. Mechanochem. Cell Motility* 2: 295.

Oschman, J. L., Hall, T. A., Peters, P. D., and Wall, B. J., 1974, Microprobe analysis of membrane-associated calcium deposits in squid giant axon, *J. Cell Biol*. 61: 156.

Packham, M. A., Guccione, M. A., Chang, P.-L., and Mustard, J. F., 1973, Platelet aggregation and release: effects of low concentrations of thrombin or collagen, *Amer. J. Physiol*. 225: 38.

Packham, M. A., Kinbough-Rathbone, R. L., Riemers, H.-J., Scott, S., and Mustard, J. F., 1977, Mechanisms of platelet aggregation independent of adenosine diphosphate, *in* "Prostaglandins in Hematology" (M. J. Silver, J. B. Smith, and J. J. Kocsis, eds.), pp. 247-276, Spectrum Publications, Inc., New York.

Papahadjopoulos, D., Vail, W. J., Newton, C., Nir, S., Jacobson, K., Poste, G., and Lazo, R., 1977, Studies on membrane fusion. III. The role of calcium-induced phase changes, *Biochim. Biophys. Acta* 465: 579.

Pickett, W. C., and Cohen, P., 1976, Mechanism of the thrombin-mediated burst in oxygen consumption by human platelets, *J. Biol. Chem*. 251: 2536.

Pickett, W. C., Jesse, R. L., and Cohen, P., 1977, Initiation of phospholipase A_2 activity in human platelets by the calcium ion ionophore A23187, *Biochim. Biophys. Acta* 486: 209.

Pollard, T. D., Fujiwara, K., Niederman, R., and Maupin-Szamier, P., 1976, Evidence for the role of cytoplasmic actin and myosin in cellular structure and motility, *in* "Cell Motility. Cold Spring Harbor Conference on Cell Proliferation," Vol. 2 (R. Goldman, T. Pollard, J. Rosenbaum, eds.), pp. 475-485, Cold Spring Harbor, New York.

Poulsen, J. H., and Williams, J. A., 1977, Effects of the calcium ionophore A23187 on pancreatic acinar cell membrane potentials and amylase release, *J. Physiol*. 264: 323.

Puszkin, E., Puszkin, S., and Aledort, L. M., 1971, Colchicine-binding protein from human platelets and its effect on muscle myosin and platelet myosin-like thrombosthenin-M, *J. Biol. Chem*. 246: 271.

Puszkin, S., Kochwa, S., and Rosenfield, R. E., 1975, Regulatory complex of human platelet actomyosin, *J. Cell Biol*. 67: 346a.

Puszkin, S., Lin, E., Kochwa, S., and Rosenfield, R. E., 1976, Immunological, physiochemical, and Ca^{2+} binding properties of

platelet and muscle regulatory proteins bound by lytron particles, *Fed. Proc.* 35: 299.

Ray, K. P., and England, P. J., 1976, Phosphorylation of the inhibitory subunit of troponin and its effect on the calcium dependence of cardiac myofibril adenosine triphosphatase, *FEBS
Letters* 70: 11.

Reddy, Y. S., and Wyborny, L. E., 1976, Phosphorylation of guinea
pig cardiac natural actomyosin and its effect on ATPase activity,
Biochem. Biophys. Res. Commun. 73: 703.

Reed, P. W., 1977, Calcium ionophore activity of prostaglandin
endoperoxides and stabilized analogues of PGH_2, *Fed. Proc.*
36: 673.

Ridgway, E. B., Gilkey, J. C., and Jaffe, L. F., 1977, Free calcium
increases explosively in activating medaka eggs, *Proc. Nat.
Acad. Sci. U. S. A.* 74: 623.

Robblee, L. S., Shepro, D., Belamarich, F. A., and Towle, C.,
1973, Platelet calcium flux and the release reaction, *Ser.
Haemat.* 6: 311.

Robblee, L. S., Shepro, D., and Belamarich, F. A., 1973, Calcium
uptake and associated adenosine triphosphatase activity of
isolated platelet membranes, *J. gen. Physiol.* 61: 462.

Rodan, G. A., and Feinstein, M. B., 1976, Interrelationships
between Ca^{2+} and adenylate and guanylate cyclases in the control of platelet secretion and aggregation, *Proc. Nat. Acad.
Sci. U. S. A.* 73: 1829.

Rubin, R. P., 1974, "Calcium and the Secretory Process," Plenum
Press, New York.

Russell, J. T., Hansen, E. L., and Thorn, N. A., 1974, Calcium
and stimulus-secretion coupling in the neurohypophysis. III.
Ca^{2+} ionophore (A-23187)-induced release of vasopressin from
isolated rat neurohypophyses, *Acta Endocrinol. (Kbh)* 77: 443.

Salganicoff, L., Hebda, P. A., Yandrasitz, J., and Fukami, M.
H., 1975, Subcellular fractionation of pig platelets, *Biochim.
Biophys. Acta* 385: 294.

Salzman, E. W., 1972, Cyclic AMP and platelet function, *New Eng.
J. Med.* 286: 358.

Sato, T., Herman, L., Chandler, J. A., Stracher, A., and Detwiler,
T. C., 1975, Localization of a thrombin-sensitive calcium
pool in platelets, *J. Histochem. Cytochem.* 23: 103.

Scarpa, A., Baldassare, J., and Inesi, G., 1972, The effect of
calcium ionophore on fragmented sarcoplasmic reticulum, *J.
gen. Physiol.* 60: 735.

Schoene, N., and Iacono, J. M., 1973, Metabolism of linoleic
and arachidonic acids in blood platelets, *Fed. Proc.* 32: 119.

Schroeder, T. E., and Strickland, D. L., 1974, Ionophore A23187,
calcium and contractility in frog eggs, *Exp. Cell Res.* 83: 139.

Seegers, W. H., 1971, Role of platelets in blood clotting, *in* "The Circulating Platelet" (S. A. Johnson, ed.), pp. 301-354, Academic Press, New York.

Seegers, W. H., Heene, D., Marciniak, E., Ivanovic, N., and Caldwell, M. J., 1965, Sensitivity of thrombin and autothrombin C to selected enzyme inhibitors, *Life Sci.* 4: 425.

Silver, M. J., Smith, J. B., Ingerman, C., and Kocsis, J. J., 1973, Arachidonic acid-induced human platelet aggregation and prosta-glandin formation, *Prostaglandins* 4: 863.

Skaer, R. J., Peters, P. D., and Emmines, J. P., 1974, The locali-zation of calcium and phosphorus in human platelets, *J. Cell. Sci.* 15: 679.

Smith, J. B., and Willis, A. L., 1971, Aspirin selectively inhi-bits prostaglandin production in human platelets, *Nature (New Biol.)* 231: 235.

Smith, J. B., Ingerman, C. M., Kocsis, J. J., and Silver, M. J., 1973, Formation of prostaglandins during the aggregation of human blood platelets, *J. Clin. Invest.* 52: 965.

Smith, J. B., and Macfarlane, D. E., 1974, Platelets, *in* "The Prostaglandins" (P. W. Ramswell, ed.), pp. 293-343, Plenum Press, New York.

Smith, J. B., Silver, M. J., Ingerman, C. M., and Kocsis, J. J., 1974, Prostaglandin D_2 inhibits the aggregation of human plate-lets, *Thrombosis Res.* 5: 291.

Smith, J. B., Ingerman, C. M., and Silver, M. J., 1976, Malondial-dehyde formation as an indication of prostaglandin production by human platelets, *J. Lab. Clin. Med.* 88: 167.

Smith, M. J. H., Walker, J. R., Ford-Hutchinson, A. W., and Penington, D. G., 1976, Platelets, prostaglandins and inflamma-tion, *Agents and Actions* 6: 701.

Sneddon, J. M., 1972, Divalent cations and the blood platelet re-lease reaction, *Nature (New Biol.)* 236: 103.

Solaro, R. J., Moir, A. J. G., and Perry, S. V., 1976, Phosphory-lation of troponin I and the inotropic effect of adrenaline in the perfused rabbit heart, *Nature* 262: 615.

Statland, B. E., Heagen, B. M., and White, J. G., 1969, Uptake of calcium by platelet relaxing factor, *Nature* 223: 521.

Steiner, M., 1975, Endogenous phosphorylation of platelet mem-brane proteins, *Archiv. Biochem. Biophys.* 171: 245.

Steiner, M., and Tateishi, T., 1974, Distribution and transport of calcium in human platelets, *Biochim. Biophys. Acta* 367: 232.

Steinhardt, R. A., and Epel, D., 1974, Activation of sea urchin eggs by Ca^{++} ionophore, *Proc. Nat. Acad. Sci. U. S. A.* 71: 1915.

Stuart, M., 1975, Inherited defects of platelet function, *Sem. Hematol.* 12: 233.

Svensson, J., Hamberg, M., and Samuelsson, B., 1975, Prostaglandin endoperoxides. 1X characterization of rabbit aorta contracting substance (RCS) from guinea pig lung and human platelets, *Acta Physiol. Scand.* 94: 222.

Tada, M., Kirchberger, M. A., Repke, D. I., and Katz, A. M., 1974, The stimulation of calcium transport in cardiac sarcoplasmic reticulum by cyclic adenosine 3':5'-monophosphate-dependent kinase, *J. Biol. Chem.* 249: 6174.

Takaya, K., 1975, Electron probe microanalysis of the dense bodies of human blood platelets, *Arch. Histol. jap.* 37: 335.

Tateson, J. E., Moncada, S., and Vane, J. R., 1977, Effects of prostacyclin (PGX) on cyclic AMP concentrations in human platelets, *Prostaglandins* 13: 389.

Thorens, S., and Endo, M., 1975, Calcium-induced calcium release and "depolarization-induced" calcium release: their physiological significance, *Proc. Japan Acad.* 51: 473.

Thorens, S., Schaub, M. C., and Lüscher, E. F., 1973, A calcium-sensitizing system from human platelets and its activity on muscle and platelet actomyosin, *Experientia* 29: 349.

Vanaman, T. C., Sharief, F., Awramik, J. L., Mendel, P. A., and Watterson, D. M., 1976, Chemical and biological properties of the ubiquitous troponin-c like protein from non-muscle tissue a multifunctional Ca^{2+} dependent regulatory protein, *in* "Contractile Systems in Non-Muscle Tissues) (S. V. Perry, A. Magreth, and R. S. Adelstein, eds.), pp. 165-176, Elsevier/North Holland Biomedical Press, New York.

Vane, J. R., 1971, Inhibition of prostaglandin synthesis as a mechanism of action for aspirin-like drugs, *Nature (New Biol.)* 231: 232.

Vargaftig, B. B., and Zirinis, P., 1973, Platelet aggregation induced by arachidonic acid is accompanied by release of potential inflammatory mediators distinct from PGE_2 and $PGF_{2\alpha}$, *Nature (New Biol.)* 244: 114.

Vargaftig, B. B., and Dao Hai, N., 1975, Selective inhibition by mepacrine of the release of "rabbit aorta contracting substance" evoked by the administration of bradykinin, *J. Pharm. Pharmacol.* 24: 159.

Vargaftig, B., 1977, Carrageenan and thrombin trigger prostaglandin synthetase-independent aggregation of rabbit platelets: inhibition by phospholipase A_2 inhibitors, *J. Pharm. Pharmacol.* 29: 222.

Vigdahl, R. L., Marquis, N. R., and Tavormina, P. A., 1969, Platelet aggregation: II. Adenyl cyclase, prostaglandin E_1, and calcium, *Biochem. Biophys. Res. Commun.* 37: 409.

Wallach, D. F. H., Surgenor, D. M., and Steele, B. B., 1958, Calcium-lipid complexes in human platelets, *Blood* 13: 589.

Walsh, P. N., 1974, Platelets, blood coagulation and hemostasis, *in* "Platelets and Thrombosis" (S. Sherry, and A. Scriabine, eds.), pp. 23-43, University Park Press, Baltimore.

Weber, K., 1976, Biochemical anatomy of microfilaments in cells in tissue culture using immunofluorescence microscopy, *in* "Contractile Systems in Non-Muscle Tissues" (S. V. Perry, A. Margreth, and R. S. Adelstein, eds.), pp. 51-66, Elsevier/North Holland

Press, New York.

Weber, K., and Groeschel-Stewart, W., 1975, Antibody to myosin: the specific visualization of myosin-containing filaments in non-muscle cells, *Proc. Nat. Acad. Sci. U. S. A.* 71: 4561.

Wells, A. W., 1972, A kinetic study of the phospolipase A$_2$ (Crotalus adamanteus) catalyzed hydrolysis of 1,2-dibutyryl-sn-glycero-3-phosphorylcholine, *Biochemistry* 11: 1030.

Wells, A. W., 1974, A phospholipase A$_2$ model system. Calcium enhancement of the amine-catalyzed methanolysis of phosphatidylcholine, *Biochemistry* 13: 2258.

Weiss, H., 1975, Platelet physiology and abnormalities of platelet function, *New Eng. J. Med.* 293: 580.

White, J. G., 1971, Platelet morphology, *in* "The Circulating Platelet" (S. A. Johnson, ed.), pp. 45-121, Academic Press, New York.

White, J. G., 1972a, The sarcoplasmic reticulum of platelets, *Fed. Proc.* 31: 654.

White, J. G., 1972b, Interaction of membrane systems in blood platelets, *Amer. J. Pathol.* 66: 295.

White, J. G., and Krivit, W., 1965, Fine structural localization of adenosine triphosphatase in human platelets and other blood cells, *Blood* 26: 554.

White, J. G., and Krivit, W., 1967, The canalicular system of blood platelets: a possible sarcoplasmic reticulum, *J. Lab. Clin. Med.* 49: 60.

White, J. G., Rao, G. H. R., and Gerrard, J. M., 1974, Effect of the ionophore A23187 on blood platelets. I. Influence on aggregation and secretion, *Amer. J. Pathol.* 77: 135.

Whittle, B. J. R., 1976, Calcium and inhibition of histamine release from rat peritoneal mast cells by non-steroid anti-inflammatory agents, *Brit. J. Pharmacol.* 58: 446P.

Willis, A. L., Vane, F. M., Kuhn, D. C., Scott, C. G., and Petrin, M., 1974, An endoperoxide aggregator (LASS) formed in platelets in response to thrombotic stimuli, *Prostaglandins* 8: 453.

Wolfe, S., and Shulman, N. R., 1970, Inhibition of platelet energy production and release reaction by PGE$_1$, theophylline and cAMP, *Biochem. Biophys. Res. Commun.* 41: 128.

Wormer, P., and Brossmer, R., 1975, Platelet aggregation and the release reaction induced by ionophores for divalent cations, *Thrombosis Res.* 6: 295.

Yuen, M., and Macey, R., 1974, Platelet aggregation induced by calcium ionophore, *Fed. Proc.* 33: 269.

Zieve, P. D., and Greenough, W. B., III, 1969, Adenyl cyclase in human platelets: activity and responsiveness, *Biochem. Biophys. Res. Commun.* 35: 462.

Zucker, M. B., and Peterson, J., 1970, Effect of acetylsalicylic acid, other non-steroidal anti-inflammatory agents and dipyridamole on human blood platelets, *J. Lab. Clin. Med.* 76: 66.

CHAPTER 10

EFFECTS OF OPIATE DRUGS ON THE METABOLISM

OF CALCIUM IN SYNAPTIC TISSUE

David H. Ross

Departments of Pharmacology and Psychiatry
The University of Texas Health Science Center
San Antonio, Texas 78284

NEUROCHEMICAL MECHANISMS FOR OPIATE ACTIONS

Pharmacological actions of opiate drugs are characterized by analgesia, respiratory depression and sedation or CNS depression. These parameters together with changes in body temperature may be observed after a single dose of the opiate agonist. However, repeated administration of the drug at a constant dose or the necessity to increase the dose to achieve the same degree of response produces an effect commonly referred to as tolerance. This effect, although easily produced by opiate drugs, is clearly one of the least understood events in all of narcotic research.

It is currently believed that metabolic tolerance to narcotics is not a primary factor in the mechanism involved since no evidence is available to suggest that alterations in absorption, distribution or metabolism of opiates take place (Hug, 1972). Earlier proposals (Axelrod, 1956; Cochin and Axelrod, 1959) suggested that the enzymes responsible for metabolism were altered; however, these studies have not been generally accepted nor do they adequately account for adaptation to repeated drug exposure or physical dependence (Dole, 1970). A more functional approach attempts to explain tolerance development based on some neurochemical adaptation by the nerve cell to repeated exposure to the opiate.

Since the majority of opiate actions are believed to originate in the central nervous system, it might be expected that changes in neurotransmitters could be correlated with the time course of development of analgesia tolerance or tolerance to some other parameter. Various theories offered by Schuster (1961), Goldstein

and Goldstein (1961, 1968), and Collier (1966) have defined tolerance (i.e., neurochemical adaptation) in terms of enzyme activity,
membrane receptor expansion and neurotransmitter feedback mechanisms
Perhaps the most plausible of these theories (Collier, 1966; Goldstein and Goldstein, 1961; 1968) view adaptation in terms of an
increase in "receptive" sites (either for neurotransmitter binding
or for substrate binding to enzymes), thus implving a change in
membrane or soluble protein synthesis.

   With the recent advent of opiate receptor isolation, it was
expected that an increase in receptor sites for opiate ligands
would be found. However, several laboratories (Klee and Streaty,
1974; Hitzeman *et al.*, 1974; Hollt *et al.*, 1975) have reported no
increase in the number of opiate receptor sites. Without direct
demonstration of a change in receptor sites, we may consider an
alternative hypothesis. This is that the binding sites for neuro-
hormones (transmitters) remains constant but binding of the opiate
ligand may cause an activation of intracellular biochemical events
which, in turn, prepares the cell for continuing exposure to
opiates and, in doing so, produces tolerance to the pharmacological
effects of opiates. This type of activation process may be quite
similar to the activation of adenylate cyclase by hormones, neurotransmitters or inorganic cations. Recent advances in opiate
receptor isolation and characterization have offered a molecular
approach to both membrane events and the coupling processes between
the binding of pharmacologically active ligands and their physiological functions. We can therefore effectively relate binding
phenomena to pharmacologic responses by more attention to those
parameters of the cell which may couple binding to response.

CELL CALCIUM AS A PHARMACOLOGIC COUPLING AGENT

   Calcium ion has recently been suggested as a regulator for
a number of key enzymes in cellular metabolism including cyclic
nucleotide enzymes, enzymes responsible for rate limiting steps
in neurotransmitter metabolism and in the translation events of
proteins. Examples of this are adenylate and guanylate cyclase
and cyclic nucleotide phosphodiesterase (Brostrom *et al.*, 1975;
Ferrendelli *et al.*, 1973; Olson *et al.*, 1976; Kakiuchi *et al.*,
1975) tyrosine and tryptophan hydroxylase (Morgenroth *et al.*, 1975;
Knapp *et al.*, 1975) and aminoacyl t-RNA synthetase (Roy, 1971;
Rao, 1974).

   Probably two more important areas for Ca^{2+} regulation are
found in this ligand's ability to stabilize membranes and to
function in secretion coupling events. Calcium ion, by nature
of its optimum hydrated radius, may bind to a variety of anionic
subsites on the membrane, regulate ion flux, and serve as a charge

carrier (Seeman, 1972). Calcium ion is an obligatory requirement
for excitation-contraction coupling (see Somlyo and Somlyo, 1968)
and excitation-secretion coupling in adrenal tissue (Douglas,
1968). This concept is of major importance in the release of
neurotransmitters (Katz and Miledi, 1965; Llinas and Nicholson,
1974) from peripheral pre-synaptic terminals. More recently,
Blaustein (Blaustein *et al.*, 1972; Blaustein, 1975) has provided
very sound data demonstrating Ca^{2+} dependent neurotransmitter
release for synaptosomes isolated from whole brain homogenates.

Since activation of biochemical and/or pharmacological
responses after opiate administration depends on the initial
opiate receptor interactions, this receptor mediated response
must be in some way coupled to intracellular events preparing the
cell for adaptive measures. Calcium ion may, in all likelihood,
function in one or more of these adaptive roles due to its close
involvement in many of the above listed events.

CALCIUM INVOLVEMENT IN OPIATE ACTIONS

Much evidence now exists to implicate a role for Ca^{2+} in the
in vivo actions of narcotic agents. Much of the work was based
on the original findings of Kakunaga *et al.*, 1966, that Ca^{2+}
when administered intra-cerebrally antagonized morphine-induced
analgesia. This report was strengthened by the fact that EDTA
or sodium citrate but not other divalent ions (Ba^{2+}, Zn^{2+}, Mn^{2+},
Mg^{2+}) were effective in antagonizing analgesia.

More recently, Mulé (1971) postulated an involvement at the
membrane level between opiates, phospholipids and Ca^{2+} based on
the chemical similarity between the cationic charge of Ca^{2+} and
the quarternary nitrogen of the opiate. He suggested that acidic
phospholipids such as phosphatidic acid may serve as binding sites
for these two positively charged species. This hypothesis was
supported by the work of Abood (1969), who suggested a similar
triangular relationship between ATP-Ca^{2+} and phospholipid structures present on the membrane. It is interesting to note that
the Ca^{2+} hypothesis was already beginning to take shape as one
year earlier Tasaki (1968) had suggested that membranes may
exist in two states, a Ca^{2+} associated or resting state and a
Ca^{2+} dissociated or active state.

Evidence for a biochemical relationship between opiates and
Ca^{2+} was later provided by Hano *et al.* (1968) and more recently
by Ross *et al.* (1974) demonstrating the administration of opiates
in analgesic doses could produce a loss of brain Ca^{2+} in either
mice or rats, respectively. This loss of Ca^{2+} was uniform throughout eight regional brain areas, was stereospecific, and was

antagonized by the narcotic antagonist naloxone (Cardenas and Ross, 1975). Hano *et al.* (1968) first reported that tolerance to repeated administration of morphine developed over a period of four weeks; however, Ross (1975) was able to demonstrate single dose tolerance as early as four hours (Ross and Lynn, 1975) and that cycloheximide was able to attenuate this tolerance development over a period of seven days (Ross, 1975). Similar studies for analgesia had been reported earlier by Cox and Osman (1970).

An examination of the analgesia studies reported earlier by Kakunaga *et al.* (1966) prompted Harris *et al.* (1975) to employ the specific Ca^{2+} ionophore A23187 in order to facilitate entry of Ca^{2+} into nerve cells and these workers were very successful in demonstrating Ca^{2+} antagonism of analgesia. These investigators also demonstrated that La^{3+}, a well-known Ca^{2+} antagonist (Weiss, 1974), may have a neuroanatomical site of action similar to morphine in producing analgesia and, in fact, may substitute for morphine in a cross tolerance fashion to supplement analgesia (Harris *et al.*, 1975, 1976). Recent advances in the isolation of opiate receptor material prompted Ross *et al.* (1976) to examine the subcellular locus for Ca^{2+} loss in brain and to determine the degree of cation specificity which may be present. The loss of Ca^{2+} was confined to synaptic fractions from brain while the levels of Na^+, K^+, or Mg^{2+} did not appear altered (Cardenas and Ross, 1976). These findings have been recently observed by Harris *et al.* (1977) who, after administration of ^{45}Ca *in vivo*, measured the content of Ca^{2+} after an acute dose of morphine and found the loss confined to synaptic fractions.

The initial opiate drug-receptor interaction, while stereospecific in nature, still relies quite heavily on electrostatic interaction between the quarternary nitrogen and a negative subsite on the membrane. It is necessary that the membrane retain as much of an optimum conformational state as possible to facilitate the ligand-receptor interaction. The environmental milieu around the opiate binding site is very sensitive to osmotic variation and ionic concentration (Simon *et al.*, 1973; Pert and Snyder, 1974). Calcium ion and Mg^{2+} as well as Na^+ and Li^+ have been reported to inhibit opiate ligand binding (Hitzeman *et al.*, 1974). Calcium ion as well as Mg^{2+} were initially found to have inhibitory effects against opiate ligand binding (Pert and Snyder, 1973); however these investigators later reported Ca^{2+} was without effect at physiological levels (Pert and Snyder, 1974). However, Na^+ and Mn^{2+} appear in *in vitro* experiments to have preferential effects on opiate ligand binding. Pert and Snyder (1974) and Simon *et al.* (1973, 1975) reported that Na^+ influences the opiate receptor to increase antagonist binding while Pasternak *et al.* (1975) report that Mn^{2+} increases the binding of opiate agonists to the receptor. If Na^+ regulates the opiate receptor conformation *in vivo*, it may be expected that opiate administration may in some fashion alter the levels of Na^+ *in vivo*. This is not the case in one series of experiments where Cardenas and Ross (1976) found Na^+ levels unchanged in seven subcellular fractions after acute administration of morphine.

Cardenas and Ross (1976) have suggested that the Na^+ effect *in vitro* is due to an initial Na^+-Ca^{2+} exchange or Na^+-induced Ca^{2+} displacement from synaptic tissue as has been observed by previous investigators (Stahl and Swanson, 1971; Swanson *et al.*, 1974; Yoshida and Ichida, 1974). The loss of agonist binding affinity with addition of 100 mM Na^+ would result from disorganization of the opiate receptor as a result of Na^+-induced Ca^{2+} depletion from membranes. This would imply that the receptor exists in a Ca^{2+}-associated state (Ross *et al.*, 1976) and explain why naloxone readily reverses the Ca^{2+} loss after opiate treatment.

Similar results with Mn^{2+} (Pasternak *et al.*, 1975) may be explained in this fashion. Manganese ion is reported to be a potent inhibitor of Ca^{2+} binding to synaptosomes (Kamino *et al.*, 1974). Substitution of Mn^{2+} for Ca^{2+} would still allow the membrane receptor to remain in a divalent ion associated state which appears to be easily recognized by the opiate agonist ligand.

The outcome of this monovalent/divalent cation manipulation of opiate ligand binding may have as its basis alterations in membrane Ca^{2+} which would, in turn, change the conformation of the opiate receptor. Lacking in the Na^+/Mn^{2+} *in vitro* hypothesis is the fact that no cooperative binding of opiate ligands has been demonstrated. Further, if the receptor protein (Pasternak and Snyder, 1974) does exist in more than one form, does the binding of the agonist or antagonist induce a cooperative interaction of the subunits? To date no cooperative binding kinetics have been reported; however, explanation for the Na^+-Mn^{2+} manipulation of the receptor for antagonist or agonist affinities may be found in a model for opiate agonist-antagonist binding to cerebroside sulfate (CS; Cho *et al.*, 1976). These investigators postulate that agonist CS complexes are more hydrophobic (facilitated by divalent cations) while antagonist-CS complexes are more hydrophillic (facilitated by monovalent cations). This hypothesis suggests that the agonists bind more readily to the divalent cation form of the receptor while antagonists more readily bind to the monovalent form. If, in fact, Ca^{2+} regulates the agonist-antagonist interconversion, then perturbation of the Ca^{2+}-receptor interaction by competitive interaction with Mn^{2+} or non-competitive interaction with Na^+ would account for the effects of Mn^{2+} and Na^+ in *in vitro* model systems.

Further support for this idea is given in Table I. This
table represents the inhibitory potency of a series of divalent
ions together with Na^+ against Ca^{2+} binding to synaptic membranes.
Each of the ions was tested at a dose which was approximately
equal to their ID_{50} in the presence or absence of naloxone. Each
of the ions produced a significant loss of Ca^{2+} binding activity;
however, only Mn^{2+} followed by Mg^{2+} is reversed in the presence
of naloxone. This suggests that Mn^{2+} and, to a lesser extent,
Mg^{2+} holds the Ca^{2+} form of the membrane in a similar conformation
as it does the agonist form of the receptor such that reversal by
naloxone of Ca^{2+} or opiate agonist binding capacity suggests that
naloxone recognizes the Ca^{2+} depleted state of the membrane. In
the presence of Na^+, the membrane is non-specifically depleted
of Ca^{2+} and held in a fixed non-convertible form due to the non-
competitive interaction of Na^+ with Ca^{2+} binding sites. The result
is that naloxone, while having affinity for the more hydrophilic
form of the receptor, is unable to reverse the non-competitive
induced Ca^{2+} depletion.

Recent studies by Ross and Cardenas (1977) have demonstrated
a Ca^{2+} receptor site on synaptic membranes containing a high
affinity for Ca^{2+} (K_D = 0.85 μM) and a saturable binding capacity
of 350 pmol/mg protein. This Ca^{2+} site is selectively affected
by opiate ligands and satisfies the criteria of stereospecificity
and antagonism of opiate agonist effects by naloxone. The K_i for
levorphanol inhibition is 9 nM, which is well within the range of
ED_{50} values for opiate agonist inhibition of ^3H-agonist binding
(Simon *et al.*, 1973) and with agonist binding to a model opiate
receptor composed of cerebroside sulfate (Cho *et al.*, 1976).

More importantly, the binding of Ca^{2+} to this high affinity
site is of a cooperative nature with a Hill coefficient of 2.2.
Figure 1 represents a series of doses of levorphanol from 0.5 to
10 nM and their inhibitory effect on Ca^{2+} binding. Increasing
the dose of levorphanol produces a sigmoid to hyperbolic shift
in the Ca^{2+} binding curves suggesting that levorphanol inhibits
the cooperative binding of Ca^{2+}. This finding is further illustrated by the Hill plot in Figure 2. This data demonstrates a
progressive shift in H_N from 2.2 to 1.1 as the concentration of
levorphanol increases.

The question often arises in experiments using CNS depressants
as to whether the parameter being measured is a response to primary
non-specific CNS depression rather than to a direct receptor
mediated response. It is well known that local anesthetic agents
including procaine, chlorpromazine and tetracaine readily absorb
to biomembranes and, in so doing, compete with or displace calcium
from fixed negative sites on the membrane. It is believed that
the majority of membrane-bound Ca^{2+} is associated with membrane

TABLE I. EFFECTS OF CATIONS[a] ON CALCIUM BINDING

| Cation (conc.) | Ca^{2+} Bound (pmol/mg membrane, mean ± SEM[b]) | |
	-Naloxone (10^{-7} M)	+Naloxone (10^{-7}M)
Control	339.6 ± 18.1	342.4 ± 14.2
Sodium (100 mM)	140.3 ± 10.6	144.3 ± 13.8
Magnesium (100 μM)	166.8 ± 15.6	207.4 ± 18.2[c]
Manganese (100 μM)	168.3 ± 9.6	276.4 ± 14.2[c]
Barium (500 μM)	167.5 ± 8.6	173.2 ± 15.7
Lanthanum (10 μM)	166.8 ± 16.1	150.7 ± 17.5

[a]Concentrations of cations approximately equal to ID_{50} for each ion. Naloxone (10^{-7} M) was present for two min prior to addition of ions to incubation media.

[b]Means represent values obtained from three separate tissue preparations. Each tissue preparation was assayed three times using triplicate points for each assay.

[c]Significantly different from values without naloxone at $P < .01$.

protein (Frank, 1968; Seeman, 1972); there are few studies describing the interaction of anesthetic amines with protein-Ca^{2+} interactions. Considerable evidence is available to suggest agents such as propranolol, narcotic amines and other anesthetic amines displace Ca^{2+} from phospholipid bilayers (Seeman, 1972). Anionic or neutral anesthetics appear to increase the binding of Ca^{2+} to phospholipids (Blaustein and Goldman, 1966; Blaustein, 1967).

Evidence supporting the receptor mediated specificity of the narcotic amines in inhibiting Ca^{2+} binding is outlined in Table II. These results suggest that while both pentobarbital and chlorpromazine at 10^{-7} M produce a small but significant decrease in Ca^{2+} binding, naloxone does not affect this binding loss. Previous studies have also demonstrated that the pentobarbital-induced decrease in brain calcium was not reversed by naloxone (Ross et al., 1976).

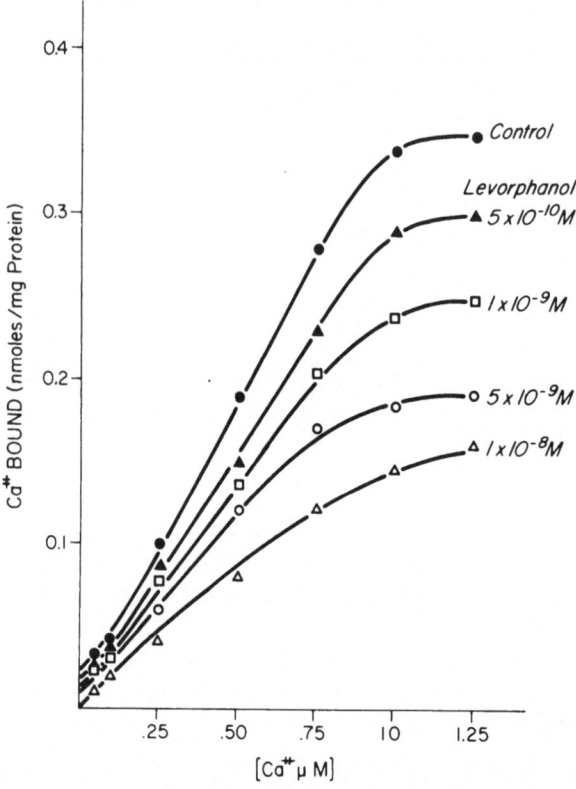

Figure 1. Relationship between synaptic membrane binding of Ca^{2+} and free Ca^{2+} in media in presence of levorphanol. Levorphanol concentration added in suspension media. ▲, 0.5 nM; □, 1.0 nM; o, 5.0 nM; △, 10.0 nM. Suspending media is 100 mM Tris·HCl buffer (pH 7.3).

FUNCTIONAL SIGNIFICANCE OF ALTERED Ca^{2+} METABOLISM

Recent studies by Harris *et al.* (1976, 1977) Ross *et al.* (1976) and Ross (1977) have demonstrated that chronic exposure of mice to opiates produces an increase in net Ca^{2+} content of synaptosomes. Harris *et al.* report this increase is principally found in synaptic vesicles isolated after the synaptosomes are lysed. Ross *et al.* report the increase in Ca^{2+} is due to an increase in synaptic membrane as well as synaptic vesicle Ca^{2+} content. Furthermore, these investigators have measured Ca^{2+} binding to SPM and found a decrease in ability to bind Ca^{2+}, presumably a reflection of more sites occupied during the adaptive

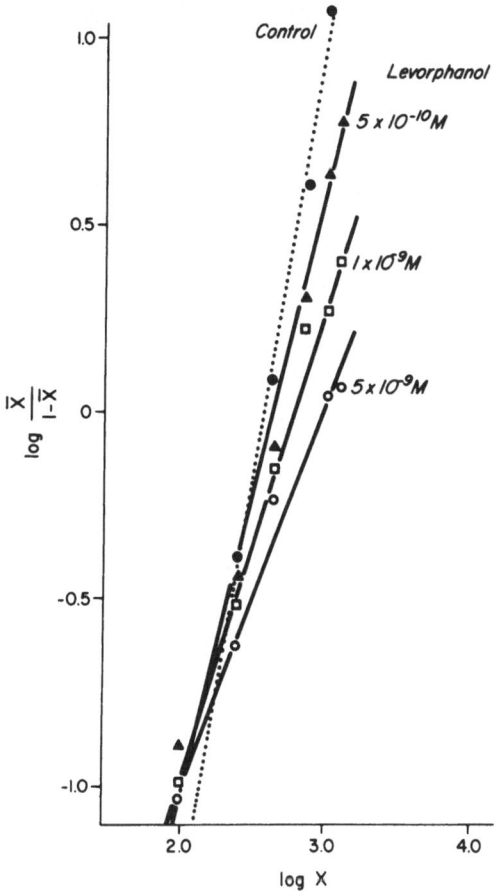

Figure 2. Hill plot of Ca^{2+} receptor binding by synaptic membranes in presence of levorphanol. Levorphanol concentrations are 0.5, 1.0 and 5.0 nM in binding media of 100 mM Tris·HCl buffer (pH 7.3).

accumulation process. Both of these studies (employing atomic absorption, fluorescent chelators of Ca^{2+}, and ^{45}Ca binding, and intraventricular injections to localize Ca^{2+} movements) are in close agreement that the locus of opiate effects in altering Ca^{2+} metabolism resides at the synaptosomal level.

The question arises as to what adaptive changes are taking place in the synaptosome to allow for an increase in Ca^{2+} content. Data presented by Ross and Cardenas (1977) establishes the

TABLE II. EFFECT OF NON-ANALGESIC CNS DEPRESSANTS ON CALCIUM/
RECEPTOR BINDING

CNS depressant (conc.)	Ca^{2+} bound (pmol/mg membrane, mean $\pm$ SEM[a])	
	-Naloxone (10^{-7}M)	+Naloxone[b] (10^{-7}M)
Control	345 $\pm$ 15	340 $\pm$ 18
Pentobarbital (10^{-7}M)	313 (10%) $\pm$ 10	283 (16%) $\pm$ 16
Chlorpromazine (10^{-7}M)	291 (16%) $\pm$ 14	285 (17%) $\pm$ 18

[a]*Means of three separate experiments. Ecah experiment run in triplicate.*

[b]*Naloxone (10^{-7}M) was present in incubation media two minutes prior to addition of pentobarbital or chlorpromazine. Values in parenthesis are % inhibition of calcium binding to synaptic membranes.*

similarity of kinetics between opiate and Ca^{2+} binding sites and the fact that opiate ligands may inhibit and/or displace Ca^{2+} from these binding sites. As pointed out by Ross (1977), the increase in Ca^{2+} content of the vesicles may be due to an increase in the actual number of vesicles or to an increase in Ca^{2+} binding sites per vesicle. Either way, this data together with the work of Harris *et al.* (1976, 1977) offer an attractive basis for a number of opiate-induced changes in enzyme and neurotransmitter functions.

The most direct explanation for the increase in synaptosomal Ca^{2+} content observed by Harris *et al.* (1977) and Ross (1977) may be in altered Ca^{2+} uptake/efflux studies. To date, no studies have been reported which directly demonstrate changes in either of these mechanisms, although indirect support for altered transport of Ca^{2+} is present. Ray *et al.* (1968) reported that acute morphine sulfate treatment produced a decrease in neurotransmitters in adrenal cells with an increase in ATPase activity and Ca^{2+} content. Chronic treatment produced a depression of ATPase and Ca^{2+} content. Earlier, Kakunaga (1966) had suggested that the analgesic action of morphine may be due to changes in Ca^{2+} flux. This suggestion has been very nicely extended by the work of Harris *et al.* (1975) using Ca^{2+} ionophores to demonstrate that apparent intracellular uptake of Ca^{2+} antagonizes analgesia.

TABLE III. EFFECTS OF OPIATE LIGANDS IN VITRO ON SYNAPTOSOMAL Ca^{2+} UPTAKE

Opiate Ligands	K^+ Stimulated Ca^{2+} Uptake (μmol/g protein, mean $\pm$ SEM[a])
Control	5.85 ± 0.23
Levorphanol (10^{-7}M)	$4.46^b \pm 0.20$ (+24.7%)
Dextrorphan (10^{-7} M)	6.16 ± 0.26
Naloxone (10^{-7}M)	5.36 ± 0.15
Naloxone + Levorphanol (10^{-7}M)	5.74 ± 0.18

[a]Means of 3 separate determinations, each determination was run in triplicate.

[b]Significantly different from control at P < 0.01.

Recently, Ho and Desiah (1976) reported changes in Na^+/K^+ and Mg^{2+} ATPase after chronic morphine treatment.

Studies in this laboratory have followed Ca^{2+} uptake in intact presynaptic nerve terminals (isolated from crude mitochondrial fractions by sucrose density gradients) after in vitro and in vivo opiate treatments. Levorphanol (10^{-7}M) was effective in reducing the K^+ stimulated Ca^{2+} uptake in rabbit synaptosomes (Table III), while dextrorphan at equimolar concentrations was ineffective. Naloxone was an effective antagonist of levorphanol while exhibiting no effects alone. Similar studies observing K^+-induced Ca^{2+} uptake as a function of $\{Ca\}_o$ in the presence or absence of levorphanol suggests the decrease in Ca^{2+} uptake is due to a non-competitive inhibition reducing the capacity for Ca^{2+} uptake with no significant change in K_M values (Table IV). Calcium uptake was linear over 60 sec and was linearly reduced by the addition of 10^{-7} M levorphanol (Table III).

These studies would suggest that at least one phase of the Ca^{2+} accumulation observed is altered by in vitro additions of opiate ligands. In order to account for an increase in Ca^{2+} content in the tolerant animal, studies were performed treating mice with levorphanol or dextrorphan (100 μg/day) for 3 days in order

*TABLE IV.   EFFECTS OF LEVORPHANOL ON SYNAPTOSOMAL CALCIUM UPTAKE
              AT DIFFERENT CALCIUM CONCENTRATIONS*

$CaCl_2$ (conc.)	Ca^{2+} Uptake (μ/mol/g protein, mean $\pm$ SEM[a])	
	Control + K^+ (50 mM)	Levorphanol (10^{-7}M) + K^+ (50 mM)
2.0 mM	15.80 $\pm$ 1.32	11.58 $\pm$ 1.13
1.25 mM	9.48 $\pm$ 0.21	6.84 $\pm$ 0.61
0.50 mM	4.84 $\pm$ 0.32	3.79 $\pm$ 0.54
0.25 mM	3.05 $\pm$ 0.11	2.42 $\pm$ 0.31

[a]*Means represent studies from three separate determinations.   Each
 determination was run in triplicate.*

to produce tolerance to analgesia as tested by the hot plate technique and dependence as evidenced by jumping phenomena following a
2 mg/kg injection of naloxone. Table V outlines the results of
these studies. Chronic treatment with levorphanol produced a
significant increase in the K^+-depolarized Ca^{2+} uptake while chronic
dextrorphan treatment was not significantly different from controls.

From a functional aspect, the adaptive increase in synaptosomal Ca^{2+} content may relate to changes in various Ca^{2+} dependent
enzymes. The induction of tyrosine hydroxylase, an enzyme activated by Ca^{2+} (Morgenroth *et al.*, 1976), has been reported follow
ing chronic opiate treatment (Reis *et al.*, 1970) with changes
observed in rat striatum and hypothalamus (Clouet and Iwatsubo,
(1975). Cardenas and Ross (1975) have suggested that the acute
loss of brain Ca^{2+} after opiates may be responsible for the increase
in acetylcholine levels by altering the Ca^{2+} dependent release of
this neurotransmitter. Further evidence for this idea has been
offered by Harris *et al.* (1976, 1977) and Ross (1977), who demonstrated that acute doses of opiates alter the vesicular Ca^{2+}
content and, in this manner, may interfere with neurotransmitter
release. Inhibition of this mechanism could set in motion feedback
loops activating enzymes (such as typosine hydroxylase) which are
responsible for neurotransmitter synthesis. The ability of the
synaptosome to accumulate excess Ca^{2+} may be related to continued
optimum levels of neurotransmitter synthesis and release.

A second focal point and probably one of equal importance
is the involvement of opiates, adenylate cyclase and Ca^{2+}. Sharma

TABLE V.   EFFECT OF CHRONIC OPIATE ADMINISTRATION
ON SYNAPTOSOMAL CALCIUM UPTAKE

Opiate[a]	Ca^{2+} *Uptake (μmol/g protein, mean ± SEM[b])*		
	$Na^{+}+5K$	*←K^{+} (50 mM)*	*ΔK*
Control	*6.01 ± 0.58*	*13.9 ± 0.32*	*7.90 ± 0.26*
Levorphanol	*7.68 ± 1.13*	*17.61 ± 1.46*	*9.93 ± ˙0.33*
Dextrorphan	*7.23 ± 0.86*	*14.72 ± 1.41*	*7.49 ± 0.55*

[a]*Drugs were administered every eight hours for three days.   Each day total dosage was 100 mg/kg.*

[b]*Values represent means of 3-5 separate determinations.   Each determination was run in triplicate.*

et al., 1975, have reported that opiate receptors may be linked to adenylate cyclase in neuroblastoma X glioma hybrid cell line. In addition, adenylate cyclase activity was inhibited by acute opiate exposure while chronic exposure led to an increase in enzyme activity above basal level (Klee *et al.*, 1974). In view of the fact that adenylate cyclase is regulated by Ca^{2+}, Ross and Cardenas (1977) have suggested that opiate inhibition of adenylate cyclase followed by activation is the result of opiate-induced changes in Ca^{2+}. While opiate agonists did not bind cooperatively to the neuroblastoma X glioma cell surface, the agonists did produce a cooperative inhibition of the enzyme. Opiate inhibition of cooperative Ca^{2+} binding may serve to remove the Ca^{2+} regulation of adenylate cyclase allowing cooperative inhibition of the enzyme. Further support for the Ca^{2+} involvement may be found in the studies of Iverson and Minneman (1977) and Bonnet and Gusik (1977) who reported that Ca^{2+} in physiological concentrations must be present in order to observe inhibitory effects of opiates or endogenous opiate peptides on adenylate cyclase activity. It is also of interest that enkephalin and opiate drugs produce an increase in cyclic GMP in the neostriatal region (Minneman and Iverson, 1976; Racogni *et al.*, 1976) and the Ca^{2+} is thought to activate guanylate cyclase as well (Olson *et al.*, 1976).

From an adaptation standpoint, the involvement of Ca^{2+} with various cellular functions such as neurotransmitter and cyclic nucleotide metabolism provides many directions through which the cell may respond to opiate treatment. Two principle mechanisms for which the most information is available are alterations in

neurotransmitter synthesis and release and regulation of adenylate
cyclase and/or guanylate (which, in turn, changes the C-AMP/C-GMP
levels).

POSSIBLE DIRECTIONS FOR FUTURE RESEARCH

The role of Ca^{2+} in the behavioral, pharmacological and biochemical actions of opiates is now well documented. Neurochemical
adaptation to the chronic administration of opiate, drugs may relate
to changes which take place both at the membrane receptor level
and at sites within the synaptosome. By virtue of the role of
Ca^{2+} in excitation-contraction and excitation-secretion coupling
mechanisms, it is reasonable to suggest that Ca^{2+} may also act to
couple the binding stimulus of opiates with the pharmacological
response. Evidence of two systems which adapt to opiates, neurotransmitter metabolism and cyclic nucleotide metabolism, and in
which Ca^{2+} plays a regulatory role, have been presented here.

A third area which may prosper in the future relates to the
interaction of Ca^{2+} dependent regulator proteins of the type
isolated by Wolff and Siegel (1972) with key enzymes which have
been shown to be regulated by Ca^{2+}. Calcium dependent regulators
(Wolff and Siegel, 1972; Wolff et al., 1972; Brooks and Siegel,
1973; Childers and Siegel, 1975) have become increasingly implicated in regulation of many cellular functions. Wolff and Siegel
(1972) and, more recently, Mahendran et al. (1974) have suggested
this class of proteins is involved in neurotransmitter release.
Wolff and Brostrom (1974) reported this protein mediates the Ca^{2+}
dependent regulation of brain cyclic nucleotide phosphodiesterase
(PDE), the activation of which is reversed by EGTA and subsequently
reactivated by the addition of Ca^{2+}. Brostrom et al. (1975) have
recently observed this protein activates adenylate cyclase as
well. More important are the observations of Kakiuchi et al. (1973,
1975); Teshimi and Kiuchi (1974) and Teo and Wang (1973) who suggested that intracellular Ca^{2+} may activate a complex of Ca^{2+}
phosphodiesterase-protein modulator to regulate its activity toward
C-AMP or C-GMP. Increased Ca^{2+} activates the enzyme while decreased
Ca^{2+} reverses this activation (Teshima and Kakiuchi, 1974). The
low concentrations of Ca^{2+} required for activation of tyrosine
hydroxylase and cyclic nucleotide phosphodiesterase provide a
basis for suggesting their activities in vivo may be regulated
by variations in intracellular Ca^{2+} content. The data presented
by Kakiuchi et al. (1973) suggests that phosphodiesterase activated
by the Ca^{2+} dependent regulator protein has a preferential affinity
for C-GMP (which would increase the intracellular C-AMP/C-GMP ratio).
From the standpoint of cellular adaptation, the Ca^{2+} binding proteins may participate in a variety of Ca^{2+}-dependent features of

cell metabolism and may be easily modified by intracellular Ca^{2+} fluxes. A particular area of relevance would be the cyclic nucleotide dependent phosphorylation of chromosomal and synaptic membrane proteins, which may play important adaptation roles in chronic opiate treatment.

REFERENCES

Abood, L. G., 1969, Calcium-adenosine tri-phosphate-lipid interactions and their significance in the excitatory membrane, *Neurosci. Res.* 2: 42.

Axelrod, J., 1956, The enzymatic N-demethylation of narcotic drugs, *J. Pharmacol. Exp. Ther.* 117: 322.

Blaustein, M. P., 1975, Effects of potassium, veratridine, and scorpion venom on Ca accumulation and transmitter release by nerve terminal *in vitro*, *J. Physiol. (London)* 247: 617.

Blaustein, M. P., 1967, Phospholipids as ion exchanges: Implications for a possible role in biological membranes excitability and anesthesia, *Biochim. Biophys. Acta* 135: 653.

Blaustein, M. P., and Goldman, D. E., 1966, Competitive action of calcium and procaine on lobster axon, *J. gen. Physiol.* 49: 1043.

Blaustein, M. P., Johnson, E. M., and Needleman, P., 1972, Calcium dependent norepinephrine release from presynaptic nerve endings *in vitro*, *Proc. Nat. Acad. Sci. U. S. A.* 69: 2237.

Bonnet, K. A., and Gusik, S., 1977, Enkephalin and morphine: Brain adenylate cyclase effects and calcium ion, *Trans. Amer. Soc. Neurochem.* 8: 84.

Brostrom, C. O., Huang, Y. C., Breckenridge, B. McL., and Wolff, D. J., 1975, Identification of a calcium binding protein as a calcium dependent regulator of brain adenylate cyclase, *Proc. Nat. Acad. Sci. U. S. A.* 72: 64.

Brooks, J. C., and Siegel, F. L., 1973, Identification of a calcium binding phosphoprotein from beef adrenal medulla, *J. Biol. Chem.* 248: 4189.

Cardenas, H. L., and Ross, D. H., 1976, Calcium depletion of synaptosomes after morphine treatment, *Brit. J. Pharmacol.* 57: 521.

Cardenas, H. L., and Ross, D. H., 1975, Morphine-induced depletion of calcium in discrete regions of rat brain, *J. Neurochem.* 24: 487.

Childers, S. R., and Siegel, F. L., 1975, Isolation and purification of a calcium binding protein from electroplax of electrophorus electricus, *Biochim. Biophys. Acta* 405: 99.

Cho, T. M., Cho, J. S., and Loh, H. H., 1976, ^{3}H-cerebroside sulfate redistribution induced by cation opiate or phosphatidyl serine, *Life Sci.* 19: 117.

Clouet, D. H., and Iwatsubo, E., 1975, Mechanisms of tolerance to and dependence on narcotic analgesic drugs, *Annu. Rev. Pharmacol.* 15: 49.

Cochin, J., and Axelrod, J., 1959, Biochemical and pharmacological changes in the rat following chronic administration of morphine, nalorphine and normorphine, *J. Pharmacol. Exp. Ther.* 125: 105.

Collier, H. O. J., 1966, Tolerance, physical dependence and receptors, *Adv. in Drug Res.* 3: 171.

Cox, B. M., and Osman, O., 1970, Inhibition of the development of tolerance to morphine in rats by drugs which inhibit ribonucleic acid or protein synthesis, *Brit. J. Pharmacol.* 38: 157.

Dole, V. P., 1970, The biochemistry of addiction, *Annu. Rev. Biochem.* 39: 821.

Douglas, W. W., 1968, Stimulus-secretion coupling, the concept and clues from chromaffin and other cells, *Brit. J. Pharmacol.* 34: 451.

Ferrendelli, J. A., Kinscherf, D. A., and Chang, M. M., 1973, Regulation of levels of guanosine cyclic 3' 5' monophosphate in the central nervous system: Effects of depolarizing agents, *Mol. Pharmacol.* 9: 445.

Frank, G. B., 1968, Drugs which modify membrane excitability, *Fed. Proc.* 27: 132.

Goldstein, A., and Goldstein, D. B., 1968, Enzyme expansion theory of drug tolerance and physical dependence, *in* "The Addictive States" (A. Wikler, ed.) pp. 265-267, Williams and Wilkins, Baltimore.

Hano, K., 1968, Calcium content in mouse brain after exposure to morphine, *Jpn. J. Pharmacol.* 17: 135.

Harris, R. A., Loh, H. H., and Way, E. L., 1976, Antinociceptive effects of lanthanum and cerium in non-tolerant and morphine tolerant-dependent animals, *J. Pharmacol. Exp. Ther.* 196: 288.

Harris, R. A., Loh, H. H., and Way, E. L., 1975, Effects of divalent cation, cation chelators and an ionophore on morphine analgesia and tolerance, *J. Pharmacol. Exp. Ther.* 195: 488.

Harris, R. A., Yamamoto, H., Loh, H. H., and Way, E. L., 1976, Alterations in brain calcium localization during the development of morphine tolerance and dependence, *in* "Opiates and Endogenous Opioid Peptides", (H. W. Kosterlitz, ed.), pp. 361-368, Elsevier-North Holland Biomed. Press, Amsterdam.

Harris, R. A., Yamamoto, H., Loh, H. H., and Way, E. L., 1977, Discrete changes in brain calcium with morphine analgesia, tolerance-dependence and abstinence, *Life Sci.* 20: 501.

Hitzeman, R. J., Hitzeman, B. A., and Loh, H. H., 1974, Binding of ^{3}H-naloxone in the mouse brain: Effects of ions and tolerance development, *Life Sci.* 14: 2393.

Ho, I. K., and Desaiah, D., 1977, Effect of morphine on mouse brain ATPase activity, *Biochem. Pharmacol.* 26: 89.

Hollt, V., Dum, J., Blasig, J., Schubert, P., and Herz, A., 1975, Comparison of *in vivo* and *in vitro* parameters of opiate receptor binding in naive and tolerant/dependent rodents, *Life Sci.* 16: 1823.

Hug, C. C., 1972, Characteristics and theories related to acute and chronic tolerance development, *in* "CRC Chemical and Biological Aspects of Drug Dependence, (S. J. Mulé and H. Brill, eds.) pp. 307–359, CRC Press, Cleveland.

Iverson, L. L., and Minneman, K. P., 1977, Interaction of dopamine receptors and opiate drugs in mammalian brain, *Trans. Amer. Soc. Neurochem.* 8: 108.

Kakiuchi, S., Yamazaki, R., Teshima, Y., and Uenishi, K., 1973, Regulation of nucleoside cyclic 3':5' monophosphate phosphodiesterase activity from rat brain by a modulator and Ca^{++}, *Proc. Nat. Acad. Sci. U. S. A.* 70: 3526.

Kakiuchi, S., Yamazaki, R., Teshima, Y., Uenshi, K., and Miyamoto, E., 1975, Multiple cyclic nucleotide phosphodiesterase activities from rat tissues and occurrence of a Ca^{++} + Mg^{++} ion dependent phosphodiesterase and its protein activator, *Biochem. J.* 146: 109.

Kakunaga, T., Kaneto, H., and Hano, K., 1966, Pharmacologic studies on analgesia significance of the calcium ion in morphine analgesia, *J. Pharmacol. Exp. Ther.* 153: 134.

Kamino, K., Uyesaka, N., Ogawa, M., and Inonye, A., 1975, Ca^{++} binding of synaptosomes isolated from rat brain cortex II. Inhibitory effects of magnesium and other cations, *J. Memb. Biol.* 21: 113.

Katz, B., and Miledi, R., 1965, The effect of calcium on acetylcholine release from motor nerve terminals, *Proc. R. Soc. Biol. London, Ser. B* 161: 496.

Klee, W. A., Sharma, S. K., and Nirenberg, M., 1975, Opiates receptors as regulators of adenylate cyclase, *Life. Sci.* 16: 1869.

Klee, W. A., and Streaty, R. A., 1974, Narcotic receptor sites in morphine dependent rats, *Nature* 248: 61.

Knapp, S., Mandell, A. J., and Bullard, W. P., 1975, Calcium activation of brain tryptophan hydroxylase, *Life Sci.* 16: 1583.

Llinas, R., and Nicholson, C., 1975, Calcium role in depolarization-secretion coupling: an aequorin study in the squid giant synapse, *Proc. Nat. Acad. Sci. U. S. A.* 72: 187.

Mahendran, C., Nicklas, W. J., and Berl, S., 1974, Evidence for calcium-sensitive components in brain actomyosin-like protein (neurostenin), *J. Neurochem.* 23: 497.

Minneman, K. P., and Iverson, L. L., 1976, Enkephalin and opiate narcotics increase cyclic GMP accumulation in slices of rat neostriatum, *Nature* 262: 313.

Morgenroth, V. H., Boadle-Biber, M. C., and Roth, R. H., 1975, Activation of tyrosine hydroxylase from central noradrenergic neurons by calcium, *Mol. Pharmacol.* 11: 427.

Mulé, S. J., 1971, Phospholipid metabolism in narcotic drugs, *in* "Biochemical Pharmacology (D. H. Clouet, ed.) pp. 190-214, Plenum Press, New York.

Olson, D. R., Kon, C., and Breckenridge, B. McL., 1976, Calcium ion effects on guanylate cyclase of brain, *Life Sci.* 18: 935.

Pasternak, G. W., Snowman, A. M., and Snyder, S. H., 1975, Selective enhancement of {^{3}H} opiate agonist binding by divalent cations, *Mol. Pharmacol.* 11: 735.

Pert, C. B., and Snyder, S. H., 1974, Opiate receptor binding of agonist and antagonists affected differentially by sodium, *Mol. Pharmacol.* 10: 868.

Pert, C. B., and Snyder, S. H., 1973, Properties of opiate receptor binding in rat brain, *Proc. Nat. Acad. Sci. U. S. A.* 70: 2243.

Racagni, G., Zsilla, G., Giudotli, A., and Costa, E., 1976, Accumulation of cGMP in striatum of rats injected with narcotic analgesics: Antagonism by naltrexone, *J. Pharm. Pharmacol.* 28: 258.

Rao, K. N., deSmit, M., Howells, A. J., and Bygrave, F. L., 1974, Inhibition of Ca^{++} of t-RNA amino-acylation in preparation of rat liver, *FEBS Lett.* 41: 185.

Ray, A. K., 1971, Inhibition of the alanine t-RNA amine acylation by Ca^{++}, *Biochim. Biophys. Acta* 246: 349.

Ray, A. K., Mukherji, M., and Ghosh, J. J., 1968, Adrenal catecholamines and related changes during different phases of morphine administration -- A histochemical study, *J. Neurochem.* 15: 875.

Reis, D. J., Hess, P., and Azmitia, E. C., 1970, Changes in enzymes subserving catecholamine metabolism in morphine tolerance and withdrawal in rats, *Brain Res.* 20: 309.

Ross, D. H., 1977, Calcium content and binding in synaptosomal subfractions during chronic morphine treatments, *Neurochemical Res.* 2: 581.

Ross, D. H., 1975, Tolerance to morphine induced calcium depletion, *Brit. J. Pharmacol.* 55: 431.

Ross, D. H., and Cardenas, H. L., 1977, Levorphanol inhibition of Ca^{++} binding to synaptic membranes *in vitro, Life Sci.* 20: 1455.

Ross, D. H., and Lynn, S. C., 1975, Characterization of acute tolerance to morphine using reserpine and cycloheximide, *Biochem. Pharmacol.* 24: 1135.

Ross, D. H., Lynn, S. C., and Cardenas, H. L., 1976, Selective control of calcium levels by naloxone, *Life Sci.* 18: 789.

Ross, D. H., Medina, M. A., and Cardenas, H. L., 1974, Morphine and ethanol: selective depletion of regional brain calcium, *Science* 186: 63.

Seeman, P., 1972, The membrane actions of anesthetics and tranquilizers, *Pharmacol. Rev.* 24: 583.

Sharma, S. K., Nirenberg, M., and Klee, W. A., 1975, Morphine receptors as regulators of adenylate cyclase activity, *Proc. Nat. Acad. Sci. U. S. A.* 72: 590.

Shuster, L., 1961, Repression and de-repression of enzyme synthesis as a possible explanation of some aspects of drug action, *Nature* 189: 314.

Simon, E. J., Hiller, J. M., and Edelman, I., 1973, Stereospecific binding of the potent narcotic analgesic {^{3}H}-etorphine to rat brain homogenate, *Proc. Nat. Acad. Sci. U. S. A.* 70: 1947.

Simon, E. J., Hiller, J. M., Groth, J., and Edelman, I., 1975, Further properties of stereospecific opiate binding sites in rat brain on the nature of the sodium effect, *J. Pharmacol. Exp. Ther.* 192: 531.

Somlyo, A. V., and Somlyo, A. P., 1968, Vascular smooth muscle I. normal structure pathology, biochemistry and biophysics, *Pharmacol. Rev.* 20: 197.

Stahl, W. L., and Swanson, P. D., 1971, Movements of calcium and other cations in isolated cerebral tissue, *J. Neurochem.* 18: 415.

Swanson, P. D., Anderson, L., and Stahl, P. D., 1974, Uptake of calcium ions by synaptosomes from rat brain, *Biochim. Biophys. Acta* 356: 174.

Tasaki, I., 1968, "Nerve excitation: A macromolecular approach", Thomas Inc., Springfield.

Teo, T. S., and Wang, J. H., 1973, Mechanism of activation of cyclic adenosine 3':5'-monophosphate phosphodiesterase from bovine heart by calcium ions, *J. Biol. Chem.* 248: 5950.

Teshima, Y., and Kakiuchi, S., 1974, Mechanism of stimulation of Ca^{+2} plus Mg^{+2} dependent phosphodiesterase from rat cerebral cortex by the modulator protein and Ca^{+2}, *Biochem. Biophys. Res. Comm.* 56: 489.

Weiss, G. B., 1974, Cellular pharmacology of lanthanum, *Annu. Rev. Pharmacol.* 14: 343.

Wolff, D. J., Huebner, J. A., and Siegel, F. L., 1972, Calcium binding phosphoprotein of pig brain effects of cations on the calcium binding, *J. Neurochem.* 19: 2855.

Wolff, D. J., and Siegel, F. L., 1972, Purification of a calcium-binding phosphoprotein from pig brain, *J. Biol. Chem.* 247: 4180.

Yoshida, H., and Ichida, S., 1974, Effects of Na^+ on Ca^{++} uptake of the synaptic plasma membrane, *Life Sci.* 15: 685.

CHAPTER 11

CALCIUM AND NEUROMUSCULAR TRANSMISSION

William Van der Kloot

Department of Physiology and Biophysics
Health Sciences Center, SUNY
Stony Brook, New York 11794

INTRODUCTION

The importance of Ca^{2+} in the release of ACh at the neuro-muscular junction was shown by experiments of such lucid design and clever execution that they became instant classics (summarized by Katz, 1969). The general opinion is that depolarization of the nerve terminal opens a voltage-gated Ca^{2+} channel. Ca^{2+} enters the terminal to initiate quantal release which ends when the Ca^{2+} is sequestered or ejected from the terminal. This clear picture, naturally enough, hides uncertainties and unanswered questions which will be uncovered as the evidence for the Ca^{2+} hypothesis is described.

ROLE OF CALCIUM ION

Neuromuscular transmission requires a small amount of Ca^{2+} in the extracellular solution (Locke, 1894). When Ca^{2+} is absent, impulses are still conducted down the motor terminals, the end-plate is sensitive to ACh, but release is blocked (del Castillo & Katz, 1954; Katz & Miledi, 1965a). In Ca^{2+}-free solutions, release can be restored within milliseconds by ejecting a pulse of Ca^{2+} from a micropipette poised over the terminal. The Ca^{2+} pulse must precede the action potential. At $25^{\circ}C$, there is a minimum delay of 5 msec between the passing of the action potential and the start of the end-plate potential (e.p.p.). Ca^{2+} applied during this latent period has no effect (Katz & Miledi, 1967b).

    In a nerve-muscle preparation placed in isotonic $CaCl_2$, the
nerves are unable to conduct, owing to the absence of Na^+. Never-
theless, ACh is released when a length of the nerve terminal is
depolarized by a current passed through an extracellular microelectrode. The ACh combines with its receptor on the end-plate
opening a channel in the membrane through which cations flow down
their electrochemical gradients. In isotonic $CaCl_2$, both electrical
and chemical gradients favor Ca^{2+} influx, the inward flow of the
positive charges depolarizes the end-plate (Katz & Miledi, 1969).
Calcium ion alone is sufficient for quantal ACh release.

    An attractive hypothesis is that the Ca^{2+} enters the nerve
terminal by way of a voltage-gated channel, as the first step in
the quantal release process. Such Ca^{2+} channels have been found
in nerve cells and also in smooth and cardiac muscle. Excitable
Ca^{2+} entry systems have been extensively studied in the squid
giant axon (reviewed by Baker, 1972, 1974). Some Ca^{2+} enters the
axon following stimulation because the Na^+ channel is imperfectly
selective. This path is blocked by tetrodotoxin (TTX). There is
a second, delayed phase of Ca^{2+} entry. The late phase is blocked
by Mn^{2+} or Co^{2+}, and by the drugs D-600 or prenylamine. The opening of the gates is detectable following a depolarization to
-45mV; a depolarization to -39mV gives an e-fold conductance increase. The peak conductance is reached at about 0 mV.

    Calcium ion conductance declines if the membrane is held de-
polarized, with a time constant of seconds. But the inactivation
is never complete. Recovery from inactivation takes minutes. In
cardiac muscle the threshold for activation of Ca^{2+} conductance
is about -30mV and the inactivation time constant is in the tens
of milliseconds range (Noble, 1975).

    The motor nerve terminal is too small to permit insertion of
an intracellular electrode, so indirect methods must be used.
Katz & Miledi (1967a) treated frog nerve-muscle preparations with
TTX to block Na^+ channels, and with tetraethylammonium (TEA) to
block K^+ channels. A length of motor nerve terminal was depolarized
with current pulses from an extracellular electrode. ACh release
was monitored by a microelectrode inserted in the underlying end-
plate. There is a sharp threshold for ACh release and a further,
small rise in depolarizing current produces a maximal release. A
depolarization just above the threshold appears to cause a regenerative Ca^{2+} influx to give a maximal release, under these unusual experimental circumstances where drugs block the univalent
cation fluxes that normally dominate the electrical behavior of
the membrane.

    The release of ACh from stimulated motor nerve terminals is
blocked by Mn^{2+} (Meiri & Rahamimoff, 1972; Kajimoto & Pirpekar,

1972), Co^{2+} (Weakley, 1973; Kita & Van der Kloot, 1973). It is also blocked by the "organic Ca^{2+} inhibitors" prenylamine and verapamil (an analogue of D-600). However these drugs have diverse actions on excitable membranes and cannot be regarded as highly specific for the Ca^{2+} channel (Van der Kloot & Kita, 1975; Van der Kloot *et al.*, 1975). All of the inhibitor studies support the idea of a voltage-gated Ca^{2+} channel.

The arguments presented above are somewhat circular. Calcium ion entry is assumed to regulate ACh release and ACh release is used as an index of Ca^{2+} entry. But further evidence will support both suppositions. At this stage it is worth turning to a consideration of the quantitative relation between $[Ca^{2+}]_o$ and quantal release, since this is necessary background for what will follow.

If Ca^{2+} enters by way of a channel, other factors being equal, influx will be proportional to extracellular concentration. The relation between $[Ca^{2+}]_o$ and e.p.p. amplitude, in the range from 0.2-1.0 mM, is highly non-linear; small increases in $[Ca^{2+}]_o$ give large increases in the number of quanta released (del Castillo & Stark, 1952; Jenkinson, 1957). Plots of log (e.p.p. amplitude) as a function of log $[Ca^{2+}]_o$, in the range between 0.15-1.0 mM, fall close to a straight line. For the frog, the slope of the line is almost 4 (Dodge & Rahamimoff, 1967). For the rat it is 2.7 (Hubbard *et al.*, 1968), for larval *Drosophila* it is 4 (Jan & Jan, 1977), for crustacean neuromuscular junction it is close to 1 (Bracho & Orkand, 1970; Zucker, 1974). The interpretation of the relation will be deferred to the final part of this section.

A steady change in the potential of the nerve terminal membrane can be produced with a current from an extracellular micro electrode in the presence of TTX (Katz & Miledi, 1965b, 1976a). Hyperpolarizing currents sometimes produce fast bursts of miniature end-plate potentials (min. e.p.p.s.). In the frog, the bursts usually only occur in response to strong hyperpolarizing currents, so they may be elicited by injury to the membrane. But in mammals they are set off by modest hyperpolarizations (Cooke & Quastel, 1973a). If the terminal is depolarized in elevated K^+, a hyperpolarizing current decreases min.e.e.p. frequency.

Even slight depolarizing currents increase min.e.p.p. frequency. A depolarization estimated to be 18 mV increases frequency 10-fold (Cooke & Quastel, 1973a). Frequency continues to rise exponentially with depolarization until the counting of individual miniatures becomes impossible--more than 500/sec.

There is an obvious discrepancy between the voltage dependence of the Ca^{2+} channel of the squid axon or of cardiac muscle and that of ACh release caused by focal depolarization. As will be discussed shortly, depolarization with elevated K^+ leads to a similar conclusion.

Another characteristic feature of Ca^{2+} channels is that they, at least partially, inactivate. When a motor nerve is depolarized for several seconds, the quantal release is sustained. In fact, there may be two phases in the response: a fast initial increase following the depolarization, and a slower growth over the next 10 to 20 msec. The second phase accounts for about one-third of the total increase (Cooke & Quastel 1973b). These experiments were performed with a rapid flow of fresh solution from a pipette positioned at the end-plate, so extracellular solution could be changed abruptly. The first phase is markedly affected by changes in $[Ca^{2+}]_0$; the second phase is almost insensitive to changes in extracellular Ca^{2+}. One possible explanation is that there is a rapid Ca^{2+} influx with depolarization, and then intracellular Ca^{2+} remains high because its disposal is prevented by the continued depolarization. This would also account for the absence of marked inactivation.

The motor nerve terminal can be uniformly depolarized by raising $[K^+]_0$. When Ca^{2+} is also present there is a notable increase in min.e.p.p. frequency, which is sustained for hours (del Castillo & Katz, 1954a). A stepwise increase in $[K^+]_0$ gives a rapid increase in frequency, followed by a second, slower rise. The maximum is reached only after 40 seconds (Cooke & Quastel, 1973c). Following a step-wise decrease in the $[K^+]_0$, back to the normal level, the fall in min.e.p.p. frequency also follows a delayed time course. All or part of the delay is probably caused by a diffusion barrier.

In elevated $[K^+]_0$, increases in $[Ca^{2+}]_0$ decrease the min. e.p.p. frequency. For example, shifting abruptly from 8 mM to 0.125 mM Ca^{2+} within a minute or two increases the frequency of the miniatures. On the other hand, elevated Ca^{2+} does not inhibit release from electrically depolarized terminals. Viewing this dichotomy, Cooke and Quastel (1973a) postulated that K^+ has some sort of special effect--other than its depolarizing action-- on the terminal.

There is another explanation, invoking a concept that will appear several times in these pages. Biological membranes have an excess of fixed negative surface charges, so there is a negative potential at the membrane-solution interface. Consequently, ions are attracted to the interface. Their concentration at the surface, $(I\pm n)_S$, is given by the Boltzmann distribution.

$$(I\pm n)_S = (I\pm n)_\infty \cdot EXP\ (\pm n\psi F/RT)$$

where $(I \pm n)_\infty$ is the concentration in the bulk solution, n is the valence, ψ is the surface potential, R, the gas constant, T, the absolute temperature, and F, the Faraday.

The potential difference between the solutions on the two sides of the membrane is divided into three steps; the potential gradient through the membrane itself and the surface potentials at the two interfaces (Figure 1).

Increasing the divalent cation concentration in the external solution brings more of them close to the membrane where they shield the fixed charges and decrease the negative surface potential. The overall potential between the two bulk solutions is unchanged, but now it is subdivided differently. The surface potential is decreased while the potential gradient within the membrane is increased. The hyperpolarization of the membrane tends to shut voltage-dependent gates. Therefore, increasing $[Ca^{2+}]_0$ may decrease conductance and therefore decrease influx (Matthews & Winkelgren, 1977).

Using plausible values (one negative charge/154 $\overset{o}{A}^2$; [univalent ions] = 0.12M; see Muller and Finkelstein, 1974), a rise in divalent cation concentration from 0.1 to 8 mM will decrease the voltage gradient in the membrane by 16 mV. Therefore the binding of Ca^{2+} to anionic surface groups may account for the inhibitory effect of raised concentrations on min.e.p.p. frequency in preparations depolarized in high K^+; when stimulation is by an electric current, elevated Ca^{2+} merely shifts the depolarization-response curve. If this is the explanation, min.e.p.p. frequency should not be inhibited with increasing $[Ca^{2+}]_0$ as long as the total divalent cation concentration in the Ringer ($[Mg^{2+}]_0$ + $[Ca^{2+}]_0$) is constant. With constant divalent cation concentrations, min.e.p.p. frequency, in preparations slightly depolarized with elevated K^+, is a monotonically increasing function of $[Ca^{2+}]_0$ (Madden & Van der Kloot, in press).

Min.e.p.p. frequencies increase progressively, over a period of hours, when preparations are soaked in isotonic $CaCl_2$ solutions (Katz & Miledi, 1969). There is a high electrochemical gradient for Ca^{2+} influx, and the outward transport of Ca^{2+} may also be depressed, because the exchange of intracellular Ca^{2+} for extracellular Na^+ is important in many types of cells (Baker, 1974). A peak frequency is reached after some hours, this is followed by a decline to low levels. After the decline, focal depolarization of the terminals no longer elicits release. A return to normal Ringer's solution restores a low min.e.p.p. frequency, but not stimulated release. After prolonged exposure to high Ca^{2+}, the vesicles in the terminal are clumped together like grapes on a stalk (Heuser et al., 1971).

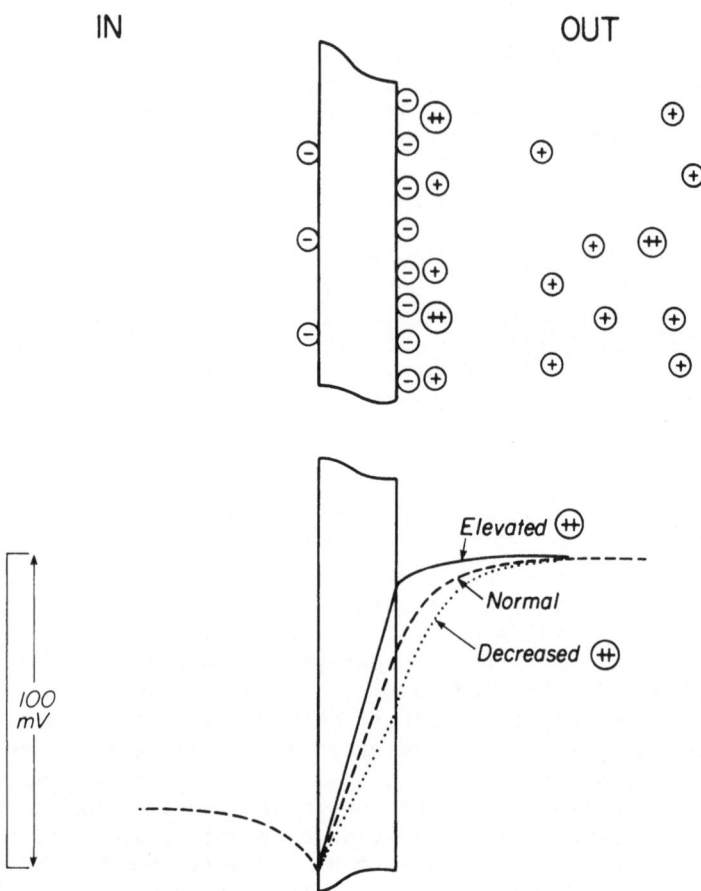

*Figure 1.   The total potential difference between the extracell-
ular and the intracellular solutions includes the negative surface
potentials at the two solution-membrane interfaces.   The surface
potentials attract cations to the solution just outside of the
membrane.   An increase in the extracellular divalent cation
concentration will diminish the surface potential, by screening,
but will increase the voltage gradient within the membrane.   Decreased divalent cation concentrations cause the opposite effects.*

The experiments described so far have been interpreted by assuming that $[Ca^{2+}]_{in}$ controls the rate of quantal release. There are other possible interpretations, some of which were used by those doing the experiments. With the discovery of ionophores, it became feasible to change intracellular divalent cation concentrations.

The first ionophore to be studied extensively was X-537A, which transports both uni- and di-valent cations through lipid bilayers and cellular membranes. In divalent cation-free solutions, X537A has no effect on min.e.p.p. frequencies. The addition of Ca^{2+} causes a substantial rise in min.e.p.p. frequencies, with a time course in minutes, followed by a decline to vanishingly low rates. When the min.e.p.p. frequency is depressed, simulated release is also blocked (Kita & Van der Kloot, 1974; 1976). The sequence of events in X537A plus Ca^{2+} is strikingly like that of isotonic $CaCl_2$ (pp. 264-265), but with a compressed time scale.

In Ca^{2+}-Ringer X-537A also markedly potentiates the effect of nerve stimulation. This increase in quantal release lasts for a few minutes and is followed by a complete block. There is a problem in interpreting the action of X-537A. It depolarizes muscle fibers, perhaps by permitting Na^+ influx (Devore & Nastuk, 1975). If the nerve terminal.is also somewhat depolarized, this could account for the rise in min.e.p.p. frequency; it would not account for the ensuing fall. In the frog, slight depolarizations of the nerve with elevated K^+ do not potentiate stimulated release, so this effect is also unlikely to be accounted for by depolarization (Kita & Van der Kloot, 1976). In the rat, X537A causes only a slight increase in min.e.p.p. frequency, with little change in e.p.p. amplitude. Soon transmission in the motor nerve terminal is blocked (Jansson *et al.*, 1976). The reasons for the differences between the rat and the frog are obscure.

A23187 is an ionophore that transports only divalent cations and it does not depolarize. In the frog, A23187 has almost no effects at temperatures below 20°C; at 25°C it causes a large increase in min.e.p.p. frequency. Stratham and Duncan (1976) propose that at the lower temperature the ionophore promotes Ca^{2+} entry, but at rates that are easily matched by the cellular mechanisms for removing Ca^{2+}. Higher temperatures favor Ca^{2+} influx but are unfavorable for the frog's metabolism, so Ca^{2+} accumulation occurs. A similar interpretation has been proposed for the X-537A dose-response curve, which appears to have a sharp threshold for stimulating min.e.p.p. release. Even low doses of the ionophore must promote Ca^{2+} influx, but high doses are needed to overwhelm the cell's machinery for bailing out Ca^{2+}.

In the rat, A23187 produces a slowly increasing min.e.p.p. frequency that reaches high levels in an hour. In preparations blocked by pretreatment with botulinum toxin, A23187 plus elevated $[Ca^{2+}]_0$ leads to high min.e.p.p. frequencies, (Cull-Candy *et al.*, 1976). The toxin appears to markedly reduce the Ca^{2+} sensitivity of the release process.

The evidence from the use of ionophores most strongly favors the idea that an elevation of intracellular Ca^{2+} is responsible for promoting quantal release.

Following each e.p.p. there is an interval during which the min.e.p.p. frequency is elevated above normal (del Castillo & Katz, 1954). In the first 0.15 sec following an e.p.p., miniature frequency is elevated about 7-fold (Rahamimoff & Yaari, 1973). The delayed release is enhanced at low temperatures. Because of the relatively small numbers of miniatures involved, it is hard to be certain of the time course of the fall-off of the delayed release. Rahamimoff & Yaari (1973) suggest that there are two phases, separated by a dip.

Essentially the same sequence is observed following a brief tetanus. There is a notable after-discharge, lasting for somewhat less than a second. The time course of the fall cannot be described as a single exponential process (Hubbard, 1963). A fall described by a single exponential would be expected if min.e.p.p. frequency is proportional to the $[Ca^{2+}]^4$, and if Ca^{2+} removal follows first-order kinetics.

An after-discharge also follows a focal depolarizing pulse in TTX-Ringer. Cooke and Quastel (1973b) found that during the after-discharge a second depolarization had less than the expected effect and that the slope of the relation between current and log (min.e.p.p. frequency) was decreased. This behavior resembles the persisting inactivation shown by the Ca^{2+} channels (p. 262). Longer after-discharges appear to decay in two exponential phases.

If the motor nerve is stimulated twice in close succession, the second action potential causes a substantially higher quantal output. The extent of the facilitation depends upon the interval between the stimuli. Katz & Miledi (1968) proposed that facilitation depends upon a residue of "active Ca^{2+}" in the nerve terminal.

Facilitation follows a complex time course. Intense early facilitation is seen only in experiments in the presence of TTX when the membrane potential is controlled by a focal electrode. At $4^{\circ}C$, the second of a pair of 1 msec depolarizing pulses, separated by 25 µsec, releases 50x as many quanta. The same effect can be seen when a one msec pulse is simply extended to 2 msec: the longer pulse releases 50x as many quanta. Obviously if Ca^{2+} entry reached a maximum at the moment of depolarization and then remained steady, twice as much Ca^{2+} would enter with the pulse of double duration. If the model is correct, quantal release should be increased by $2^4=16$ times. The obvious explanation is that there is an appreciable time lag between depolarization and the increase in Ca^{2+} conductance.

When the motor nerve is stimulated twice with a 5 msec interval, the second stimulus gives twice the quantal output. This facilitation falls off with a time constant of about 35 msec. After 100 msec the facilitation of a second release is only about 1.05 times the first. Then facilitation begins to increase with still longer intervals, reaching a second peak at 180 msec when the second release is 1.15 times the first. The second phase decays with a time constant of 250 msec (Mallart & Martin, 1967).

Katz & Miledi (1968) tested the effects of changing $[Ca^{2+}]_o$ on paired action potentials. A Ca^{2+}-containing micropipette was placed over a point on the nerve terminal so $[Ca^{2+}]_o$ could be altered between the first and second stimulus. The preparation was in a Ca^{2+}-free solution. A pulse of Ca^{2+} always preceded the second stimulus, so enough quanta were released to give meaningful results. The first stimulus, even in very low Ca-Ringer, facilitated the second by a factor of 1.1 There is no evidence for or against the idea that this slight facilitation results from intracellular Ca^{2+} release.

If the first stimulus is also preceded by a Ca^{2+} pulse, the second is facilitated two-fold. The facilitation might result from the persistence of active Ca^{2+} within the terminal, or it might mean that the properties of the terminal are in some ways changed as a result of quantal release. Elevated $[Ca^{2+}]_o$ increases the duration of this early phase in facilitation (Rahamimoff, 1968). The decay of facilitation is slowed by low temperatures (Balnave & Gage, 1970). If the active-Ca^{2+} hypothesis is correct, the long tail on facilitation means that Ca^{2+} cannot be removed from the active sites by a first order process (Katz & Miledi, 1968; Barrett & Stevens, 1972; Younkin, 1974). Possible explanations will be considered in the final section.

With a short train of stimuli, each e.p.p. is larger than its predecessor. Often the growth of the facilitation fits the predictions of a model in which each stimulus produces the same incremental jump, which then decays exponentially (Mallart & Martin, 1968). An exception is seen in the toad where facilitation grows more rapidly than this model predicts (Balnave & Gage, 1977).

One problem in interpreting the data on facilitation is that it is hard to be sure that there are not changes in the shape of the action potential or in the extent of the terminal invaded by the action potential. It would be worth repeating many of the observations in TTX-Ringer, using focal depolarization.

Following a tetanus there is a period, lasting from seconds to minutes depending on the conditions, in which an additional stimulus is facilitated. The extent of this post-tetanic potentiation depends on $[Ca^{2+}]_O$ during the tetanus, so Ca^{2+} accumulation interpretations are reasonable, but not exclusive (Gage & Hubbard, 1966; Rosenthal, 1969).

Over a limited range of Ca^{2+} concentrations,

$$\log \text{ (e.p.p. amplitude)} \propto n \cdot \log [Ca^{2+}]_O$$

so Dodge and Rahamimoff (1968) suggested that release depends on a cooperative interaction between four activated Ca^{2+} complexes, CaX,

$$\text{(e.p.p. amplitude)} \propto (CaX)^4,$$

and that $\quad Ca + X \rightleftarrows CaX$,

with a limited amount of X available. Therefore the relationship is formally analogous to an enzyme-substrate interaction, and a Lineweaver-Burke plot of (e.p.p. amplitude)$^{-\frac{1}{4}}$ as a function of $[Ca^{2+}]_O^{-1}$ should give a straight line. Over the limited range, this is true. The cooperative interaction of 4 active complexes has an appealing simplicity, but like most attempts to interpret data from complicated systems with kinetic models, there are alternatives.

To choose just one of the other possibilities, suppose that there is an energy barrier that must be overcome before any given quantum can be released. The available quanta have an energy distribution such that, at rest, only an occasional quantum has sufficient kinetic energy to breach the barrier to be released. Any reduction in the barrier will result in a marked increase in the release rate in a highly non-linear fashion. Cooke *et al.*, (1973) showed that release at the mammalian neuromuscular junction fits well with a model that assumes that each Ca^{2+} combining at an effective site decreases the energy barrier. A similar model, with a more specific identification of the possible components of the barrier, was described by Van der Kloot and Kita (1973).

There are good reasons to seriously doubt the cooperative interaction model. The values of n varies from 1 to 5, depending upon the species studied (see p. 263). In a single preparation,

n is altered in different experimental circumstances. In frog
Ringer made hypertonic with added sucrose, n is reduced to about
1.5 (Kita & Van der Kloot, 1971). Treating rats with botulinum
toxin shifts the slope from 3 to about 1.3 (Cull-Candy et al.,
1976).

    In the frog, the 4th-power relation fails at $[Ca^{2+}]_o = 0.1$ mM;
at lower concentrations n is about 1 (Crawford, 1974). When the
solution contains Co^{2+} as an inhibitor of Ca^{2+} influx, the points
change from a 4th-power to a 1st-power function of $[Ca^{2+}]_o$ at
about 2 mM (Crawford, 1974). It seems clear that both the effects
of hypertonic solution and botulinum toxin on n could be accounted
for by a lowering of the level of effective intracellular Ca^{2+}.
A variety of models can account for the shift to lower slopes at
lower $[Ca^{2+}]$; one of them is the energy barrier model.

NON-QUANTAL ACh RELEASE

    Only a small fraction of the normal leakage of ACh from rest-
ing nerve terminals is in the form of quanta (Potter, 1969). There
is a steady background of molecular ACh efflux that depolarizes
the end-plate by about 70 μV (Katz & Miledi, 1977). The action
of Ca^{2+} on this release is unexplored.

DIVALENT METALS AS INHIBITORS

    The number of quanta released from a stimulated nerve termi-
nal is reduced when $[Mg^{2+}]_o$ is increased. One interpretation is
that Mg^{2+} competes with Ca^{2+} for the receptor, X (Jenkinson, 1957).
Lineweaver-Burke plots of (e.p.p. amplitude)$^{-1/4}$ as a function of
$[Ca^{2+}]_o^{-1}$ at different $[Mg^{2+}]_o$ fit with the idea of a competitive
inhibitor. If this analysis is correct, either X is on the outside
of the terminal, or the $[Mg^{2+}]_i$ is a direct function of $[Mg^{2+}]_o$.

    There is an alternative interpretation. The concentration
of Ca^{2+} at the surface of the nerve terminal is a function of the
surface potential. Increasing the $[Mg^{2+}]_o$ screens the negative
surface charges, and thereby reduces the $[Ca^{2+}]_s$ (Muller &
Finkelstein, 1974). They assume that Ca^{2+} entry is directly proportional to $[Ca^{2+}]_s$, that quantal release is proportional to
$[Ca^{2+}]_{in}^{3.8}$, and that there is one excess negative charge/154Å^2 of
terminal surface. With these assumptions, the effects of changing
$[Mg^{2+}]_o$ on the surface potential can account for the data. The
surface charge model also predicts that decreasing $[Na^+]_o$ should
increase the surface potential--less screening--, increase $[Ca^{2+}]_s$,
and thereby increase quantal release. This prediction appears to
be true.

Divalent ions such as Co^{2+}, Mn^{2+}, and Pb^{2+} are more effective blockers than Mg^{2+}. Their effects cannot be accounted for by screening of surface charges. They may bind to anionic groups near the entrance of the Ca^{2+} channels, thereby diminishing local Ca^{2+} concentrations, or interfere with Ca^{2+} movements through the channels, or compete with Ca^{2+} for binding to X (Kita & Van der Kloot, 1973; Weakly, 1973; Manalis & Cooper, 1973).

Mercurous ion (Hg^{2+}) belongs in a class by itself. It works at low concentrations (1 μM). It causes a marked transitory potentiation of stimulated quantal release before a block is produced and the potentiation is not accompanied by any increase in min. e.p.p. frequencies (Manalis & Cooper, 1975).

DIVALENT METALS AS STIMULATORS

Strontium ion can replace Ca^{2+} in neuromuscular transmission (Dodge et al., 1969; Meiri & Rahamimoff, 1971), but Sr^{2+} is not as effective. On a plot of log (e.p.p. quantal output) as a function of log ($[Sr^{2+}]_o$), the slope is about 2.5 (from Figure 8, Dodge et al., 1969). Strontium ion may prove to be a most interesting tool for studying neuromuscular transmission. Barton and Cohen (personal communication) found that raising $[Sr^{2+}]_o$ increased the half-time ($T_{\frac{1}{2}}$) of facilitation but decreased the $T_{\frac{1}{2}}$ of delayed release.

Soaking a preparation in isotonic Mg^{2+} produces a delayed, massive increase in min.e.p.p. frequency, followed by a decline to a complete halt--much like the effects of isotonic Ca^{2+} (p. 265). But unlike $CaCl_2$, this treatment does not aggregate the vesicles and, following a return to Ringer, there is some restoration of stimulated release (Heuser et al., 1971).

In solutions containing Mg^{2+} and EDTA, but without added Ca^{2+}, tetanic stimulation at 10/sec produces an exponential increase in min.e.p.p. frequency (Blioch et al., 1968; Hurbut et al., 1971). The rate at which min.e.p.p. frequency increases is proportional to $[Mg^{2+}]_o$, so the effect cannot be attributed to traces of Ca^{2+} emerging from the muscle. Focal depolarization in Ca^{2+}-free, Mg^{2+}-Ringer produces as much as a 100-fold increase in min.e.p.p. frequency, but there is no after-discharge (Cooke & Quastel, 1973a). Qualitatively similar results are seen with tetanic stimulation in Co^{2+} and Ni^{2+} (Kita & Van der Kloot, 1973 and in preparation). The increase in min.e.p.p. frequency is an exponential function of the concentration of the metal in the solution or the number of stimuli to the nerve. Following each tetanus, there is a progressive decrease in min.e.p.p. frequency back toward normal levels. The sequence can be repeated time

after time. If these other metals are acting by releasing intracellular Ca^{2+}, then the Ca^{2+} must all be resequestered within the
terminal, ready for reuse. Min.e.p.p. frequencies are also greatly
increased when preparations depolarized in high K^+-Ringer are exposed to Ni^{2+} or Co^{2+} (Kita & Van der Kloot, 1973).

Preparations exposed to X-537A in the absence of divalent
metals show no increase in min.e.p.p. frequency. There is a
notable stimulation when a divalent metal is added to the solution.
Judging from the degree of stimulation and the concentrations of
X-537A required, the apparent sequence of effectiveness is:

$$Ba^{2+} > Sr^{2+} > Ca^{2+} > Mn^{2+} \simeq Co^{2+} \simeq Ni^{2+} > Mg^{2+}$$

(Kita & Van der Kloot, 1974; 1976). This must not be taken as the
sequence of the effectiveness of the metals in promoting quantal
release. The sequence is roughly parallel to the ability of the
ionophore to transport the metals into a hydrophobic layer. It
seems likely that the nerve terminals can either sequester or pump
out the metals. If the quantal release rate depends upon the
accumulation of free metal in the axoplasm, it will depend upon
the balance between inflow and elimination. Calcium ion, for
example, might be the most effective in causing release, but it
may not be brought in by the ionophore as rapidly as Ba^{2+} and it
may be taken out of the axoplasm far more quickly than any of the
others.

Little has been done with A23187 using metals other than Ca^{2+}.
For the frog, in conditions where the ionophore in Ca^{2+}-Ringer is
almost without effect, a steady rise in min.e.p.p. frequencies
follows the addition of the metal to ionophore-containing solutions
(Kita *et al.*, 1976). In the rat, a similar steady increase in
min.e.p.p. frequencies follows the addition of A23187 to a Ringer
that has very low Ca^{2+}, (but which presumably contains Mg^{2+})
(Cull-Candy *et al.*, 1976). The possibility that this rise depends
upon Mg^{2+} has not been tested.

TRIVALENT IONS

La^{3+}, Pr^{3+}, and Y^{3+} increase min.e.p.p. frequencies and
also block stimulated quantal release (Alnaes & Rahamimoff, 1974;
Bowen, 1972; Kajimoto & Pirpekar, 1972; Heuser & Miledi, 1971).
It seems likely that they block stimulated Ca^{2+} influx, and may
also either release Ca^{2+} within the terminal or mimic the effects
of elevated intracellular Ca^{2+}.

METABOLIC INHIBITORS

If quantal release is triggered by Ca^{2+} entry, it must be ended by Ca^{2+} removal, presumably by pumping or sequestering. The hope is that the mechanism can be identified by finding inhibitors of these processes.

Anoxia, uncouplers, antimycin A, and CN^- increase min.e.p.p. frequencies and the quantal output from stimulated terminals (Hubbard & Loyning, 1966; Glagoleva *et al.*, 1970; Katz & Edwards, 1973; Rees, 1974; Rahamimoff & Alnaes, 1973). These effects may well be an index of an elevated $[Ca^{2+}]_{in}$. However, the e.p.p.s appear to have essentially normal durations, so the mitochondria are unlikely to be playing a major role in terminating Ca^{2+} action.

Part of the mechanism for keeping $[Ca^{2+}]_{in}$ low involves an exchange of Na^+ from without for Ca^{2+} from within (Baker, 1974). Reducing the Na^+ in the Ringer slightly increases min.e.p.p. frequencies and the quantal content of the e.p.p.s (Birks & Cohen, 1968; Kelly, 1965; Gage & Quastel, 1966).

Inhibitors of the $Na^+ - K^+$ exchange pump, ouabain or low external K^+, also slowly increase min.e.p.p. frequencies and stimulated quantal release (Elmquist & Feldman, 1965; Birks & Cohen, 1968), but the increase in min.e.p.p. frequency occurs even in very low $[Ca^{2+}]_o$ (Baker & Crawford, 1975). These results and the similar stimulating effects of Li^+ currently have no clear explanation, though we can speculate about changing levels of $[Ca^{2+}]_{in}$, $[K^+]_{in}$, or the like (Baker & Crawford, 1975). To me, the most striking point is the essentially normal time course of the e.p.p.s, showing that the mechanism for rapidly terminating quantal release is almost totally untouched.

STATISTICS OF QUANTAL RELEASE

A train of stimuli produces e.p.p.s of varying amplitudes, reflecting a statistical variation in the number of quanta released from trial to trial. In many instances, this variation is best fit by a binomial distribution function in which there are two variables, the mean probability of release, and the number of quanta available for release (Johnson & Wernig, 1971; Zucker, 1973; Bennett & Florin, 1974). Increasing $[Ca^{2+}]_o$ appears to increase both the probability of release and, to a lesser extent, the number of quanta available for release (Branisteanu *et al.*, 1976; Bennett *et al.*, 1976). This emphasizes the possibility that Ca^{2+} may exert a number of complementary effects within the terminal.

MECHANISM OF CALCIUM ION ACTION

There is only preliminary speculation about how Ca^{2+} triggers quantal release. One problem in speculating is that although the evidence for quantal release is overwhelming, the evidence for the vesicle hypothesis is still inconclusive (for a brief review of alternatives, see Van der Kloot, 1977). Nonetheless, I will assume that the ACh is packaged in vesicles, that release involves the fusion of the vesicles with the nerve terminal membrane, and that following stimulation this process is initiated by Ca^{2+}.

One suggestion is that contractile systems are involved. Contractile proteins are regulated by low levels of Ca^{2+}, Actin-like and myosin-like proteins are found in nerve cells. We can imagine a contractile interaction pulling the vesicle close to the membrane, or tearing a hole for ACh escape (see the review by Bray, 1977). On the other hand, the muscle-like proteins are found in cells of all descriptions; they are not especially prominent in nerve terminals. Known contractile systems are controlled by Ca^{2+}, and most other divalent metals are poor substitutes. At the neuromuscular junction, it seems quite possible that other metals can substitute for Ca^{2+} (see p. 272), if they can get into the nerve terminal.

Another line of thought involves the mechanisms that favor the approach and then the fusion of lipid bilayers. This is a field that is just beginning to be explored experimentally and involves ideas that are unfamiliar to most neurobiologists. The bilayers will be attracted by very short-range London-van der Waal's forces. They are usually kept separated by a series of barriers. One barrier for close approach is the electrodynamic repulsion caused by the excess negative charges in the bilayers. This repulsion will be reduced by divalent metals screening the charges or binding to anionic groups (Biloch *et al.*, 1968). Increases in univalent cation concentrations will decrease repulsion by screening. It has been suggested that the increase in min.e.p.p. frequency that is produced when the nerve terminals are shrunk in hypertonic solutions may be a result of the increased intracellular cation concentrations (Kita & Van der Kloot, 1977). If negative surface charges are important in regulating release, a fall in intracellular pH should increase min.e.p.p. frequency. This prediction is fulfilled (Cohen & Van der Kloot, 1977). The magnitude of these electrostatic repulsive forces has been estimated by calculations based on model systems familiar to colloid chemistry; the repulsion may be large enough so that changes in surface potential can modulate release, but they are unlikely, by themselves, to be sufficient to keep membrane and vesicle apart (Remler, 1973; Van der Kloot & Kita, 1973).

Another factor keeping the two membranes apart is the layers of water molecules held like a hydration shell to the membrane (Bass & Moore, 1966). At present, little is known about the state of water near the membranes. Spertell (1976) suggests that the fluid layer separating the two membranes will be broken by the movement of the heads of the phospholipid molecules which will exert a traction on the film of water leading to instability and then fusion of the outer layer of the vesicle and the inner layer of the nerve membrane. When the two opposing layers have fused, the other halves of the bilayer will follow.

It is probably not enough to bring the two bilayers close together. Lipid bilayers vesicles can be attached to one another without fusing (Papahadjopoulos *et al.*, 1974). Fusion is promoted by elevated Ca^{2+} but the levels required (0.2 mM) are high by intracellular standards. The fusion critically depends upon the fluidity of the bilayers. Calcium ion may act by causing a phase transition, in which some of the phospholipids are bound together by Ca^{2+} chelation producing solid islands and leaving other patches of the membrane highly fluid, ready to fuse.

In biological membranes, the proteins may be more influential in fusion than the phospholipids (Poste & Allison, 1973; Ahkong *et al.*, 1975). An aggregation of membrane proteins precedes the clumping of isolated chromaffin granules (Schoher *et al.*, 1977). It is uncertain whether the proteins are made to aggregate, thereby leaving fluid patches of membrane for fusion, or whether the membrane first becomes more fluid, which then allows the proteins to drift together. Another line of thought is that as the vesicle approaches the membrane a lipase is activated, perhaps by Ca^{2+}, which transforms phospholipids to more fluid products and thereby promotes fusion.

Hall and Simon (1976) presented an interesting model in which Ca^{2+} binds to the inner face of the nerve terminal, reducing the surface potential so the vesicles can approach. Some of the Ca^{2+} transfers to the lipids of the vesicle, which changes the surface pressure, so that the vesicle flattens out against the membrane and the two fuse, releasing the ACh. When the Ca^{2+} is removed, the change in the surface pressure on the inner face of the terminal causes budding inward of new vesicles.

This is clearly an area in which speculation has out-stripped fact. However, there are a number of new experimental approaches to the study of membrane fusion in model systems, and an increasing interest in the biophysics of fusion. I expect a rapid increase in knowledge.

SCHWANN CELLS

Even the most enthusiastic modeller or theorist must face facts like the following. At denervated muscles there are still occasional min.e.p.p.s, apparently produced by quanta released by Schwann cells (Birks *et al.*, 1960). Quantal release from the nerve terminals are increased by hypertonic Ringer, ethanol, or elevated K^+. All of these are without effect on the Schwann cells. At the nerve terminal, release is depressed in hypotonic Ringer; at the Schwann cell, release is increased. Electrical stimulation of Schwann cells causes release, but it is non-quantal and probably is initiated by momentary membrane breakdown (Dennis & Miledi, 1974). Ionophores reduce the rate of quantal release, suggesting that Ca^{2+} influx is inhibitory (Ito & Miledi, 1977) (however, note that it has not yet been shown that Ca^{2+} is necessary for the ionophore's effect). All of the evidence suggests that this system works by rules that are diametrically opposite to release at the nerve terminal.

SUMMARY AND CONCLUSIONS

It is close to certainty that the entry of Ca^{2+} into the terminal is the trigger for quantal release. The pathway for Ca^{2+} influx is unimportant, it can enter by voltage-gated channels (pp. 262, 263), by translocation with an ionophore (p. 261), or by leaking through the resting membrane (p. 265), but it always stimulates quantal release.

Calcium ion influx at the nerve terminal is blocked by the same agents that block the channels in the squid axon and in cardiac muscle - Mn^{2+}, Co^{2+}, and organic Ca^{2+} inhibitors. On the other hand, even slight depolarizations appear to enhance Ca^{2+} influx into the terminal, while the channels in squid axon and cardiac muscle open appreciably only with depolarizations of about 50 mV. There is little indication of inactivation in the terminal, unlike the other tissues. Facile assumptions about the similarities between the Ca^{2+}-channel in squid axon and the influx-mechanism in motor nerve terminals may be misleading.

The idea that there is a cooperative interaction of four CaX complexes in triggering release is widely quoted, but it is clear that at low levels of $[Ca^{2+}]_o$ the data does not fit this interpretation (p. 270). The data is fit better by models in which release is opposed by an energy barrier that is progressively diminished with a rise in $[Ca^{2+}]_{in}$ (p. 270). As pointed out by Cooke *et al.* (1973), this model also can help account for the ever-lengthening list of variables that affect quantal release rates, like Ca^{2+}, ethanol, and osmotic pressure, each of which may act on a different part of the barrier.

The recognition that the release rate is not proportional to $[Ca^{2+}]_{in}^{4}$ at all concentrations has implications for facilitation and after-discharge. At low levels, release is proportional to $[Ca^{2+}]_{in}^{1}$. The shift from a fourth-power to a first power relation as $[Ca^{2+}]_{in}$ falls produces a tail of elevated release, even if Ca^{2+} is removed by a first-order process (Figure 2). The tail will not account for all of the features of facilitation and delayed release, but it certainly adds to the possible interpretations.

Quantal release is increased following tetanic stimulation in solutions containing different metals (p. 272) or following the application of ionophores plus different metals (p. 273). Either each of the metals can stimulate release if brought into the terminal, or the metals can cause the graded release of Ca^{2+} from intracellular stores.

Intracellular stores of Ca^{2+} are frequently invoked to explain nerve terminal behavior, but there is scant evidence for their existence. The ionophores are lipid soluble, and should enter the terminal to become incorporated into intracellular membranes. Any Ca^{2+} held with intracellular membranes should be released into the axoplasm. However, the ionophores, in the absence of an extracellular divalent metal, rarely causes more than a small, transient stimulation of quantal release. If the ionophores release Ca^{2+} from a store, it must be quickly transported out of the cells.

Tetanic stimulation in the presence of divalent metals can cause prolonged enhanced quantal release. Similar prolonged stimulation occurs in high K^{+}-Ringer plus the metals. It is hard to believe that the terminal has intracellular Ca^{2+} stores that support such a sustained and massive quantal release.

One reason to be wary of the idea that divalent ions other than Ca^{2+} can stimulate release is the observation that Mg^{2+} appears to have activity. Intracellular $[Mg^{+}]$ in the squid axon is 6 mM (Baker & Crawford, 1972); in barnacle muscle it is also 6 mM (Brinley et $al.$, 1977). $[Ca^{2+}]_{in}$ is in the micromolar range. When the basal level is so high, how could tetanic stimulation or ionophores appreciably increase $[Mg^{2+}]_{i}$? Krnjevic et $al.$ (1976) iontophoresed Mg^{2+} into cat motoneurons. Elevated $[Mg^{2+}]_{in}$ increased membrane resistance, probably by decreasing K^{+} conductance. Increasing $[Ca^{2+}]_{in}$ had the opposite effect, decreasing membrane resistance. The effects are produced by the same doses of Ca^{2+} or Mg^{2+}. This striking observation lends credence to the idea

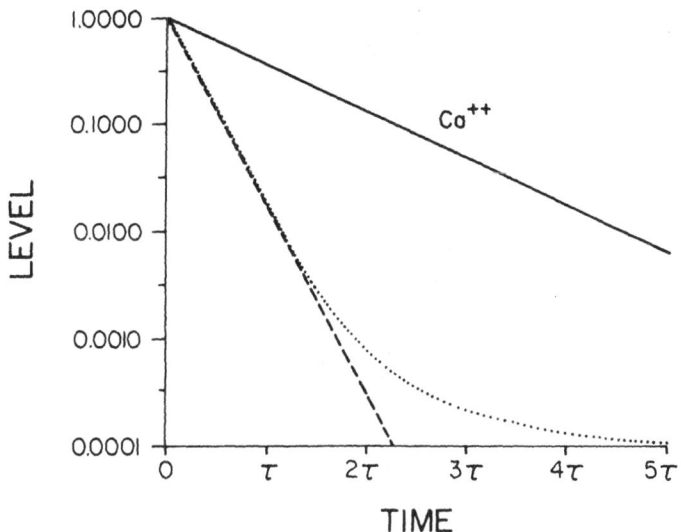

Figure 2. Suppose that following an action potential $[Ca^{2+}]_{in}$ within the nerve terminal is elevated and then declines by a first-order process. If release rate is proportional to $[Ca^{2+}]_{in}^4$, then it will decrease by a simple exponential (dashed line). If however, as $[Ca^{2+}]_{in}$ reaches low levels (in this case 1/100 of the maximum), release becomes proportional to $[Ca^{2+}]_{in}$ then release will have a long tail.

that increases in $[Mg^{2+}]_{in}$ in the motoneuron terminal stimulate quantal release. The following observations are consistent with this hypothesis.

1) Mg^{2+} + X-537A increases min.e.p.p. frequencies (p. 273).

2)   Tetanic stimulation in Mg^{2+}-Ringer increases min.e.p.p. frequencies; the increase is proportional to $[Mg^{2+}]_o$ (p. 272).

3)   Prolonged soaking in isotonic $MgCl_2$ increases min.e.p.p. frequency to a high level (p. 272).

4)   Focal depolarization in Mg^{2+}-Ringer ($[Ca^{2+}]_o = 10^{-7}$ M) produces large increases in min.e.p.p. frequency. In Ringer without Mg^{2+}, with $[Ca^{2+}]_o = 10^{-10}$ M, the depolarization is without effect (p. 263). The difference might be owing to the change in $[Ca^{2+}]_o$, but this seems to be a strained interpretation.

IN   OUT

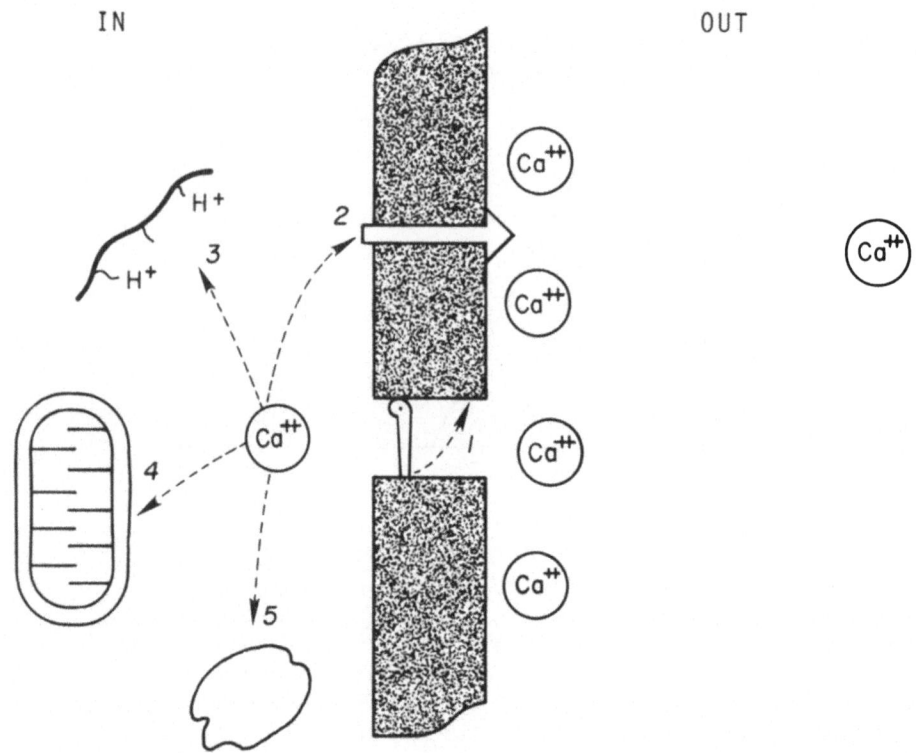

Figure 3. Some of the major events and possible events in neuro-muscular transmission (1.) Ca^{2+} enters the terminal through a voltage-gated channel. The elevation in intracellular Ca^{2+} triggers quantal release. The Ca^{2+} may then be eliminated by: (2.) transport out of the terminal, (3.) binding to proteins with the release of H^+, (4.) sequestration in mitochondria or (5.) in other unidentified membrane-bounded structures.

5) After treatment with diamine, min.e.p.p. frequency becomes proportional to $[Mg^{2+}]_o$ (Carlen *et al.*, 1976). Perhaps the diamine increases the leak conductance for Mg^{2+}.

6) Some facilitation is produced in EDTA-Mg^{2+}-Ringer. This may reflect Mg^{2+} influx (p. 269).

7) In increases in min.e.p.p. frequencies seen in preparations in low Ca^{2+}-Ringer, normal Mg^{2+}-treated with ouabain or Li^+ may come about by Mg^{2+} entry (Baker & Crawford, 1974; Crawford, 1975).

There is strong evidence that Mg^{2+} can enter by a voltage-sensitive system and stimulate quantal release. This adds weight to the proposition that a variety of divalent metals can serve as the release trigger. Until we have a better estimate of their intracellular concentrations during the experiment, we can say nothing about relative potency. It is possible that the specificity for extracellular Ca^{2+} is a measure only of the ability to enter the stimulated terminal. It is also possible that Mg^{2+} entry plays a physiological role in synaptic transmission, both by modest enhancement of the release rate and by changing the K^+ conductance and therefore the excitability and the action potential duration in the terminal. The elevated min.e.p.p. frequency persists for minutes after the end of a long tetanus in Mg^{2+}-Ringer, so such changes might have a relatively long time course.

Almost nothing is known about the mechanism that terminates the greatly enhanced quantal release that follows Ca^{2+} entry (Figure 3). No inhibitor has yet been found that markedly prolongs the period of quantal release. Meech and Thomas (1977) observed that intracellular Ca^{2+} injections cause only a short rise in $[Ca^{2+}]_{in}$, followed by a rise in $[H^+]_{in}$. The Ca^{2+} appears to be bound to molecules that release the H^+. It should be noted that a rise in $[H^+]_{in}$ increases min.e.p.p. frequencies (Cohen & Van der Kloot, 1977), so this might account for a part of the after-discharge. At present there is also no information beyond speculation about the way in which a rise in $[Ca^{2+}]_{in}$ triggers quantal release. This remains one of the most intriguing problems in biological science.

Acknowledgements

The preparation of this chapter was assisted by Grant 10320 from the NINCDS. I thank Kathleen Shaver Madden and Lorraine Brandwein for help in the preparation of the manuscript.

REFERENCES

Ahkong, Q. F., Fisher, D., Tampion, W., and Lucy, J. A., 1975, Mechanisms of cell fusion, *Nature* 253: 194.
Alnaes, E., & Rahamimoff, R., 1975, On the role of mitochondria in transmitter release from motor nerve terminals, *J. Physiol. (London)* 248: 285.
Alnaes, E., & Rahamimoff, R., 1974, Dual action of Praseodymium (Pr^{+++}) on transmitter release at the frog neuromuscular synapse, *Nature* 247: 478.
Baker, P. F., 1972, Transport and metabolism of calcium ions in nerve, *Progr. Biophys. Mol. Biol.* 24: 179.

Baker, P. F., 1974, Excitation - secretion coupling, *Recent Advances in Physiol.* 9: 51.

Baker, P. F., and Crawford, A. C., 1972, Mobility and transport of magnesium in squid giant axons, *J. Physiol. (London)* 227: 855.

Baker, P. F., and Crawford, A. C., 1975, A note on the mechanism by which inhibitors of the sodium pump accelerate spontaneous release of transmitter from motor nerve terminals, *J. Physiol. (London)* 209: 226.

Balnave, R. J., and Gage, P. W., 1977, Facilitation of transmitter secretion from toad motor nerve terminals during brief trains of action potentials, *J. Physiol. (London)* 266: 435.

Balnave, R. J., and Gage, P. W., 1970, Temperature sensitivity of the time course of facilitation of transmitter release, *Brain Res.* 21: 297.

Bass, L., and Moore, W. J., 1966, Electrokinetic mechanism of miniature postsynaptic potentials, *Proc. Nat. Acad. Sci. U. S. A.* 55: 1214.

Barrett, E. F., and Stevens, C. F., 1972, The kinetics of transmitter release at the frog neuromuscular junction, *J. Physiol. (London)* 227: 691.

Bennett, M. R., and Florin, T., 1974, A statistical analysis of the release of acetylcholine at newly formed synapses in striated muscle, *J. Physiol. (London)* 238: 93.

Bennett, M. R., Florin, T., and Pettigrew, A. G., 1976, The effect of calcium ions on the binomial statistic parameters that control acetylcholine release at preganglionic nerve terminals, *J. Physiol. (London)* 257: 597.

Birks, R. I., and Cohen, M. W., 1968, The action of sodium pump inhibitors on neuromuscular transmission, *Proc. R. Soc. London, Ser. B* 170: 381.

Birks, R., Katz, B., and Miledi, R., 1960, Physiological and structural changes at the amphibian myoneural junction, in the course of nerve degeneration, *J. Physiol. (London)* 150: 145.

Branisteanu, D. D., Miyamoto, M. D., and Volle, R. L., 1976, Affects of physiologic alterations on binomial transmitter release at magnesium-depressed neuromuscular junctions, *J. Physiol. (London)* 254: 19.

Blioch, Z. L., Glagoleva, I. M., Liberman, E. A., and Nenashev, V. A., 1968, A study of the mechanism of quantal transmitter release at a chemical synapse, *J. Physiol. (London)* 199: 11.

Bowen, J. M., 1972, Effects of rare earths and yttrium on striated muscle and the neuromuscular junction, *Can. J. Physiol. Pharmacol.* 50: 603.

Bracho, H., and Orkand, R. K., 1970, Effect of calcium on excitatory neuromuscular transmission in the crayfish, *J. Physiol. (London)* 206: 61.

Bray, D., 1977, Actin and myosin in neurones: a first review, *Biochimie* 59: 1.

Brinley, Jr., F. J., Scarpa, A., and Tiffert, T., 1977, The concentration of ionized magnesium in barnacle muscle fibres, *J. Physiol. (London)* 266: 545.

Carlen, P. I., Kosower, E. M., and Werman, R., 1976, The thiol-oxidizing agent diamide increases transmitter release by decreasing calcium requirements for neuromuscular transmission in the frog, *Brain Res.* 11: 257.

del Castillo, J., and Stark, L., 1952, The effect of calcium on the motor end-plate potentials, *J. Physiol. (London)* 116: 507.

del Castillo, J., and Katz, B., 1954a, Changes in end-plate activity produced by pre-synaptic polarization, *J. Physiol. (London)* 124: 586.

del Castillo, J., and Katz, B., 1954b, The membrane change produced by the neuromuscular transmitter, *J. Physiol. (London)* 125: 546.

Cohen, I., and Van der Kloot, W., 1976, The effects of pH changes on the frequency of miniature end-plate potentials at the frog neuromuscular junction, *J. Physiol. (London)* 262: 401.

Cooke, J. D., and Quastel, D. M. J., 1973a, Transmitter release by mammalian motor nerve terminals in response to focal polarization, *J. Physiol. (London)* 228: 377.

Cooke, J. D., and Quastel, D. M. J., 1973b, Cumulative and persistent effects of nerve terminal depolarization on transmitter release, *J. Physiol. (London)* 228: 407.

Cooke, J. D., and Quastel, D. M. J., 1973c, The specific effect of potassium on transmitter release by motor nerve terminals and its inhibition by calcium, *J. Physiol. (London)* 228: 435.

Cooke, J. D., Okamoto, K., and Quastel, D. M. J., 1973, The role of calcium in depolarization-secretion coupling at the motor nerve terminal, *J. Physiol. (London)* 228: 459.

Crawford, A. C., 1974, The dependence of evoked transmitter release on external calcium ions at very low mean quantal contents, *J. Physiol. (London)* 240: 255.

Crawford, A. C., 1975, Lithium ions and the release of transmitter at the frog neuromuscular junction, *J. Physiol. (London)* 246: 109.

Cull-Candy, S. G., Lundh, H., and Thesleff, S., 1976, Effects of botulinum toxin on neuromuscular transmission in the rat, *J. Physiol. (London)* 260: 177.

Dennis, M. J., and Miledi, R., 1974, Electrically induced release of acetylcholine from denervated Schwann cells, *J. Physiol. (London)* 237: 431.

Devore, D. I., and Nastuk, W. L., 1975, Effects of 'calcium ionophore' X-537A on frog skeletal muscle, *Nature* 253: 644.

Dodge, F. A., Jr., and Rahamimoff, R., 1967, Co-operative action of calcium ions in transmitter release at the neuromuscular junction, *J. Physiol. (London)* 193: 419.

Dodge, F. A., Jr., Miledi, R., and Rahamimoff, R., 1969, Strontium and quantal release of transmitter at the neuromuscular junction, *J. Physiol. (London)* 200: 267.

Elmqvist, D., and Feldman, D. S., 1965, Effects of sodium pump inhibitors on spontaneous acetylcholine release at the neuromuscular junction, *J. Physiol. (London)* 181: 498.

Gage, P. W., and Quastel, D. M. J., 1966, Competition between sodium and calcium ions in transmitter release at a mammalian neuromuscular junction, *J. Physiol. (London)* 185: 95.

Glagoleva, I. M., Liberman, Y. A., and Khashayev, Z., 1970, Effect of uncoupling agents of oxidation phosphorylation on the release of acetylcholine from nerve endings, *Biophysics (USSR)* 15: 76.

Hall, J. E., and Simon, S. A., 1976, A simple model for calcium induced exocytosis, *Biochim. Biophys. Acta* 436: 613.

Heuser, J., and Miledi, R., 1971, Effect of lanthanum ions on function and structure of frog neuromuscular junction, *Proc. R. Soc. London Ser. B* 179: 247.

Heuser, J., Katz, B., and Miledi, R., 1971, Structural and functional changes of frog neuromuscular junction in high calcium solutions, *Proc. R. Soc. London Ser. B* 178: 407.

Hubbard, J. I., 1963, Repetitive stimulation at the mammalian neuromuscular junction and the mobilisation of transmitter, *J. Physiol. (London)* 169: 641.

Hubbard, J. I., and Løyning, Y., 1966, The effects of hypoxia on neuromuscular transmission in a mammalian preparation, *J. Physiol. (London)* 185: 205.

Hubbard, J. J., Jones, S. F., and Landau, E. M., 1968, On the mechanism by which calcium and magnesium affect the release of transmitter by nerve impulses, *J. Physiol. (London)* 196: 75.

Hurlbut, W. P., Longenecker, H. B., and Mauro, A., 1971, Effects of calcium and magnesium on the frequency of end-plate potentials during prolonged tetanization, *J. Physiol. (London)* 219: 17.

Ito, Y., and Miledi, R., 1977, The effect of calcium-ionophores on acetylcholine release from Schwann cells, *Proc. R. Soc. London, Ser. B* 196: 51.

Jan, L. Y., and Jan, Y. N., 1976, Properties of the larval neuromuscular junction in Drosophila melanogaster, *J. Physiol. (London)* 262: 189.

Jansson, S. E., Heinonen, E., Heinänen, V., Gripenberg, J., Tolppanen, E. M., and Salmi, T., 1976, On the effect of the ionophore X-537A on neuromuscular transmission in the rat, *Life Sci.* 18: 1359.

Jenkinson, D. H., 1957, The nature of the antagonism between calcium and magnesium ions at the neuromuscular junction, *J. Physiol. (London)* 138: 434.

Johnson, E. W., and Wernig, A., 1971, The binomial nature of transmitter release at the crayfish neuromuscular junction, *J. Physiol. (London)* 218: 757.

Kajimoto, N., and Pirpekar, S. M., 1972, Effects of manganese and lanthanum on spontaneous release of acetylcholine at frog motor nerve terminals, *Nature (New Biol.)* 235: 29.

Katz, B., 1969, "The release of neural transmitter substances," Charles C. Thomas, Springfield, 60 pp.

Katz, B., and Miledi, R., 1965a, The effect of calcium on acetyl-choline release from motor nerve terminals, *Proc. R. Soc. London, Ser. B* 161: 496.

Katz, B., and Miledi, R., 1965b, Release of acetylcholine from a nerve terminal by electric pulses of variable strength and duration, *Nature* 207: 1097.

Katz, B., and Miledi, R., 1967a, The release of acetylcholine from nerve endings by graded electric pulses, *Proc. R. Soc. London, Ser. B* 167: 23.

Katz, B., and Miledi, R., 1967b, The timing of calcium action during neuromuscular transmission, *J. Physiol. (London)* 189: 535.

Katz, B., and Miledi, R., 1968, The role of calcium in neuro-muscular facilitation, *J. Physiol. (London)* 195: 481.

Katz, B., and Miledi, R., 1969, Spontaneous and evoked activity of motor nerve endings in calcium Ringer, *J. Physiol. (London)* 203: 689.

Katz, B., and Miledi, R., 1977, Transmitter leakage from motor nerve endings, *Proc. R. Soc. London, Ser. B* 196: 59.

Katz, N., and Edwards, C., 1973, Effects of metabolic inhibitors on spontaneous and evoked transmitter release from frog nerve terminals, *J. gen. Physiol.* 61: 259.

Kelly, J. S., 1965, Antagonism between Na^+ and Ca^{2+} at the neuro-muscular junction, *Nature* 205: 296.

Kita, H., and Van der Kloot, W., 1971, The effects of changing the osmolarity of the Ringer on acetylcholine release at the frog neuromuscular junction, *Life Sci.* 10: 1423.

Kita, H., and Van der Kloot, W., 1973, The quantitative relation between extracellular calcium and acetylcholine release at the frog neuromuscular junction, *Brain Res.* 49: 205.

Kita, H., and Van der Kloot, W., 1973, Action of Co and Ni at the frog neuromuscular junction, *Nature (New Biol.)* 245: 52.

Kita, H., and Van der Kloot, W., 1974, Calcium ionophore X-537A increases spontaneous and phasic quantal release of acetylcholine at frog neuromuscular junction, *Nature* 250: 658.

Kita, H., and Van der Kloot, W., 1976, Effects of the ionophore X-537A on acetylcholine release at the frog neuromuscular junction, *J. Physiol. (London)* 259: 177.

Kita, H., and Van der Kloot, W., 1977, Time course and magnitude of effects of changes in tonicity on acetylcholine release at frog neuromuscular junction, *J. Neurophysiol.* 40: 212.

Kita, H., Madden, K, and Van der Kloot, W., 1976, Effects of the "Calcium ionophore" A-23187 on transmitter release at the frog neuromuscular junction, *Life Sci.* 17: 1837.

Krnjevic, K., Puil, E., and Werman, R., 1976, Intracellular Mg^{2+} increases neuronal excitability, *Can. J. Physiol. Pharmacol.* 54: 73.

Locke, F. S., 1894, Notiz uber den Einfluss physiologischer Kochsalz-losung auf die elektrische Erregbarkeit von Muskel and Nerv., *Zentralbl. Physiol.* 8: 166.

Mallart, A., and Martin, A. R., 1967, An analysis of facilitation of transmitter release at the neuromuscular junction of the frog, *J. Physiol. (London)* 193: 679.

Manalis, R. S., and Cooper, G. P., 1973, Presynaptic and post-synaptic effects of lead at the frog neuromuscular junction, *Nature* 243: 354.

Manalis, R. S., and Cooper, G. P., 1975, Evoked transmitter re-leased increased by inorganic mercury at frog neuromuscular junction, *Nature* 257: 690.

Matthews, G., and Wickelgren, W. O., 1977, On the effect of calcium on the frequency of miniature end-plate potentials at the frog neuromuscular junction, *J. Physiol. (London)* 266: 91.

Meech, R. W., and Thomas, R. C., 1977, The effect of calcium injection on the intracellular sodium and pH of snail neurones, *J. Physiol. (London)* 265: 867.

Meiri, U., and Rahamimoff, R., 1972, Neuromuscular transmission: inhibition by manganese ions, *Science* 176: 308.

Meiri, U., and Rahamimoff, R., 1971, Activation of transmitter release by strontium and calcium ions at the neuromuscular junction, *J. Physiol. (London)* 215: 709.

Muller, R. U., and Finkelstein, A., 1974, The electrostatic basis of Mg^{++} inhibition of transmitter release, *Proc. Nat. Acad. Sci. U. S. A.* 71: 923.

Noble, D., 1975, "The initiation of the heart beat", *Clarendon Press*, Oxford, 150 pp.

Papahadjopoulos, D., Poste, G., Schaeffer, B. E., and Vail, W. J., 1974, Membrane fusion and molecular segregation in phospholipid vesicles, *Biochim. Biophys. Acta* 352:10.

Poste, G., and Allison, A. C., 1973, Membrane fusion, *Biochim. Biophys. Acta* 300: 421.

Potter, L. T., 1969, Synthesis, storage and release of (^{14}C) acetyl-choline in isolated rat diaphragm muscles, *J. Physiol. (London)* 206: 145.

Rahamimoff, R., 1968, A dual effect of calcium ions on neuromuscu-lar facilitation, *J. Physiol. (London)* 195: 471.

Rahamimoff, R., and Alnaes, E., 1973, Inhibitory action of Ruthenium red on neuromuscular transmission, *Proc. Nat. Acad. Sci. U. S. A.* 70: 3613.

Rahamimoff, R., and Yaari, Y., 1973, Delayed release of transmitter at the frog neuromuscular junction, *J. Physiol. (London)* 228: 241.

Rees, D., 1974, The effect of metabolic inhibitors on the cockroach nerve-muscle synapse, *J. Exp. Biol.* 61: 331.

Remler, M. P., 1973, A semiquantitative theory of synaptic vesicle movements, *Biophys. J.* 13: 104.

Rosenthal, J., 1969, Post-tetanic potentiation at the neuromuscular junction of the frog, *J. Physiol. (London)* 203: 121.

Schober, R., Nitsch, C., and Rinne, U., Calcium-induced displace-ment of membrane-associated particles upon aggregation of chromaffin granules, *Science* 195: 495.

Spertell, R. B., 1976, A theoretical inquiry into the role of phospholipids in membrane fusion, *J. Theor. Biol.* 60: 197.

Stratham, H. E., and Duncan, C. J., 1976, The action of ionophores at the frog neuromuscular junction, *Life Sci.* 17: 1401.

Van der Kloot, W., 1977, Quantal acetylcholine release: vesicles or gated channels?, *Gen. Pharmacol.* 8: 21.

Van der Kloot, W., and Kita, H., 1973, The possible role of fixed membrane surface charges in acetylcholine release at the frog neuromuscular junction, *J. Memb. Biol.* 14: 365.

Van der Kloot, W., and Kita, H., 1975, The effects of the "calcium-antagonist" verapamil on muscle action potentials in the frog and crayfish and on neuromuscular transmission in the crayfish, *Comp. Biochem. Physiol.* 50C: 121.

Van der Kloot, W., Kita, H., and Kita, K., 1975, Action of the "calcium-antagonist", prenylamine, on skeletal muscle, the myoneural junction, and the adrenal of the frog, *Gen. Pharmacol.* 6: 63.

Weakly, J. N., 1973, The action of Cobalt ions on neuromuscular transmission in the frog, *J. Physiol. (London)* 234: 597.

Younkin, S. G., 1974, An analysis of the role of calcium in facilitation at the frog neuromuscular junction, *J. Physiol. (London)* 237: 1.

Zucker, R. S., 1973, Changes in the statistics of transmitter release during facilitation, *J. Physiol. (London)* 229: 787.

CHAPTER 12

ROLE OF CALCIUM IN DESENSITIZATION AT THE MOTOR

END-PLATE OF SKELETAL MUSCLE

Rodney L. Parsons

Department of Physiology and Biophysics
University of Vermont
Burlington, Vermont 05401

GENERAL CONSIDERATIONS

When acetylcholine or other depolarizing compounds are applied
to the motor end-plate region of skeletal muscle fibers, the postjunctional membrane undergoes a rapid increase in ionic conductance
as the cholinergic receptors are activated. This agonist-induced
increase in ionic conductance remains for a short period and then
reverses even though the agonist application is continued. Thesleff
(1955) initially studied this phenomenon using intracellular recordings of the drug-induced depolarization-repolarization sequence
produced in individual muscle fibers during sustained application
of depolarizing drugs. As repolarization occurred, nerve evoked
end-plate potentials were reduced progressively and subsequent
application of agonist produced no additional depolarization
(Thesleff, 1955). Under these conditions, the end-plate membrane
receptors gradually became refractory to agonist action and were
said to be "desensitized" (Thesleff, 1955).

Desensitization will develop during the sustained application
of quite low concentrations of agonist. As an example, the activation-desensitization sequence produced by local microperfusion of
25 µM carbachol, an analogue of acetylcholine resistant to hydrolysis by acetylcholinesterase, to the end-plate region of an
individual amphibian muscle fiber is shown in Figure 1. In this
experiment, the end-plate current induced by sustained agonist
application was measured with a point voltage clamp technique
(Takeuchi and Takeuchi, 1959). During the initial moments of
carbachol perfusion, an inward current developed as postjunctional
membrane receptors were activated, but after a few seconds the

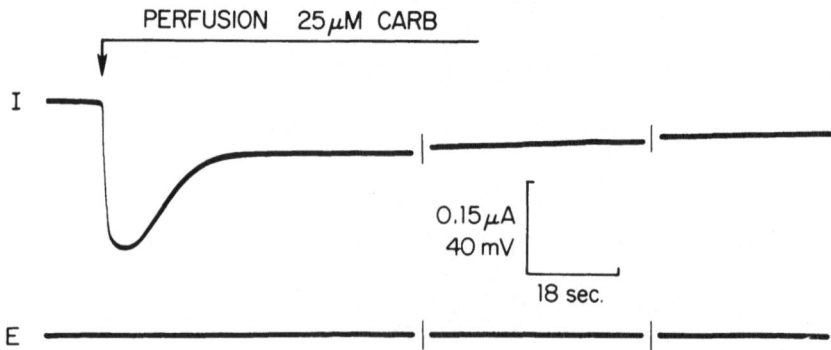

Figure 1. An example of the activation-desensitization sequence produced by the local application of 25 μM carbachol onto the end-plate region of an individual amphibian muscle fiber. The preparation was maintained in a hypertonic sodium-sucrose Ringer solution containing ~10^{-7} g/ml tetrodotoxin to minimize muscle contraction and action potential generation. The resting membrane potential was maintained at -100 mV by means of point voltage clamp technique. The E-trace represents membrane voltage and I-trace indicates current. The breaks in the record indicate 60 sec intervals when the recording camera was stopped. The vertical arrow indicates the initiation of carbachol application. Calibration: Y axis = 40 mV for E-trace and 150 nA for I-trace. X axis = 18 sec. (Parsons and Spannbauer, unpublished observation).

drug induced current declined toward the pre-agonist level although the agonist application was continued. The rate of decline of the carbachol-induced current from the peak is an index of the time course of the development of desensitization.

Although desensitization has been demonstrated during the sustained application of concentrations of agonist as low as 10 μM (Jenkinson and Terrar, 1973), it has not been shown to occur following neurally evoked release of acetylcholine even with repetitive stimulation; presumably the transient exposure to acetylcholine during transmission is too brief for desensitization to develop (Otsuka, Endo, and Nonomura, 1962). That desensitization has not been observed at the vertebrate neuromuscular junction during evoked release of acetylcholine does not preclude the possibility of a role in synaptic integration at other cholinergic synapses. For example, the conversion of synaptic excitation to inhibition during repetitive stimulation at a dual chemical synapse in *Aplysia* has been attributed in part to desensitization of excitatory receptors (Wachtel and Kandel, 1971). Curtis and Ryall (1966) have suggested desensitization as one mechanism of synaptic integration on spinal Renshaw cells. Because desensitization is involved in synaptic function at some synapses and because this process occurs with most drug-receptor interactions, it is of physiological and pharmacological interest to investigate factors influencing this process.

A considerable amount of information concerning the pharmacology of the desensitization process is available, but unfortunately the molecular mechanisms responsible for desensitization still remain unknown. Anderson and Stevens (1973) have shown that, as desensitization develops, no change in the kinetic properties of individual end-plate channels is apparent, but rather there is a decrease in the number of active channels during sustained exposure to agonist. Further, Koester (1971) and Lambert, Spannbauer and Parsons (1977) found no difference in the transmitter reversal potential at partially desensitized versus curarized motor end-plates indicating no selective change in the ionic conductances activated by acetylcholine occurs as desensitization progresses. Two fundamentally different classes of mechanisms, i.e. receptor and extrareceptor mechanisms, have been postulated to explain the phenomenon of desensitization. In the first, desensitization is viewed as resulting from an alteration in the chemical receptor or agonist binding site (Katz and Thesleff, 1957; Rang and Ritter, 1970). The second type of mechanism suggests that desensitization results from an alteration at some extrareceptor site which controls the ionic channel(s) in the end-plate membrane (Nastuk and Parsons, 1970; Magazanik and Vyskocil, 1970, 1975). The observation that Ca^{2+} markedly accelerated desensitization without altering end-plate activation led to the proposal that different macromolecular entities may be responsible for end-plate activation and desensitization (Parsons, 1969; Nastuk and Parsons, 1970; Magazanik and Vyskocil, 1970). Further, it was felt this view was strengthened by recent evidence indicating that the site of action of Ca^{2+} and other accelerators of desensitization is on the inner surface rather than the external surface of the postjunctional membrane (Magazanik and Vyskocil, 1975; DeBassio, Parsons and Schnitzler, 1976). In this view the reaction of Ca^{2+} with some anionic site on the inner surface of the postjunctional membrane was thought to alter channel gating without necessarily altering the binding properties of the agonist-recognition site. Unfortunately, the evidence is not decisive and is also compatible with the view that Ca^{2+} binds to sites on the inner surface of the membrane, changes the membrane environment, and in some unspecified manner, changes the binding properties of the agonist-receptor molecule. The answer to this question of whether receptor or extrareceptor mechanisms are responsible for desensitization awaits a better understanding of the molecular nature of the receptor-ionophore complex.

In this review I have attempted to provide a brief overview of studies concerning desensitization in skeletal muscle, pointing out some of the difficulties encountered in previous work and to discuss the role of calcium in the development of desensitization.

FACTORS AFFECTING DESENSITIZATION ONSET

The rate of desensitization onset depends to a significant extent on the nature and concentration of agonist employed. Evidence has been presented which supports the view that certain agonists are more potent desensitizers than activators. For instance, the "partial agonists", decamethonium and phenyltrimethylammonium produce limited depolarization but more effectively desensitize the frog motor end-plate than the "full agonists" carbachol and succinylcholine (Parsons, 1969; Gissen and Nastuk, 1970; Koester, 1971).

Further, for any particular agonist, a critical factor in the rate of development and equilibrium level of desensitization is drug concentration. The rate and depth of desensitization increase with increasing concentration of agonist (Katz and Thesleff, 1957; Parsons, 1969; Nastuk and Parsons, 1970; Adams, 1975). In the presence of high agonist concentration, where the rate and depth are already near some maximum level, the influence of many other factors which alter the time course of development and the equilibrium level of desensitization, is greatly diminished (Nastuk and Parsons, 1970). Consequently, it is important to study the desensitization process with moderate agonist concentration.

The rate of desensitization onset is also influenced markedly by the level of membrane potential. Magazanik and Vyskocil (1970) initially reported that the rate of desensitization onset was increased with hyperpolarization and decreased with depolarization. This voltage sensitivity of desensitization onset is illustrated in Figure 2. This example illustrates the end-plate response of two different voltage clamped frog sartorius muscle fibers during local microperfusion of 50 μM carbachol. In these examples the time course of desensitization onset was estimated from the half decay time of the carbachol-induced current from the peak value to the final level in the presence of carbachol. The estimated half-time ($T_{\frac{1}{2}}$) of desensitization onset was 42 seconds for the fiber voltage clamped at -30 mV and 11 seconds for the fiber voltage clamped at -100 mV.

Unfortunately, most experiments comparing the rate of desensitization onset by different agonists have not been done with voltage clamp techniques and need to be re-examined because some

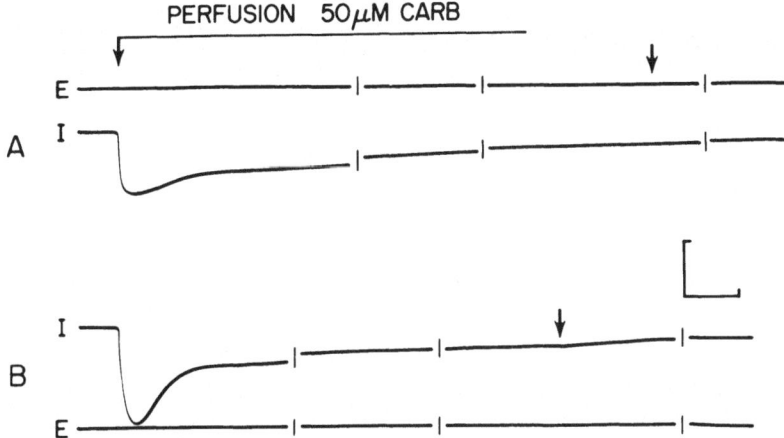

Figure 2. Influence of membrane voltage on the time course of desensitization by 50 µM carbachol in an amphibian muscle fiber maintained in the hypertonic sodium-sucrose Ringer containing ~10⁻⁷ g/ml tetrodotoxin. Carbachol-induced currents were measured with the point voltage clamp technique. A, Record of experiment in which muscle fiber was voltage-clamped at -30 mV. B, Record of experiment in which muscle fiber was voltage-clamped at -100 mV. The E-trace represents membrane potential and I-trace indicates current. The breaks in the records indicate 60 second periods when the recording was stopped. The small vertical arrows indicate when the carbachol perfusion was terminated. The half-time of decline of the agonist-induced current from the peak value to the plateau level (when desensitization appeared maximally developed) in the presence of carbachol was used as an index of the rate of development of desensitization. Estimated half-time of desensitization onset was 42 seconds in A and 11 seconds in B. Calibration: Y axis = 50 mV for E-traces and 100 nA in A and 200 nA in B for the I trace. X axis = 25 seconds (Parsons and Spannbauer, unpublished observations).

of the differences observed may have resulted, at least in part, from differences in the amount of membrane depolarization produced during the initial moments of agonist exposure.

One problem apparent from a review of the literature concerning desensitization is that the reported rates of desensitization vary markedly with the method of drug application. The time course of development of desensitization is reported to occur over a period of many minutes with bath application (Thesleff, 1955; Nastuk and Parsons, 1970; Hancock and Henderson, 1972). In contrast, values of $T_{\frac{1}{2}}$ of desensitization onset usually are tens of seconds with the local microperfusion of agonists and only a

few seconds with the iontophoretic method of drug application
(Manthey, 1966; Nastuk and Parsons, 1970; Katz and Thesleff, 1957;
Magazanik and Vyskocil, 1970). The question has been raised as
to whether these differences in onset timecourse reflect measurement of different processes or they can be explained by other
factors known to affect the rate of desensitization onset.

Many studies have utilized postjunctional membrane depolarization-repolarization during bath applied agonist to estimate the
timecourse of receptor activation and desensitization. Under
these conditions, desensitization appears to develop over a period
of many minutes (Thesleff, 1955; Nastuk and Parsons, 1970; Cochrane
and Parsons, 1972; Hancock and Henderson, 1972). Two clear complications exist with this method of agonist application. The first
is related to the voltage sensitivity discussed above. When the
postjunctional membrane is depolarized during activation, the
initial rate of development of desensitization will be slow. As
desensitization continues and the postjunctional membrane repolarizes, the rate of desensitization onset is continually changing
and therefore is a complex function of membrane voltage and time.
Secondly, during the initial depolarization with activation, there
is an influx of chloride ions which become trapped and tend to
stabilize the membrane potential at depolarized levels. This slows
repolarization and therefore also slows the apparent rate of desensitization (Nastuk and Parsons, 1970; Jenkinson and Terrar,
1973).

With the microperfusion technique agonist is applied locally
to the end-plate region of individual fibers. Recently, Scubon-
Mulieri and Parsons (unpublished observations) have demonstrated
using the quaternary ion sensitive microelectrode developed by
Dionne (1976) that the carbachol concentration was quite uniform
over the end-plate region for distances within approximately 500
μm of the perfusion pipette during microperfusion ($\sim$100 μm diameter
pipette; $\sim$15 cm H_2O hydrostatic pressure). Microperfusion techniques have been used to apply agonist while monitoring several
indices of the activation-desensitization sequence such as membrane
potential and input resistance (Manthey, 1966; Parsons, 1969;
Nastuk and Parsons, 1970). One limitation to these input resistance measurements was that the conductance changes produced by
agonists could not be measured directly because the chemosensitive
membrane is electrically coupled to the adjacent voltage dependent
conductile membrane of the muscle fiber. Hence input resistance
measurements represented the resistance of the postjunctional
membrane in parallel with that of the adjacent conductile membrane
(Nastuk and Parsons, 1970). A second problem not initially considered is the voltage dependence of desensitization onset. As
discussed above for bath application, the rate of desensitization

is continually changing as the muscle fiber repolarizes. Both
problems can be minimized either by measuring input conductance
in potassium-depolarized fibers where potential changes are
essentially eliminated by working at the agonist reversal potential or by measuring end-plate currents in voltage clamped muscle
fibers. Both of these approaches have been utilized recently
(Manthey, 1970, 1972; Adams, 1975; Scubon-Mulieri and Parsons,
1977; Lambert, Spannbauer, and Parsons, 1977).

In the iontophoretic technique initially used by Katz and
Thesleff (1957) to study the kinetics of desensitization onset and
recovery, small, transient postjunctional membrane depolarizations
were elicited by discrete application of brief test pulses of
agonist ejected from one barrel of a double-barreled pipette.
During a train of such pulses, agonist is allowed to diffuse out of
the second barrel and "condition" the postjunctional membrane.
During such a conditioning period, the test responses are reduced
rapidly with $T_{\frac{1}{2}}$ in the order of a few seconds. With this method
the agonist concentrations are unknown and are likely to be highly nonuniform over the postjunctional membrane (Katz and Thesleff,
1975; Nastuk and Parsons, 1970; Adams, 1975, 1976). The possibility of a high degree of spatial nonuniformity of agonist
concentration over the postjunctional membrane is a complicating
factor. As discussed above both rate and equilibrium level of
desensitization are concentration dependent and therefore, the
apparent rate is a complex function of time and the concentration
profile over the chemosensitive postjunctional membrane. The
very rapid onset of desensitization with this technique reflects
the fact that these experiments most often have been done at or
near the resting membrane potential; a voltage level where
desensitization onset is fast.

In summary then, the differences in rate of development of
desensitization between the initial studies utilizing iontophoretic, microperfusion or bath application can be plausibly
explained on the basis of differences in experimental conditions
such as local agonist concentration and levels of membrane potential when desensitization is developing.

Recently, Scubon-Mulieri and Parsons (1977) observed that
desensitization onset is accelerated by a prior activation-
desensitization sequence. This observation was made in a study
of desensitization onset and recovery in K^{+} depolarized muscles;
the time constant of desensitization onset being smaller in
subsequent exposures than in the initial carbachol application.
The progressive decrease of the time constant of desensitization
onset reversed as end-plate sensitivity recovered being complete
only after many minutes of washing.

The ionic composition of the bathing medium influences the time course of desensitization onset produced by many agonists (Manthey, 1966; Magazanik and Vyskocil, 1970, Nastuk and Parsons, 1970). For instance, when the external Ca^{2+} concentration is elevated, desensitization is accelerated (Manthey, 1966; Nastuk and Parsons, 1970). This effect of Ca^{2+} occurs in polarized as well as K^+-depolarized muscle fibers (Manthey, 1966; 1970; 1972; Scubon-Mulieri and Parsons, 1977). Other physiological ions such as Na^+, K^+, and Mg^{2+} are reported to have an opposite effect on the development of desensitization (Manthey, 1966, 1972; Parsons, Schnitzler, and Cochrane, 1974).

INFLUENCE OF CALCIUM ON END-PLATE DESENSITIZATION

Manthey (1966) initially reported that elevating the external Ca^{2+} increased the rate of desensitization onset. In this study, Manthey (1966) used the time course of return of the input resistance (after an initial fall) to estimate the rate of development of desensitization. Example recordings from Manthey's original study which demonstrate the influence of Ca^{2+} on desensitization are shown in Figure 3. Although the $T_{1/2}$ values for desensitization measured under these conditions are a complex function of voltage and time (see preceding discussion) and therefore the absolute values difficult to interpret, the differences clearly demonstrate the influence of the external Ca^{2+} concentration on the processes controlling the development of desensitization.

There appears to be a limited time period during which Ca^{2+} influences the desensitization process. An equilibration with Ca^{2+} prior to activation is not required. Rather, Ca^{2+} need only be present with agonist application (Manthey, 1970, 1974; Cochrane and Parsons, 1972; Scubon-Mulieri and Parsons, 1977). On the other hand, reducing the external Ca^{2+} concentration locally in the region of the end-plate by perfusing calcium chelating agents with the agonist slows the development of desensitization (Manthey, 1970). Further, Ca^{2+} need not be present during the initial period of activation and can be effective when added a few seconds after the agonist (Cochrane and Parsons, 1972; Manthey, 1974). An example of this is shown in Figure 4. In this double perfusion experiment, carbachol-induced activation of postjunctional membrane receptors occurred in the absence of Ca^{2+}. After activation had reached a maximum, 10 mM Ca^{2+} was added locally to the end-plate region with the rate of desensitization onset being noticeably increased.

The rate of development of desensitization has an upper limit and the controlling factors such as membrane voltage, agonist concentration and Ca^{2+} concentration are not independent. For

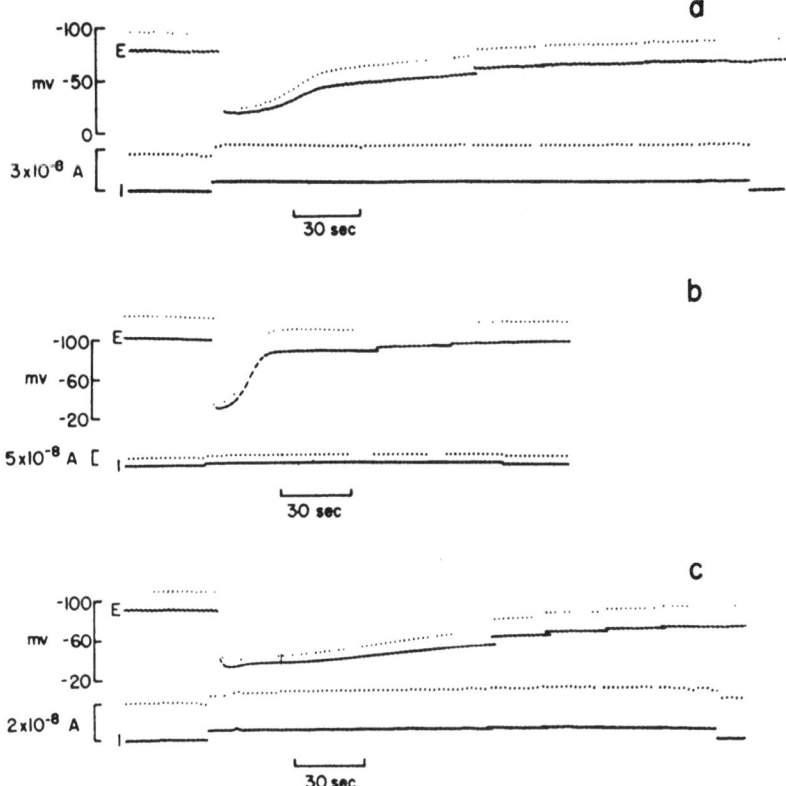

Figure 3.   Records of experiments in hypertonic sodium-sucrose solutions showing the influence of extracellular Ca^{2+} on the time course of development of desensitization produced by carbachol. In (a) the Ca^{2+} concentration was 1.8 mM, in (b) 10 mM, and in (c) 0 mM.   The traces representing membrane potential (E) appear above and those of membrane current (I) below.   Hyperpolarizing current pulses of about 200 to 400 msec duration were passed across the postjunctional membrane at 2 sec intervals producing short excursions of both potential and current which appear as a series of dots above the E and I traces.   The input resistance was calculated as the ratio of the amplitudes of the voltage and current pulses.   The duration of perfusion of the postjunctional region with 270 µM carbamylcholine is indicated by a small upward deflection of the current (I) trace.   The blank spaces in the latter parts of the traces denote periods of 60 sec during which the recording film was stopped.   The time course of desensitization was estimated from the return (after the initial decline) of the input resistance toward the plateau value during continued carbachol application.   The estimated half-time of desensitization was 35 sec in A, 12 sec in B and ~100 sec in C, respectively. Reproduced with permission from Manthey (1966).

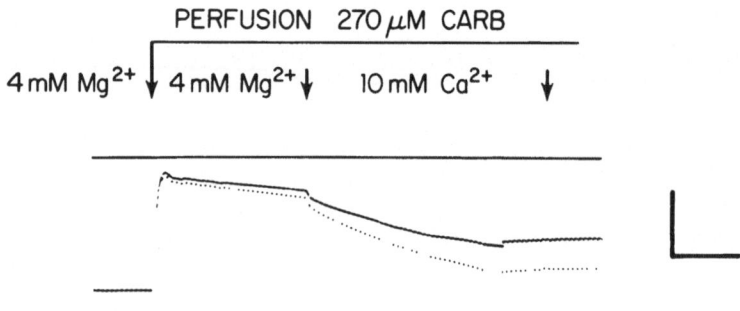

PERFUSION 270 μM CARB

4 mM Mg^{2+} 4 mM Mg^{2+} 10 mM Ca^{2+}

Figure 4. A double perfusion experiment showing the effect of Ca^{2+} on carbachol-induced desensitization. The muscle preparation was maintained in an isotonic Ca^{2+}-deficient, Ringer solution containing 4 mM Mg^{2+} and 1 mM EGTA. The first vertical arrow indicates the initial microperfusion of 270 μM carbachol in the Ca^{2+}-deficient solution. The second vertical arrow denotes the application of 270 μM carbachol along with 10 mM Ca^{2+}. The microperfusion was terminated at the third vertical arrow. The rate of development of desensitization was estimated from the time course of return of the input resistance (after the initial carbachol-induced decrease) towards the pre-agonist value. Calibration: Y axis 40 mV, X axis 30 sec. Reproduced with permission from Cochrane and Parsons (1972).

instance, as the carbachol concentration was progressively raised to higher and higher levels, the acceleration of desensitization onset due to an elevation of the external Ca^{2+} concentration from the normal level (1.8 mM) to 10 mM is diminished (Nastuk and Parsons, 1970). This demonstrated an interaction between external Ca^{2+} and agonist concentration. The extent of acceleration of desensitization onset by elevating external Ca^{2+} also is a function of membrane voltage. This interaction can be seen from inspection of the results summarized in Figure 5. In these experiments, K^{+}-depolarized muscle fibers were voltage clamped to +40, -40, or -100 mV and activated by microperfusion of 250 μM carbachol. The Ca^{2+} concentration was either 1.8 mM or 5.4 mM. Elevating the external Ca^{2+} concentration accelerated desensitization onset in fibers voltage clamped at +40 or -40 mV, but had no significant influence on the rate of desensitization onset in those fibers voltage clamped at -100 mV. Therefore when desensitization onset is accelerated by one factor, e.g. voltage or high agonist concentration, no further change in onset rate is produced by the addition of a second factor, e.g. elevating the external Ca^{2+}.

The influence of other divalent cations on carbachol-induced desensitization has been investigated to gain further insight

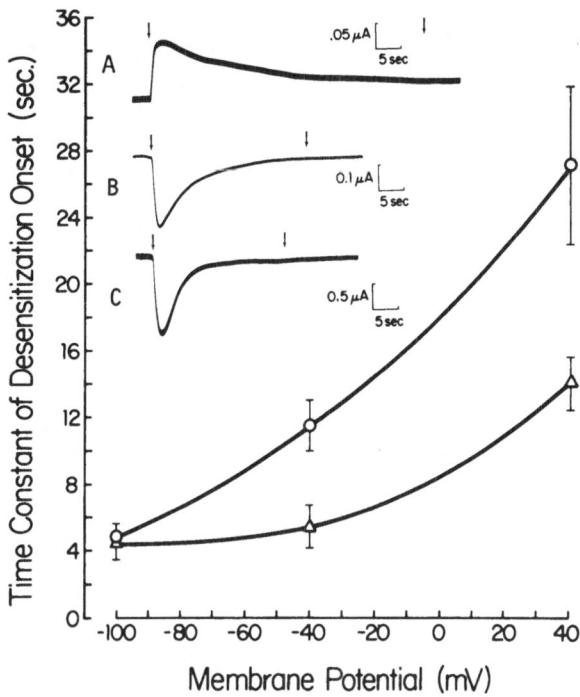

*Figure 5. Voltage dependence of desensitization onset produced
by 250 μM carbachol in K^+-depolarized muscle fibers voltage
clamped to +40, -40, or -100 mV. These data were obtained from
fibers bathed in an isotonic K^+-propionate solution containing
either 1.8 mM Ca^{2+} (0) or 5.4 mM Ca^{2+} (Δ). The time constant of
desensitization onset was determined from the time course of the
decay (after the initial peak) of the carbachol-induced currents
during sustained agonist application. Each point represents the
mean ± SE obtained from at least four fibers. The inset shows
examples of carbachol-induced currents from three different fibers
measured under voltage clamp conditions. In these examples, Ca^{2+}
was 1.8 mM; the voltage was +40 mV in A, -40 mV in B, and -100 mV
in C. Arrows indicate the onset and termination of carbachol
application. An upward deflection indicates outward current and
a downward deflection indicates inward current (Parsons, Scubon-
Mulieri and Spannbauer, unpublished observations).*

into the mechanism of action of Ca^{2+} on this process. The rate
of desensitization onset by carbachol is altered when Ca^{2+} is
replaced by many other divalent cations. For instance, Nastuk
and Parsons (1970) observed that desensitization developed much
more slowly in the presence of other divalent cations such as
Mg^{2+}, Sr^{2+} or Mn^{2+} than when Ca^{2+} was present. An example of

this specificity of Ca^{2+} is illustrated in Figure 6 which shows the effect of replacing external Ca^{2+} with Mg^{2+} on the time course of 100 μM carbachol-induced desensitization. These two records show the time course of carbachol-induced end-plate currents measured in two different frog sartorius muscle fibers voltage clamped to -100 mV. In example A the solution contained 1.8 mM Ca^{2+} and in record B the solution contained 2.0 mM Mg^{2+} with Ca^{2+} omitted. In these examples, the $T_{\frac{1}{2}}$ of decline of the agonist-induced current from the peak value to the plateau level (when desensitization appeared maximally developed) was used to estimate the time course of onset. The $T_{\frac{1}{2}}$ value was 6 sec when Ca^{2+} was present (Fig. 6A) and 18 sec (Fig. 6B) when Mg^{2+} was present.

The time course of carbachol-induced desensitization remained significantly slower when external Ca^{2+} was replaced by Mg^{2+} even when the agonist concentration was raised to very high levels (Parsons, 1969). Also Magazanik and Vyskocil (1970) found that the rate of desensitization onset induced by iontophoretic acetylcholine application was considerably slower when Mg^{2+} was substituted for Ca^{2+} in the bathing solution.

Magnesium ion appears to antagonize the action of Ca^{2+} on desensitization. Raising the extracellular Mg^{2+} concentration (up to 12 mM) in the presence of 1.8 mM Ca^{2+} slowed the rate of desensitization. Further, when the external concentration of Mg^{2+} was maintained at 12 mM, the slowing of desensitization onset was reduced by elevating the external Ca^{2+} concentration. These observations suggest that Ca^{2+} and Mg^{2+} act antagonistically on the desensitization process (Nastuk and Parsons, 1970).

From their observations, Nastuk and Parsons (1970) suggested that the relative effectiveness of the divalent cations studied as accelerators of desensitization onset was:

$$Ca^{2+} > Sr^{2+}, \; Mn^{2+} > Mg^{2+}$$

The inability of other divalent cations to exert an influence comparable to that of Ca^{2+} on the rate of desensitization onset suggests that the action of Ca^{2+} cannot be attributed to some nonspecific action of Ca^{2+} as a membrane stabilizer (Nastuk and Parsons, 1970).

An antagonistic action between Ca^{2+} and monovalent cations such as Na^+ and K^+ on the rate of desensitization onset has also been proposed. Manthey (1966) demonstrated that Na^+ antagonized the acceleration of desensitization onset by Ca^{2+} in a series of experiments in which sucrose was substituted for sodium chloride. This interaction between Ca^{2+} and Na^+ also has been studied using other Na^+ substitutes (Parsons, Schnitzler, and Cochrane, 1974).

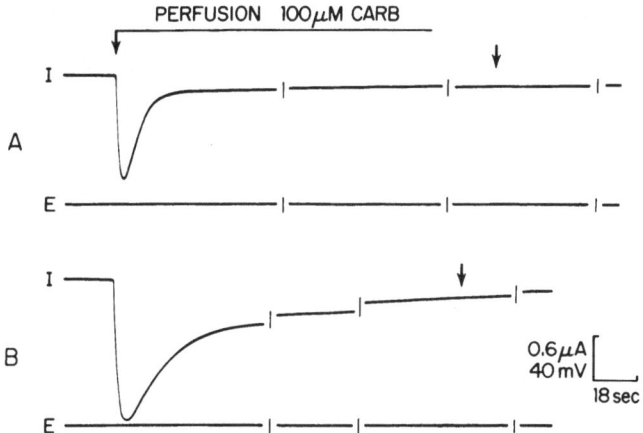

Figure 6. Alteration in the time course of development of 100 μM carbachol-induced desensitization when external Ca^{2+} is replaced by Mg^{2+}. The muscle preparation was maintained in a hypertonic sodium-sucrose Ringer solution containing ∿10^{-7} g/ml tetrodotoxin. In both examples, the membrane potential was maintained by point voltage clamp technique at -100 mV. A, Record of experiment in 1.8 mM Ca^{2+} solution. B, Record of experiment in a Ca^{2+}-deficient solution (no chelator added) containing 2.0 mM Mg^{2+}. The E-trace represents membrane potential and I-trace indicates current. The breaks in the records indicate 60 sec periods during which the recording was stopped. The small vertical arrows indicate when the carbachol perfusion was stopped. The time course of desensitization was estimated from the $T_{\frac{1}{2}}$ of decay of the carbachol-induced current from the initial peak value to the plateau level during continued agonist application. The estimated $T_{\frac{1}{2}}$ of development of desensitization was 6 sec in A and 18 sec in B (Parsons and Spannbauer, unpublished observations).

For instance, the rate of desensitization onset increased when Li^+ was progressively substituted for Na^+. Maximum acceleration of desensitization onset occurred with fifty percent substitution of Li^+ for Na^+. The addition of a similar concentration of Li^+ (60 mM) to the hundred percent sodium solution did not significantly influence desensitization onset. This observation suggested that Na^+ lack rather than the presence of Li^+ was responsible for the acceleration of desensitization. The antagonism between Ca^{2+} and Na^+ was most pronounced at low Ca^{2+} concentrations (Manthey, 1966; Parsons, Schnitzler and Cochrane, 1974). This is illustrated in Figure 7. In these experiments the time course of return of the input resistance (after the initial drop) toward the pre-carbachol level was used to estimate the time course of desensitization onset. Because membrane potential was not maintained constant throughout drug exposure, the

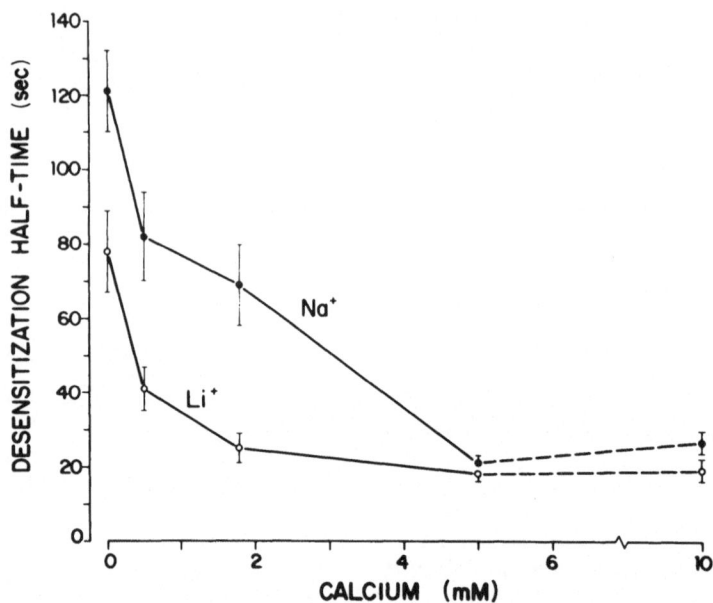

Figure 7. Comparison of effect of Ca^{2+} on the rate of desensitization produced by 270 μM carbamylcholine in amphibian muscle preparations maintained in a hypertonic sodium-sucrose or hypertonic lithium-sucrose Ringer solution. The time course of development of desensitization was approximated from the time course of return of the input resistance after the initial drop (see Figure 3) toward the plateau level during sustained agonist perfusion. Each point represents results from at least 5 fibers and vertical bars indicate standard error of the mean (Reproduced with permission from Parsons, Schnitzler, and Cochrane, 1974).

measured $T_{\frac{1}{2}}$ values of resistance return do not accurately indicate the absolute value of the rate of desensitization onset as discussed previously. However, the extent of the initial depolarization by carbachol was similar in the Li^+ or Na^+ solutions so the data can be used to illustrate the qualitative difference in the development of carbachol-induced desensitization when Na^+ was replaced by Li^+. These observations suggest that Ca^{2+} and Na^+ have opposing actions on the desensitization process; Ca^{2+} accelerating onset and Na^+ slowing onset.

An antagonism between K^+ and Ca^{2+} on desensitization onset has also been suggested (Manthey, 1966, 1972). Experiments indicating this were done using muscle fibers maintained in solutions containing different K^+ concentrations and consequently the membrane voltage ranged between -36 and -6 mV depending on the K^+ level. Magazanik and Vyskocil (1970) have argued that the slowing of desensitization with increasing K^+ was related to differences in membrane potential rather than primarily a direct influence of K^+ on the desensitization process as proposed (Manthey, 1966, 1972). Recently, Parsons, Scubon-Mulieri and Spannbauer (unpublished observations) have attempted to resolve this issue using voltage clamped, K^+-depolarized fibers. A summary of the time course of desensitization onset produced by 250 µM carbachol at +40, -40, and -100 mV when the bath Ca^{2+} concentration was either 1.8 mM or 5.4 mM was presented in Figure 5. The onset of desensitization was more rapid at -40 than at +40 mV at both levels of Ca^{2+}. Further, increasing the Ca^{2+} concentration accelerated desensitization onset at both voltages. These results suggest that the level of membrane potential could have influenced the rate of desensitization onset under the conditions of Manthey's experiments and that elevating the external Ca^{2+} concentration shifts this relationship between membrane potential and desensitization onset. Therefore, at least part of the proposed antagonism between Ca^{2+} and K^+ resulted from the voltage dependence of desensitization onset.

SITE OF CALCIUM ACTION

Although it is well established that Ca^{2+} accelerates endplate desensitization, the site of its action has been a matter of speculation. Nastuk and Parsons (1970) proposed that this site is located on the internal surface of the postjunctional membrane and therefore is distinct from the agonist-recognition site located on the external surface. In this view an increase in Ca^{2+} concentration at the internal surface of the postjunctional membrane could result from either the influx of Ca^{2+} during the agonist-induced conductance increase or the depolarization-coupled release of Ca^{2+} from internal stores. Indeed, there is considerable evidence that Ca^{2+} influx occurs during end-plate activation (Takeuchi, 1963; Katz and Miledi, 1969; Parsons and Nastuk, 1969; Parsons, Cochrane, and Schnitzler, 1973; Evans, 1974; Manthey, 1974). That this Ca^{2+} influx is the primary source of Ca^{2+} influencing desensitization onset is supported by the following observations. First, desensitization onset rate decreased markedly as the external Ca^{2+} concentration was reduced. Second, Ca^{2+} acceleration of desensitization occurs in K^+-depolarized fibers, glycerol-treated preparations, and voltage clamped muscle fibers where the depolarization-coupled release of Ca^{2+} from internal stores was reduced or eliminated (Manthey, 1966, 1970, 1972; Scubon-Mulieri and Parsons, 1977; Parsons, unpublished observations).

The Nastuk and Parsons proposal would be greatly strengthened by the demonstration that desensitization onset could be accelerated by raising the intracellular ionized Ca^{2+} level.

Experiments utilizing the calcium ionophore, X-537A, have demonstrated that the rate of desensitization onset becomes increased when the level of intracellular ionized calcium is raised (DeBassio, Parsons, and Schnitzler, 1976). These experiments were done on K^+-depolarized amphibian muscle preparations to eliminate the change in membrane potential and contraction associated with end-plate activation in polarized muscle fibers. In most experiments, the muscle preparations were maintained in a Ca^{2+}-deficient solution containing 1 mM ethylene(oxyethylenenitrilo)-tetracetic acid (EGTA). Under these conditions any ionophore-induced elevation of intracellular Ca^{2+} would result from its ability to mobilize cell Ca^{2+} from sarcoplasmic reticulum and mitochondria (Entman, Gillette, Wallick, Pressman, and Schwartz, 1972; Scarpa and Inesi, 1972; Scarpa, Baldassare and Inesi, 1973; Lin and Kun, 1973). The ability of the ionophore to induce tension development in relaxed, K^+-depolarized muscles was taken as evidence that the intracellular Ca^{2+} concentration was increasing during exposure to X-537A (DeBassio, Parsons, and Schnitzler, 1976).

Desensitization developed more rapidly in muscles treated with the ionophore. The acceleration of desensitization occurred without any effect on the conductance of the membrane in the absence of carbachol or on the extent of the carbachol-induced increase in conductance. These results are summarized in Table I. Further, the fact that desensitization onset in the presence of ionophore was maximally accelerated at concentrations which produced just noticeable muscle contraction indicated that those processes responsible for desensitization are more sensitive to intracellular Ca^{2+} than the contractile machinery.

In summary, the acceleration of carbachol-induced desensitization during the exposure to X-537A in a Ca^{2+}-deficient solution supports the hypothesis that the site of Ca^{2+} action is on the inner surface.

Vyskocil and Magazanik (1972) have reported that the onset of acetylcholine-induced desensitization can be increased by the intracellular injection of certain membrane stabilizers and snake venoms. They also suggest that the mechanisms responsible for the development of desensitization can be affected by agents acting at the inner part of the cholinergically-activated end-plate permeability system where acetylcholine recognition sites are absent (Del Castillo and Katz, 1955).

Given that the site of Ca^{2+} action in desensitization is on the inner surface of the postjunctional membrane rather than on its external surface, two mechanisms can explain the relative ineffectiveness of other divalent cations in accelerating desensitization. First, specificity may result from limited access

TABLE I. INFLUENCE OF 20 μM X-537A ON FIBER INPUT CONDUCTANCE AND TIME COURSE OF 1 mM CARBACHOL-INDUCED DESENSITIZATION IN AMPHIBIAN MUSCLE PREPARATIONS EQUILIBRATED IN Ca^{2+}-FREE, 2 mM Mg^{2+}, 1 mM EGTA, K PROPIONATE SOLUTION

Condition	Input Conductance Prior to Carbachol[a] (mho x 10^{-6})	Maximum Input Conductance During Carbachol Perfusion[a] (mho x 10^{-6})	Desensitization Half-Time ($T_{\frac{1}{2}}$)[a] (sec)	No. of Fibers
Control	4.4 ± 0.4	17.2 ± 1.4	58.8 ± 5.5[b]	16
X-537A for 30 min.	4.1 ± 0.4	15.9 ± 2.1	20.5 ± 1.4[b]	13

[a] Means ± S.E.M.

[b] Significant, $p < 0.05$

to hypothesized "desensitization sites" because of differences in mobility through the carbachol-activated postjunctional membrane. Second, the specificity may be due to differences in ability to react with the specific sites which control desensitization. To differentiate between these explanations desensitization in frog sartorius muscles has been studied in various sodium-substituted, isotonic, divalent-cation Ringer solutions, i. e. in isotonic Ca^{2+}, Mg^{2+}, Sr^{2+}, or Mn^{2+} Ringer solution (Parsons, Cochrane and Schnitzler, 1973). In muscle fibers voltage clamped at -100 mV, E_K, the agonist-induced end-plate current represents the transmembrane influx of the divalent cation. Two observations are of interest to the present discussion. Carbachol-induced end-plate currents were observed in muscle fibers maintained in all solutions studied and the peak value of the 54 μM carbachol-induced current in fibers voltage clamped to -100 mV was similar in all solutions (Table II) indicating that divalent cation influx through the carbachol-activated end-plate membrane was comparable in each case. Desensitization onset was fastest in the Ca^{2+} solution, intermediate in the Sr^{2+} and Mn^{2+} solutions and considerably slower in the Mg^{2+} solution. Sample results from one fiber maintained in the isotonic Ca^{2+} solution and from a second fiber kept in the isotonic Mg^{2+} solution are shown in Figure 8. In additional studies done to quantitatively compare the development of desensitization onset in these same divalent cation solutions, the time course of onset of 270 μM carbachol-induced desensitization was estimated from input conductance measurements in unclamped muscle fibers. The results of these experiments, summarized in Table III, show carbachol-induced desensitization developed more rapidly in the presence of Ca^{2+} than the other divalent cations studied. Therefore, the inability of these other divalent cations to accelerate desensitization as effectively as Ca^{2+} cannot be attributed to a limited mobility through the carbachol-activated postjunctional membrane, but rather must reflect the specificity of some site on the inner surface of the postjunctional membrane which is important to the desensitization process.

POSSIBLE MECHANISMS OF ACTION FOR CALCIUM IN DESENSITIZATION

A cyclic scheme such as that proposed initially by Katz and Thesleff (1957) appears to most adequately describe the kinetics of desensitization onset and recovery. This type of scheme is shown below.

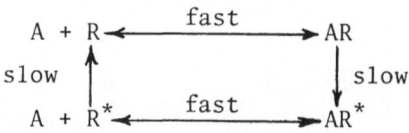

*TABLE II.   PEAK END-PLATE CURRENT PRODUCED BY 54μM CARBAMYLCHOLINE
            IN MUSCLE FIBERS VOLTAGE CLAMPED AT -100 mV AND MAIN-
            TAINED IN SODIUM-DEFICIENT, DIVALENT CATION RINGER
            SOLUTIONS*

Ringer Solution	Peak End-Plate Current $X10^{-8}A^{a}$	Number of Fibers
$CaCl_2$	3.19 ± 0.56	8
$MnCl_2$	3.93 ± 0.92	6
$SrCl_2$	3.90 ± 0.76	6
$MgCl_2$	3.14 ± 0.53	9

^{a}*Means $\pm$ SEM*

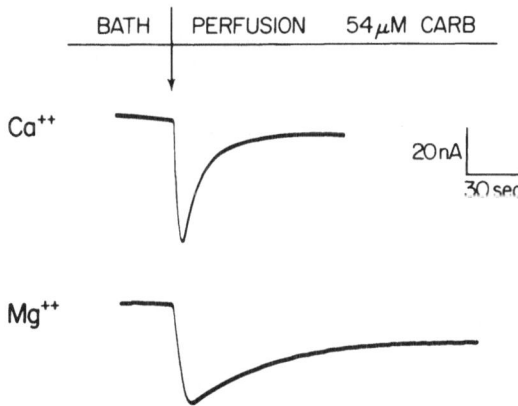

*Figure 8.   End-plate currents produced by local microperfusion
of 54 μM carbachol in two different muscle fibers voltage-clamped
to -100 mV and maintained either in an isotonic calcium solution
(Ca^{2+}) or an isotonic magnesium solution (Mg^{2+}). (Parsons and
Williams, unpublished observations).*

*TABLE III.   DESENSITIZATION PRODUCED BY 270μM CARBAMYLCHOLINE IN
            SODIUM DEFICIENT, DIVALENT CATION RINGER SOLUTIONS*

Ringer Solution	*Desensitization Half-Time[a] (seconds)*	*Number of Fibers*
$CaCl_2$	3.9 ± 2.5	4
$SrCl_2$	7.4 ± 1.8	4
$MnCl_2$	11.1 ± 2.4	4
$MgCl_2$	33.2 ± 2.8	5

[a]*Mean $\pm$ SEM*

Desensitization in this model is generally associated with a
change in receptor state, however, it would equally well describe
desensitization onset and recovery even if these result from an
alteration in some other component such as the ionic channels in
the receptor-ionophore complex (Magazanik and Vyskocil, 1974).
Consequently, it is not possible on a kinetic basis to differentiate
the receptor from subsequent steps in the permeability - activation
system as the site undergoing change during desensitization.   In
this scheme, the activated AR is slowly converted to an inactive
state AR^* with prolonged exposure to agonist and the evidence
suggest that an elevation of internal Ca^{2+} accelerates the transition between the activated AR complex to the inactive state, AR^*,
that is:

$$\text{Desensitization onset rate} = f([Ca^{2+}]_i)$$

The recovery of sensitivity after desensitization would occur as
AR^* dissociates and R^* reverts to R and is complete when all receptor has returned to the free, R, configuration.

    Although the view that Ca^{2+} acts at an internal site on the
postjunctional membrane to control desensitization is well supported,
the mechanism at the molecular level can be only a matter for speculation.   The specificity of Ca^{2+} in desensitization and the relative
ineffectiveness of common Ca^{2+} substitutes suggest that Ca^{2+} binding to some specific "Ca^{2+}-receptor" site on the inner surface of
the membrane may be the first step.

Calcium ion binding to some specific "desensitization" site in the receptor-ionophore complex may directly promote channel inactivation or increase the rate of conversion of the receptor from an activated to desensitized state.

An alternative mechanism may be that the binding of Ca^{2+} on the inner surface of the membrane neutralizes the layer of fixed surface charge (Frankenhaeuser and Hodgkin, 1957; Chandler, Hodgkin, and Meves, 1965). A rise of the internal Ca^{2+} concentration could also affect the surface potential by "screening" these charges without necessarily binding to specific sites (McLaughlin, Szato, and Eisenman, 1971). Changes in surface charge would be expected to alter the electric field across the postjunctional membrane which in turn might secondarily affect the gating molecules controlling the end-plate channels or alter the binding properties of the recognition site.

Although it is well established that Ca^{2+} affects desensitization onset, the mechanism of Ca^{2+} action requires further investigation. The studies of Ca^{2+} action in desensitization demonstrate that small changes in ionized calcium level can alter postsynaptic responsiveness. An important question is whether transient changes in intracellular Ca^{2+} occurring in postsynaptic cells during synaptic transmission might be modulators of the transmission process. For example, Scubon-Mulieri and Parsons (1977) have postulated that the acceleration of desensitization onset by prior activation is caused by a time dependent elevation of the level of intracellular ionized calcium. Intracellular Ca^{2+} accumulation in the postjunctional cell during synaptic transmission has been demonstrated at the neuromuscular junction (Marco, 1974; Evans, 1974; Pappas and Rose, 1976) and at neuronal synapses (Kusano, Miledi, and Stinnakre, 1975). An intriguing thought is that desensitization may provide one means of limiting the duration of synaptic activity such as seen during habituation.

The possibility that a Ca^{2+}-mediated change in membrane conductance may occur is not unique. Recently, many investigators have demonstrated that changes in the level of intracellular Ca^{2+} can alter membrane permeability in a variety of cell types including muscle, nerve and glands (Isenberg, 1975; Krnjevic and Lisewicz, 1972; Meech and Strumwasser, 1970; Rose and Loewenstein, 1974; see Meech 1976 for review). In these other systems, as at the muscle postjunctional membrane, Ca^{2+}-mediated changes in permeability appear to result from an elevation in the level of intracellular Ca^{2+} produced by either Ca^{2+} influx or by the release of Ca^{2+} from intracellular stores or some combination of these (Meech, 1976). Changes quite similar to those observed during desensitization at the motor end-plate have been reported to occur with light-induced desensitization in the *Limulus* photoreceptor. For instance, a Ca^{2+}-mediated decrease in conductance has been suggested as an explanation for the light adaptation (desensitization) of the *Limulus* ventral photoreceptor (Lisman and Brown, 1975; Brown and Lisman, 1975). In this preparation iontophoretic injection of Ca^{2+} decreases the amplitude of the receptor potential whereas intracellular injection of agents which buffer Ca^{2+} concentration prevents the light-induced desensitization (Lisman and Brown, 1975). Further a light-induced elevation of internal Ca^{2+} has been demonstrated with aequorin (Brown and Blinks, 1974). Brown and Lisman (1975) suggest that this action of Ca^{2+} may represent an effect on the Na^+ conductance channels in this photoreceptor.

Acknowledgements

The author's work described in this review was supported by Grant NS-07740 from the National Institutes of Health. I wish to express my sincere thanks to Drs. B. Scubon-Mulieri, V. E. Dionne and R. B. Low for their many helpful discussions and criticisms of this manuscript.

REFERENCES

Adams, P. R., 1975, A study of desensitization using voltage clamp, *Pflügers Arch.* 360: 135.

Adams, P. R., 1976, A comparison of the time course of excitation and inhibition by iontophoretic decamethonium in frog end-plate, *Brit. J. Pharmacol.* 57: 59.

Anderson, C. R., and Stevens, C. F., 1973, Voltage clamp analysis of acetylcholine produced end-plate current fluctuations at frog neuromuscular junction, *J. Physiol. (London)* 235: 655.

Brown, J. E., and Blinks, J. R., 1974, Changes in intracellular free calcium during illumination of invertebrate photoreceptors: detection with aequorin, *J. gen. Physiol.* 64: 643.

Brown, J. E., and Lisman, J. E., 1975, Intracellular Ca modulates sensitivity and time scale in Limulus ventral photoreceptors, *Nature* 258: 252.

Cochrane, D. E., and Parsons, R. L., 1972, The interaction between caffeine and calcium in the desensitization of muscle post-junctional membrane receptors, *J. gen. Physiol.* 59: 437.

Chandler, W. K., Hodgkin, A. L., and Meves, H., 1965, The effect of changing the internal solution on sodium inactivation and related phenomenon in giant axons, *J. Physiol. (London)* 180: 821.

Curtis, D. R., and Ryall, R. W., 1966, The synaptic activation of Renshaw cells, *Exp. Brain Res.* 2: 81.

DeBassio, W. A., Parsons, R. L., and Schnitzler, R. M., 1976, Effects of ionophore X-537A on desensitization rate and tension development in potassium-depolarized muscle fibres, *Brit. J. Pharmacol.* 57: 565.

Dionne, V. E., 1976, Characterization of drug iontophoresis with a fast microassay technique, *Biophys. J.* 16: 705.

Entman, M. L., Gillette, P. C., Wallick, E. T., Pressman, B. C., and Schwartz, A., 1972, A study of calcium binding and uptake by isolated cardiac reticulum: the use of a new ionophore (X-537A), *Biochem. Biophys. Res. Commun.* 48: 847.

Evans, R. H., 1974, The entry of labelled calcium into the innervated region of the mouse diaphragm muscle, *J. Physiol. (London)* 240: 517.

Frankenhaeuser, B., and Hodgkin, A. L., 1957, The action of calcium on the electrical properties of squid axons, *J. Physiol. (London)* 137: 218.

Gissen, A. J., and Nastuk, W. L., 1970, Succinylcholine and decamethonium: comparison of depolarization and desensitization, *Anesthesiology* 33: 611.

Hancock, J. C., and Henderson, E. G., 1972, Antinicotinic action of nicotine and lobeline on frog sartorius muscle, *Naunyn-Schmied. Arch. Pharmacol.* 272: 307.

Isenberg, G., 1975, Is potassium conductance of cardiac Purkinje fibres controlled by $[Ca^{2+}]_i$?, *Nature* 253: 273.

Jenkinson, D. H., and Terrar, D. A., 1973, Influence of chloride ions on changes in membrane potential during prolonged application of carbachol to frog skeletal muscle, *Brit. J. Pharmacol.* 47: 363.

Katz, B., and Miledi, R., 1969, Spontaneous and evoked activity of motor nerve endings in calcium Ringer, *J. Physiol. (London)* 203: 689.

Katz, B., and Thesleff, S., 1957, A study of the 'desensitization' produced by acetylcholine at the motor end-plate, *J. Physiol. (London)* 138: 63.

Koester, J. D., 1971, Some effects of partial agonists at the frog sartorius neuromuscular junction, Ph.D. Thesis, Columbia University, New York City, New York.

Krnjevic, K., and Lisiewicz, A., 1972, Injections of calcium ions into spinal motoneurons, *J. Physiol. (London)* 225: 363.

Kusano, K., Miledi, R., and Stinnakre, J., 1975, Postsynaptic entry of calcium induced by transmitter action, *Proc. R. Soc. London, Ser. B* 189: 49.

Lambert, D. H., Spannbauer, P. M., and Parsons, R. L., 1977, Desensitization does not selectively alter sodium channels, *Nature* 268: 553.

Lisman, J. E., and Brown, J. E., 1975, Effects of intracellular injection of calcium buffers on light adaptation in Limulus ventral photoreceptors, *J. gen. Physiol.* 66: 489.

Lin, D. C., and Kun, E., 1973, Mode of action of the antibiotic X-537A on mitochondrial glutamate oxidation, *Biochem. Biophys. Res. Commun.* 50: 820.

Magazanik, L. G., and Vyskocil, F., 1970, Dependence of acetylcholine desensitization on the membrane potential of frog
muscle fibre and on the ionic changes in the medium, *J. Physiol.
(London)* 210: 507.

Magazanik, L. G., and Vyskocil, F., 1973, Desensitization at the
motor end-plate, *in* "Drug Receptors" (H. P. Rang, ed.), pp. 105-
119, University Park Press, Baltimore.

Magazanik, L. G., and Vyskocil, F., 1975, The effect of temperature
on desensitization kinetics at the post-synaptic membrane of
the frog muscle fibre, *J. Physiol. (London)* 249: 285.

Manthey, A. A., 1966, The effect of calcium on the desensitization
of membrane receptors at the neuromuscular junction, *J. gen.
Physiol.* 49: 963.

Manthey, A. A., 1970, Further studies of the effect of calcium
on the time course of action of carbamylcholine at the neuromuscular junction, *J. gen. Physiol.* 56: 407.

Manthey, A. A., 1972, The antagonistic effects of calcium and
potassium on the time course of action of carbamylcholine at
the neuromuscular junction, *J. Memb. Biol.* 9: 319.

Manthey, A. A., 1974, Changes in Ca permeability of muscle fibers
during desensitization to carbamylcholine, *Amer. J. Physiol.*
226: 481.

Marco, L., 1972, Further findings on sarcomeric oscillations of
frog skeletal muscle, *Life Sci.* 11: 509.

Meech, R. W., 1976, Intracellular calcium and the control of
membrane permeability, *in* "Calcium in biological systems" (C. J.
Duncan, ed.) pp. 161-191, Cambridge University Press, Cambridge.

Meech, R. W., and Strumwasser, F., 1970, Intracellular calcium
injection activates potassium conductance in Aplysia nerve cells,
Fed. Proc. 29: 834.

McLaughlin, S. G. A., Szabo, G., and Eisenman, G., 1971, Divalent
cations and the surface potential of charged phospholipid
membranes, *J. gen. Physiol.* 58: 667.

Nastuk, W. L., and Parsons, R. L., 1970, Factors in the inactivation of postjunctional membrane receptors of frog skeletal
muscle, *J. gen. Physiol.* 56: 218.

Otsuka, M., Endo, M., and Nonomura, Y., 1962, Presynaptic nature
of neuromuscular depression, *Jpn. J. Physiol.* 12: 573.

Pappas, G. D., and Rose, S., 1976, Localization of calcium deposits
in the frog neuromuscular junction at rest and following stimulation, *Brain Res.* 103: 362.

Parsons, R. L., 1969, Changes in postjunctional receptors with
decamethonium and carbamylcholine, *Amer. J. Physiol.* 217: 805.

Parsons, R. L., and Nastuk, W. L., 1969, Activation of contractile
system in depolarized skeletal muscle fibers, *Amer. J. Physiol.*
217: 364.

Parsons, R. L., Cochrane, D. E., and Schnitzler, R. M., 1973,
End-plate desensitization: specificity of calcium, *Life Sci.*
13: 459.

Parsons, R. L., Schnitzler, R. M., and Cochrane, D. E., 1974, Inhibition of end-plate desensitization by sodium, *Amer. J. Physiol.* 227: 96.

Rang, H. P., and Ritter, J. M., 1970, On the mechanism of desensitization at cholinergic receptors, *Mol. Pharmacol.* 6: 357.

Rose, B., and Loewenstein, W. R., 1975, Permeability of cell junction depends on local cytoplasmic calcium activity, *Nature* 254: 250.

Scarpa, A., and Inesi, G., 1972, Ionophore mediated equilibration of calcium ion gradients in fragmented sarcoplasmic reticulum, *FEBS Lett.* 22: 273.

Scarpa, A., Baldassare, J., and Inesi, G., 1972, The effect of calcium ionophores on fragmented sarcoplasmic reticulum, *J. gen. Physiol.* 60: 735.

Scubon-Mulieri, B., and Parsons, R. L., 1977, Desensitization and recovery at the frog neuromuscular junction, *J. gen. Physiol.* 69: 431.

Takeuchi, A., and Takeuchi, N., 1969, Active phase of frog's end-plate potential, *J. Neurophysiol.* 22: 395.

Takeuchi, N., 1963, Effects of calcium on the conductance change of the end-plate membrane during the action of transmitter, *J. Physiol. (London)* 167: 141.

Thesleff, S., 1955, The mode of neuromuscular block caused by acetylcholine, decamethonium, and succinylcholine, *Acta. Physiol. Scand.* 34: 218.

Vyskocil, F., and Magazanik, L. G., 1972, The desensitization of postjunctional muscle membrane after intracellular application of membrane stabilizers and snake venom polypeptides, *Brain Res.* 48: 417.

Wachtel, H., and Kandel, E. R., 1971, Conversion of synaptic excitation to inhibition at a dual chemical synapse, *J. Neurophysiol.* 34: 56.

CHAPTER 13

EFFECT OF PHARMACOLOGICAL AGENTS ON CALCIUM STORES

IN AMPHIBIAN FAST AND SLOW MUSCLE FIBERS

C. Paul Bianchi

Department of Pharmacology
Jefferson Medical College
Thomas Jefferson University
Philadelphia, Pennsylvania 19107

COMPARISON OF PHYSIOLOGICAL PROPERTIES OF AMPHIBIAN SLOW AND FAST SKELETAL MUSCLE

Amphibian fast and slow muscles muscle fibers differ in regard to structure, innervation, and contractile response. These differences can be utilized to study drug effects on cellular Ca^{2+} metabolism. The amphibian slow muscle fiber contains multiple end plates, is innervated by small nerve fibers, and gives a graded tonic response to repetitive neural stimulation. Tension is regulated by graded levels of depolarization of the surface membrane (Kuffler and Williams, 1953a, 1953b). Identical contractures produced by K^+ depolarization or acetylcholine are associated with a sustained increase in Ca^{2+} influx, a transient increase in Ca^{2+} efflux and a net gain of Ca^{2+} which amounts to 0.24 μmol/g for the KCl contracture and 0.27 μmol/g for the acetylcholine contracture (Bianchi, 1968a). During relaxation the Ca^{2+} becomes sequestered within the sarcoplasmic reticulum of the slow muscle fibers. The sarcoplasmic reticulum of the amphibian slow muscle fiber lacks the triad structure of the amphibian fast muscle fiber, but does contain invaginations of the cell membrane which extend into the cell interior and run in a longitudinal fashion parallel to the fiber axis (Page, 1965). The primary function of the sarcoplasmic reticulum present in the amphibian slow muscle fiber is to allow for rapid relaxation following the shutting off of Ca^{2+} influx during repolarization of the surface membrane. In the relaxed state Ca^{2+} efflux must exceed influx in order to restore the fiber Ca^{2+} content to steady state conditions.

The amphibian fast muscle fiber responds with a twitch to each conducted action potential; increases in stimulus frequency leads to potentiation of the muscle twitch, incomplete relaxation of the twitches and finally at a sufficiently high frequency, a fused tetanic response is observed (Giese, 1973). Fatigue of the amphibian fast muscle fiber (decreased ability to contract in response to the muscle action potential) develops during repetitive stimulation, especially at high frequencies. Fatigue develops at two rates when the frog sartorius muscle is stimulated at a frequency of one per second. Twitch tension drops by 60% within 4 minutes and is followed by a slower decline. The relaxation time of the twitch doubles after 3 minutes of stimulation and then rises to 4 times the initial value by the end of 9 minutes (Eberstein and Sandow, 1961). Upon cessation of stimulation a rapid partial restoration of twitch tension occurs in 15 seconds. Potassium induced contracture of the frog sartorius fast muscle is characterized by a transient contraction of 2 to 3 minutes which spontaneously relaxes even though the plasmalemma is still depolarized. The function of the well developed sarcoplasmic reticulum of amphibian fast muscle fibers is to serve both as a source of Ca^{2+} for contraction as well as a sink for Ca^{2+} removal during muscle relaxation.

Studies on the removal of surface Ca^{2+} from slow muscle fibers reveal that EDTA causes a sustained contracture in frog rectus abdominis (30% slow muscle fibers, 70% fast fibers) and a translocation of 70 nmoles/g of Ca^{2+} from a superficial fiber site into the myoplasm. Calcium efflux rises during the sustained contracture and then declines as the muscle relaxes to pre-contracture level. The increased loss of Ca^{2+} during the contracture amounts to 77 nmols/g slow muscle fiber which is in good agreement with the translocated Ca^{2+}. In contrast, EDTA applied to frog sartorius muscle fiber causes a marked increase in Ca^{2+} efflux without any tension being developed (Bianchi, 1965). In both cases removal of surface Ca^{2+} by EDTA leads to a release of Ca^{2+} to the myoplasm; the amphibian slow muscle fiber develops tension since the Ca^{2+} cannot be sequestered sufficiently by the poorly developed intracellular sarcoplasmic reticulum. Relaxation is governed by Ca^{2+} removal from the slow muscle fiber interior by transport from the muscle fiber to the cell exterior. In the case of the fast muscle fiber, the myoplasmic Ca^{2+} level is not allowed to reach a concentration necessary for contraction presumably because of resequestration of the released Ca^{2+} by the well developed sarcoplasmic reticulum (internal resequestration). The effect of surface Ca^{2+} removal in frog slow muscle fibers by EDTA is independent of membrane depolarization. Procaine (0.34 mM) and lidocaine (0.5 mM) both prevent the membrane depolarization associated with Ca^{2+} removal from the surface of slow muscle fibers but do not prevent the EDTA induced contracture (Bianchi, 1965).

Drugs that release Ca^{2+} from the sarcoplasmic reticulum in muscle may or may not cause contraction to take place. If resequestration by an intracellular storage site (fast fiber) is sufficient to maintain myoplasmic Ca^{2+} below the level necessary for contraction i.e. less than 10^{-7} M, Ca^{2+} release can occur in the absence of contraction. If internal resequestration is deficient, and myoplasmic free Ca^{2+} rises to above 10^{-7} M, contracture occurs until myoplasmic free Ca^{2+} is restored below 10^{-7} M (amphibian slow fiber).

In frog sartorius muscle the sarcoplasmic reticulum consists of two continuous portions: 1) the terminal and intermediate cisternae adjacent to the transverse tubular element and 2) the longitudinal reticulum with its fenestrated collar which extends over the sarcomere (Peachey, 1965). The terminal cisternae are the primary locus for Ca^{2+} release in response to electrical coupling. Translocation of Ca^{2+} from the terminal and intermediate cisternae to the longitudinal reticulum occurs during tetanus. At rest intracellular Ca^{2+} labeled by prolonged exchange with extracellular Ca^{2+} is located in the terminal cisternae; following cessation of stimulation (tetanic) the ^{45}Ca is observed in the longitudinal reticulum. The Ca^{2+} in the longitudinal reticulum becomes restored to the terminal cisternae during recovery with a half time ($T_{\frac{1}{2}}$) of about 9 seconds (Winegrad, 1970). Thus, fatigue in directly stimulated fast muscle fibers can be thought of as being due to translocation of Ca^{2+} from a storage and release site tightly coupled to the action potential to a storage site loosely coupled to the action potential, hence uncoupling of the action potential from contraction eventually occurs.

The amount of Ca^{2+} released from the terminal cisternae appears to vary as a function of stimulus frequency. In muscle fibers stimulated at infrequent intervals (> 2 min) the Ca^{2+} release from terminal cisternae as measured by the intracellular aequorin blue light response to released Ca^{2+} remains essentially unchanged. When a train of stimuli occurs the aequorin light response to released Ca^{2+} is greatest in the first twitch and declines during subsequent twitches in the series. The decline in Ca^{2+} release can be observed even though the twitch response increases during the train (frequency 1/sec) (Taylor et al., 1975).

A possible interpretation of the above results can be as follows. The first stimulus in a series of stimuli, or a single stimulus at infrequent intervals releases Ca^{2+} from a readily releasable pool of Ca^{2+} in the terminal cisternae and serves as a priming source of Ca^{2+} to saturate Ca^{2+} binding sites in the myoplasm in addition to the tropomyosin sites related to contraction. Once these sites are saturated, contraction and relaxation is regulated by the binding or removal of Ca^{2+} from the tropomyosin sites (Orentlicher *et al.*, 1974). With continued stimulation Ca^{2+} release declines as the readily releasable pool of Ca^{2+} becomes depleted. However, tension increases since a greater fraction of the released Ca^{2+} becomes available to tropomyosin. As the initial phase of fatigue occurs the readily releasable pool declines and contraction becomes more dependent upon a second pool of Ca^{2+} of relatively large magnitude but with a much smaller quanta of Ca^{2+} released per impulse. The second stage of fatigue observed by Eberstein and Sandow (1961) would be associated with the disappearance of Ca^{2+} from this secondary pool.

There are two basic mechanisms of release of Ca^{2+} from the sarcoplasmic reticulum; (1) by depolarization (electrical coupling of sarcoplasmic reticulum to the transverse tubular element in response to the membrane action potential or K^+ depolarization) and (2) a Ca^{2+} induced release of Ca^{2+} which does not require depolarization of the transverse tubular element. The conditions of Ca^{2+} release of Ca^{2+} are a high concentration of Ca^{2+} in the S-R and a sufficiently high myoplasmic Ca^{2+}. Caffeine in concentrations that produce reversible caffeine contracture causes the low myoplasmic Ca^{2+} level consistent with resting muscle ($< 10^{-8}$ M) to trigger off the release of Ca^{2+} stored in the terminal or intermediate cisternae. The contracture produced by intermediate caffeine concentrations in amphibian fast muscle fibers is not sustained, suggesting depletion of the Ca^{2+} pool affected by intermediate levels of caffeine and resequestration of the released Ca^{2+} by the longitudinal reticulum. Procaine (10 mM) blocks the caffeine induced Ca^{2+} release of Ca^{2+} from the sarcoplasmic reticulum but does not block the electrically coupled release of Ca^{2+}, suggesting that the two pools of Ca^{2+} in the terminal or intermediate cisternae may be released by separate mechanisms (Endo, 1975; Thorens and Endo, 1975).

Sandow (1973), in his discussion of electromechanical transforms and mechanism of excitation-coupling in amphibian fast muscle fiber, distinguishes between the effects of the rise phase of the action potential and the falling phase of the action potential on the early phase of tension development during the muscle twitch. Electrical stimulation of sartorius muscle leads to an action potential in which the membrane potential reverses from -90 mV to +20 mV within 1 msec after the initial shock, repolarizes to -60 mV 1.8 msec after the initial shock, and slowly repolarizes to -90 mV over the next 50 msec. Tension relaxes 2 msec after stimulation (latency relaxation) and then rises after 3 msec; the maximal rate of rise in tension is reached after 14 msec, peak tension occurs at 25 msec and tension declines back to baseline after 100 msec. The rise phase of the action potential is related to the initial rate of change of tension (dp/dt) between 2.5 and 3.5 msec,

the falling phase is associated with rate of change of tension between 3.5 and 4.5 msec. After 4.5 msec the rate of tension change
slowly increases to a maximum at 14 msec. Sandow suggests that the
slow rise in dp/dt following the rapid repolarization of the muscle
action potential may be due to Ca^{2+} release of Ca^{2+} from the sarcoplasmic reticulum. The action potential causes electrically coupled
release of Ca^{2+} which in turn triggers off a further release of
Ca^{2+}. Under physiological conditions a concentration of 3×10^{-4} M
Ca^{2+} is required to cause a net release of Ca^{2+} from the sarcoplasmic reticulum. Caffeine at a concentration of 0.5 mM lowers
the concentration of Ca^{2+} required for the release of Ca^{2+} from
3×10^{-4} M to 3×10^{-5} M; at 5 mM caffeine the required Ca^{2+} concentration is lowered to $5 \cong 5 \times 10^{-7}$ M (Endo, 1975). Caffeine at 0.5 mM
markedly enhances the electrically elicited muscle twitch while
5 mM caffeine causes a muscle contracture without causing a membrane depolarization (Bianchi, 1968a).

If the Ca^{2+} released from the terminal cisternae at the junc-
ture between terminal cisternae and the transverse tubular element
accumulates transiently because of restricted diffusion to the sarcoplasm, a local high concentration of Ca^{2+} can occur ($> 10^{-5}$) which
may further enhance Ca^{2+} release from the sarcoplasmic reticulum
and thus contribute to shaping the Ca^{2+} pulse related to twitch
tension.

SUBMECHANICAL POTASSIUM STIMULATION OF OXYGEN UPTAKE
IN FROG SARTORIUS MUSCLE

Depolarization of frog sartorius muscles by 20 mM K_o^+ causes a
sustained release of Ca^{2+} from the sarcoplasmic reticulum, an increase in oxygen utilization, and a potentiation of the electrically
elicited muscle twitch (Bianchi *et al.*, 1975; Bianchi, 1975;
Chirandini and Stefani, 1974). The release of Ca^{2+} and enhanced
O_2 uptake caused by submechanical threshold levels of external K_o^+
is enhanced by low levels of caffeine and is blocked by procaine,
which can be interpreted to mean that the mechanism of Ca^{2+} release
of Ca^{2+} from the sarcoplasmic reticulum is the major factor related
to increase in O_2 uptake (Van der Kloot, 1969; Novotny and Vyskocil,
1966). Vos and Frank (1972) demonstrated that exposure of frog
muscle fibers to subthreshold concentrations of K^+ (17 mM) enhanced
subsequent K^+ induced contractures (K_o^+, 27 mM). The Ca^{2+} released
by subthreshold levels of K^+ may serve a priming function by binding to non-specific sites in the sarcoplasm and thus increase the
effectiveness of binding to troponin C of Ca^{2+} released by higher
K^+ levels.

Brief treatment of sartorius muscle with 400 mM glycerol
causes the myoplasm to become hypertonic to normal Ringer's solution, restoration of the muscle to normal Ringer's results in

rapid water movement across the cell membrane and leads to disruption of the transverse tubular elements. Upon recovery, the resting potential and action potential are normal but the action potential is no longer able to elicit contraction. Submechanical threshold levels of K^+ are also no longer able to increase oxygen uptake or Ca^{2+} release from the sarcoplasmic reticulum; K^+ contractures are no longer possible (Ebashi, 1976; Van der Kloot, 1969). The procedures that can restore K^+ stimulation of respiration in glycerol "shocked" muscle are priming the muscle with either low levels of caffeine, dibutyrl C-AMP, or C-GMP (10^{-9} M). Thus it would appear that glycerol "shock" produces a biochemical lesion that leads to uncoupling of submechanical levels of depolarization from Ca^{2+} release from the sarcoplasmic reticulum, preventing the subsequent increase in respiration; C-GMP appears to be able to remedy the biochemical lesion (Dawson and Bianchi, 1975; Bianchi *et al.*, 1975).

EFFECT OF RYANODINE ON OXYGEN UPTAKE IN FROG SARTORIUS MUSCLE

Ryanodine, a nonbasic alkaloid of empirical composition $C_{25}H_{35}NO_9$, has pharmacological actions on frog sartorius muscle similar to caffeine. Ryanodine causes a marked increase in oxygen uptake in frog sartorius muscle; this declines as tension develops. Ryanodine also increases Ca^{2+} efflux from frog sartorius muscle without causing membrane depolarization.

In recent studies we have found that ryanodine in concentrations as low as 10^{-11} M causes a transient 10-fold increase in oxygen uptake in sartorius muscle (Table I), the effect is optimal at 10^{-10} M (Figure 1 and Table I) and declines to a five-fold increase at concentrations between 10^{-9} M and 10^{-5} M. Benzocaine (2.5 mM) blocks a caffeine-induced contracture and efflux of Ca^{2+} from the frog sartorius muscle (Bianchi, 1968) and also blocks the effect of ryanodine on oxygen uptake in sartorius muscle (Table I). Ryanodine at 10^{-8} M causes a transient increase in O_2 uptake; enhances the increase in O_2 uptake produced by K^+ depolarization (Figure 2), and increases Ca^{2+} efflux from frog sartorius muscle (Figure 3). The increase in oxygen uptake was attributed to an increase in Ca^{2+} release from the terminal cisternae and an increase in ATP utilization by the calcium ATPase of the sarcoplasmic reticulum associated with intracellular resequestration of Ca^{2+}. The efflux of Ca^{2+} across the transverse tubular element associated with low levels of membrane depolarization (7 to 25 mM K_o^+) is blocked by replacement of Na^+ of the Ringer's solution by $Tris^+$ or choline ions (Bianchi *et al.*, 1975). Replacement of Na^+ by choline markedly increases the sensitivity of the muscle to a ryanodine-induced contracture; 10^{-7} M ryanodine

TABLE I.   PEAK OXYGEN UPTAKE IN FROG SARTORIUS MUSCLE

| Ryanodine Conc., M | Oxygen Uptake (μmol O_2/g hr) | |
	Ryanodine	Ryanodine + Benzocaine (2.5 mM)
0	2.3	2.5
10^{-11}	23.4	---
10^{-10}	27.1	---
10^{-9}	10.3	---
10^{-8}	10.7	2.3
10^{-7}	----	3.7
10^{-6}	----	2.4
10^{-5}	12.0	2.4

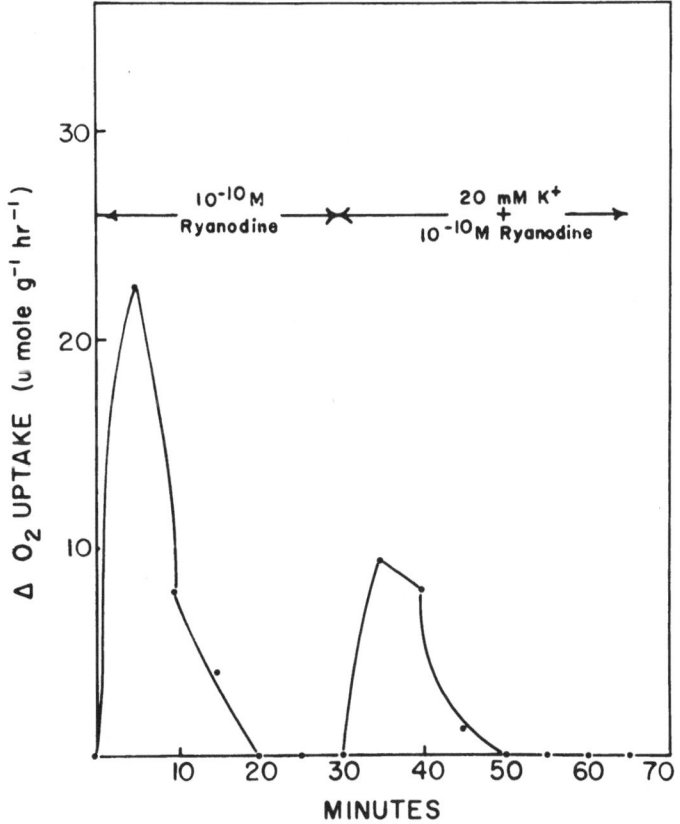

Figure 1.   Effect of 10^{-10} M ryanodine and potassium on oxygen uptake by frog sartorius muscle.

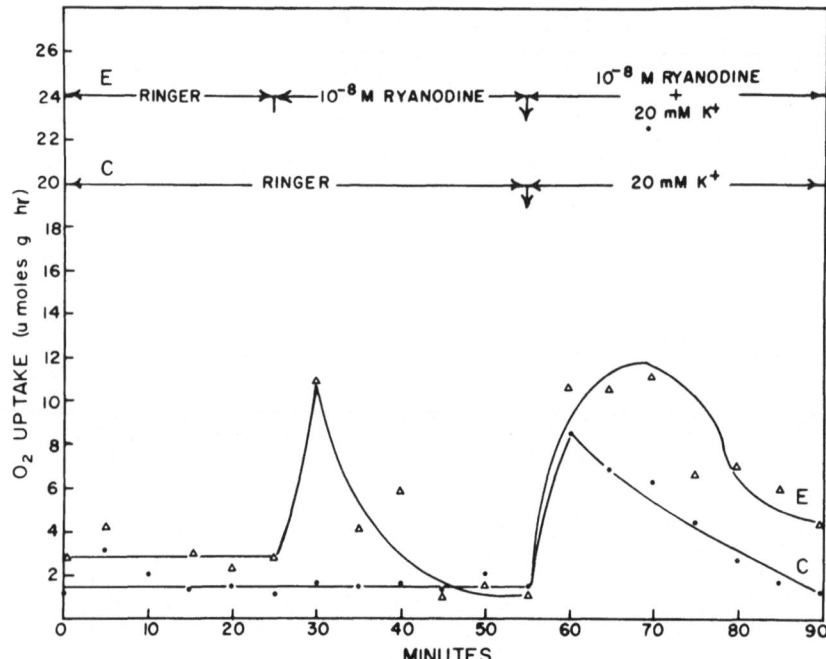

Figure 2. Effect of 10^{-8} M ryanodine on potassium stimulation of oxygen uptake.

doubles the O_2 uptake of muscle and causes a slight contracture to take place (Table II). In the presence of sodium the threshold for ryanodine contracture (at 20^0 C) is 10^{-4} M with a delay of onset of 30 to 40 minutes. In the presence of choline, 10^{-4} M ryanodine causes an immediate development of contracture.

In normal Ringer solution (111 mM NaCl, 2.5 mM KCl, 1.0 mM $CaCl_2$, 10 mM Tris buffer, pH 7.2) neither 10^{-6} M ryanodine nor 1 mM caffeine cause a contracture of frog sartorius muscle. Pre-equilibration of the sartorius muscle with 10^{-6} M ryanodine for 30 minutes, allows 1 mM caffeine to produce a weak contracture; pre-equilibration for 70 minutes results in a marked increase in contracture tension upon addition of 1 mM caffeine. Ryanodine is a hydrophilic molecule whose action on muscle can be demonstrated to occur within the time necessary to diffuse to a surface membrane site (Bianchi, 1968); consequently it is postulated that ryanodine is exerting its effect by acting on a surface receptor to increase the synthesis of a second messenger, which in turn enhances the release of Ca^{2+} from the sarcoplasmic reticulum. Since cyclic-GMP at 10^{-9} M has been shown to recouple K^+ depolarization of glycerol "shocked" muscles with stimulation of

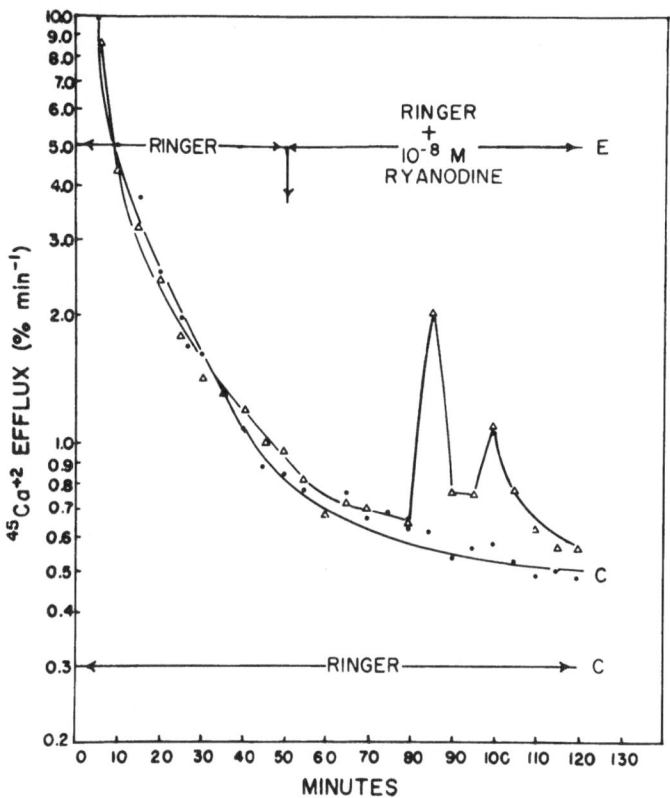

Figure 3. Effect of 10^{-8} M ryanodine on ^{45}Ca efflux.

TABLE II.   EFFECT OF RYANODINE ON O_2 UPTAKE IN FROG SARTORIUS
IN CHOLINE RINGER

N	Condition	Tension Increase (%)	O_2 Uptake ($\mu mol\ g^{-1}\ hr^{-1}$)
6	Ringer (Sodium)	0	2.8 ± 0.2
6	Ringer (Choline)[a]	0	3.4 ± 0.2
4	10^{-9} M Ryanodine	0	5.0 ± 0.3
7	10^{-8} M "	0	6.1 ± 0.3
7	10^{-7} M "	5	7.0 ± 0.2
6	10^{-6} M "	28	7.3 ± 0.2
6	10^{-5} M "	60	7.4 ± 0.3
6	10^{-4} M "[b]	210	7.0 ± 0.3

[a]Sodium in the Ringer solution is replaced by choline.

[b]Threshold for contracture in normal Ringer's is 10^{-4} M with a 30
to 40 min delay. In Choline Ringer onset of contracture is
immediate.

O_2 uptake (Bianchi *et al.*, 1975) and an increase in cyclic AMP was associated with a depression of K^+ stimulated respiration (Bianchi, 1975), the second messenger formed in response to ryanodine is postulated to be C-GMP. Addition of 10^{-9} M C-GMP and 10^{-6} M ryanodine to a sartorius muscle equilibrated in choline Ringer causes a contracture to develop which reaches a peak tension of 26 g/g wet weight of muscle with a $T_{\frac{1}{2}}$ of 35 minutes. Neither agent by itself caused a contracture to develop. Pre-equilibration of the muscles with 10^{-9} M C-GMP for 30 minutes prior to the addition of 10^{-6} M ryanodine increased tension to 30 g/g wet weight muscle, and reduced the $T_{\frac{1}{2}}$ to peak tension to 25 minutes. The contracture curves for this series of experiments (Table III, solutions 4, 5, 6) is shown in Figure 4 (C, B, A).

If ryanodine were acting at a receptor site on the transverse tubular element, the glycerol "shocked" muscles with impaired T-system should be less responsive to ryanodine. In glycerol "shocked" muscles the threshold concentration for ryanodine necessary to increase O_2 uptake was increased to 10^{-4} M (Figure 5) and benzocaine markedly depressed the enhancement of O_2 uptake by 10^{-4} M ryanodine (Table IV). Ryanodine (10^{-4} M) causes a weak contracture to occur in glycerol "shocked" muscle and increases Ca^{2+} efflux (Figure 6). Glycerol "shocked" muscles show a net gain of Ca^{2+}, the Ca^{2+} content of sartorius muscle is increased from 1.95 μmol/g to 2.62 μmol/g (Bianchi and Bolton,

TABLE III.   EFFECT OF cGMP AND CAFFEINE ON RYANODINE INDUCED CONTRACTURE OF FROG SARTORIUS MUSCLE

Solution	Peak tension (g/g wet weight muscle)	Time to half-peak tension (min)
1. *Normal Ringer + 10^{-6} M ryanodine*	*no contracture*	
2. *Normal Ringer + 10^{-6} M ryanodine 30'; then 1 mM caffeine*	*5*	*18'[b]*
3. *Normal Ringer + 10^{-6} M ryanodine 70'; then 1 mM caffeine*	*20*	*28'[b]*
4. *Choline Ringer + 10^{-6} M ryanodine*	*18*	*40'*
5. *Choline Ringer + 10^{-9} M cGMP + ryanodine 10^{-6} M*	*26*	*35'*
6. *Choline Ringer + 10^{-9} M cGMP 30'; then 10^{-6} M ryanodine*	*30*	*25'*

[a]*Temp. $21°$ C*
[b]*Time to half peak tension measured from addition of caffeine.*

1974). The weak contracture produced by ryanodine (10% of tetanus tension) cannot be due to low intracellular Ca^{2+} stores which are high in glycerol "shocked" muscles but must be due to impairment of the steps between ryanodine binding to a receptor and Ca^{2+} release from the sarcoplasmic reticulum. Cyclic GMP (10^{-6} M) increases Ca^{2+} efflux from glycerol "shocked" sartorius muscle in a manner similar to ryanodine (Figure 7).

The data from the above experiments are in keeping with the hypothesis that submechanical threshold levels of K^+ depolarization or ryanodine cause mobilization of Ca^{2+} from the sarcoplasmic reticulum by a C-GMP dependent process. The increased mobilization of Ca^+ is reflected by 1) increased O_2 uptake due to resequestration of Ca^{2+} by the sarcoplasmic reticulum and 2) increased Ca^{2+} efflux across the transverse tubular element and the plasmalemma. In fast striated muscle the loss or resequestration of Ca^{2+} leads to an uncoupling of the muscle action potential from the twitch (ryanodine depression of twitch tension) and eventually Ca^{2+} released from the sarcoplasmic reticulum causes the ryanodine contracture. In amphibian slow muscle fibers, ryanodine releases Ca^{2+} from internal stores; however, tension develops without any delay which indicates that internally released

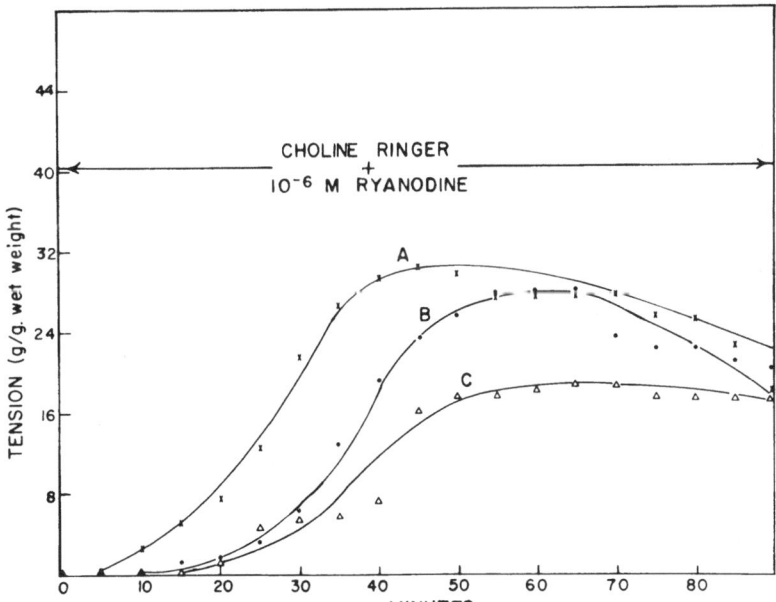

Figure 4. Cyclic-GMP enhancement of ryanodine induced contracture by muscles soaked in Choline Ringer. A) The sartorius muscle was exposed to 5 x 10^{-9} C-GMP before administration of ryanodine. B) Muscle was exposed to 5 x 10^{-9} C-GMP and ryanodine at the same time. C) Control muscle exposed only to ryanodine.

TABLE IV.   EFFECT OF RYANODINE ON O_2 UPTAKE IN GLYCEROL
                "SHOCKED" SARTORIUS MUSCLES

N	Ryanodine	O_2 Uptake ($\mu mol \ g^{-1} \ hr^{-1}$)
5	0	2.2 ± 0.4
4	10^{-6} M	2.3 ± 0.2
5	10^{-5} M	2.4 ± 0.2
4	10^{-4} M	12.4 ± 0.3
4	10^{-4} M + 2.5 mM Benzocaine	4.2 ± 0.3

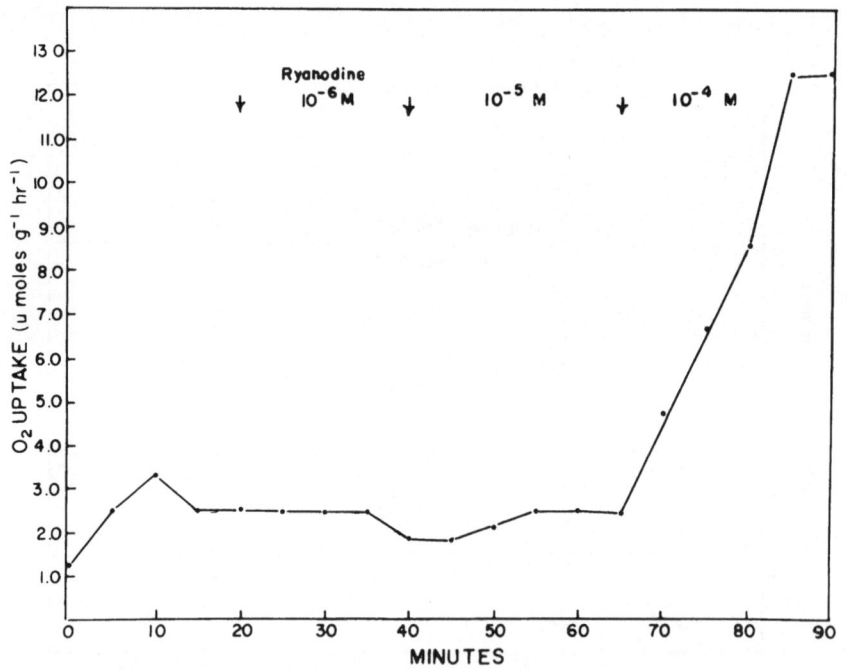

Figure 5.   Enhancement of ^{45}Ca efflux from glycerol "shocked"
muscle by C-GMP.

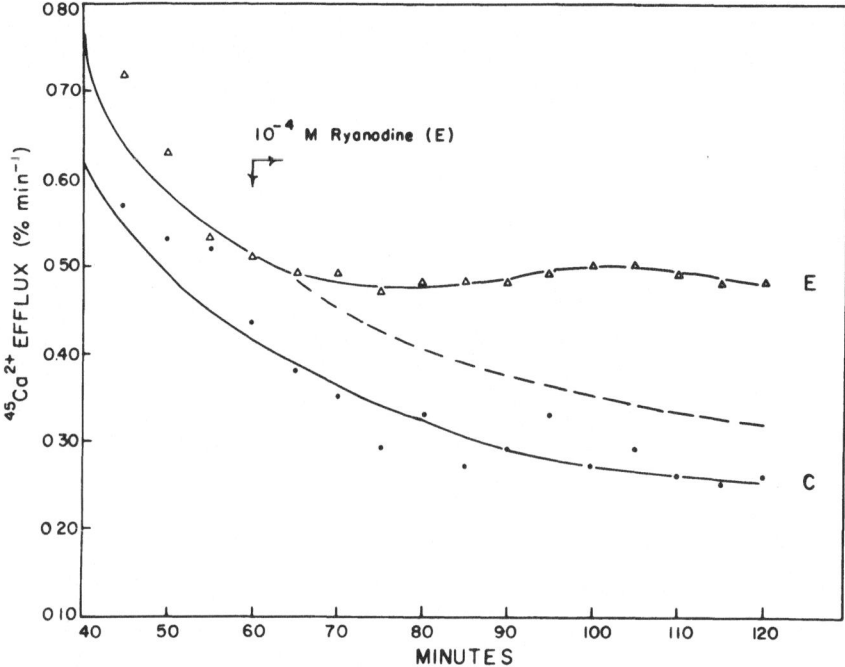

Figure 6. Enhancement of ^{45}Ca *efflux from glycerol "shocked" muscle by ryanodine.*

Ca^{2+} is not being sequestered internally as occurs in the amphibian twitch fiber. The functional role of sarcoplasmic reticulum varies with muscle fiber type, and the pharmacological action of drugs on the sarcoplasmic reticulum can lead to uncoupling of electrical events from contraction if the Ca^{2+} store becomes depleted. If depletion occurs with the myoplasmic level of free Ca^{2+} being below 10^{-7} M no tension develops, if it rises above this level then tension development will occur.

The complex action of ryanodine on different types of muscle [contracture of amphibian slow muscle fiber, uncoupling of the action potential from the muscle twitch in fast muscle fiber followed by a delayed contracture, or uncoupling of the cardiac potential from contraction (Jenden and Fairhurst, 1969)] appears to depend upon the manner in which the calcium released from the internal calcium store is handled. If the sarcoplasmic reticulum cannot maintain intracellular free calcium below 10^{-7} M a contracture can ensue; translocation to either the extracellular phase by Na^{+}-Ca^{2+} exchange across the transverse tubular element combined with resequestration in the longitudinal reticulum can lead to uncoupling of the action potential from muscle contraction.

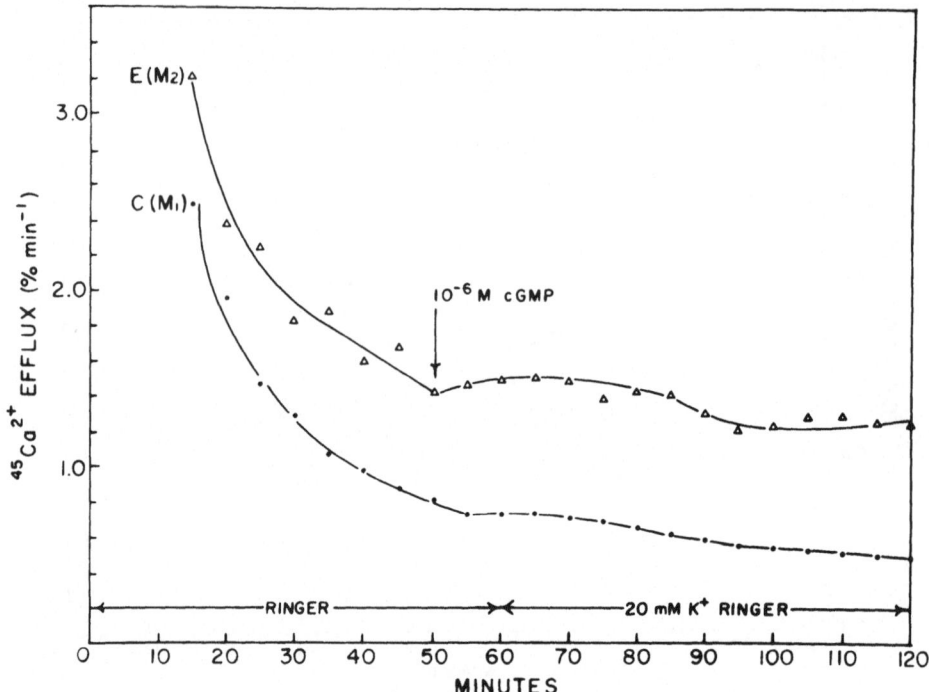

Figure 7.   Effect of ryanodine on oxygen uptake in glycerol "shocked" muscle.

Thus, the data presented strongly suggests an interaction between ryanodine and cyclic GMP. However, only further experimentation will answer the question: Does ryanodine exert its action on muscle by increasing intracellular levels of cyclic-GMP?

REFERENCES

Bianchi, C. P., 1975, Calcium fluxes in skeletal muscle and integration of metabolic and contractile events in concepts of membrane regulation and excitation, *in* "Concepts of Membranes in Regulation and Excitation" (M. Rocha e Silva and G. Suarez-Kurtz, eds.), pp. 1-6, Raven Press, New York.
Bianchi, C. P., 1968a, Cell Calcium, Butterworths, London.
Bianchi, C. P., 1968b, Pharmacological actions on excitation-contraction coupling in striated muscle, *Fed. Proc.* 27: 126.
Bianchi, C. P., 1965, The effect of EDTA and SCN on radiocalcium movement in frog rectus abdominis muscle during contractures induced by calcium removal, *J. Pharmacol. Exp. Ther.* 147: 360.

Bianchi, C. P., and Bolton, T. C., 1974, Effect of hypertonic
  solutions and "glycerol treatment" on calcium and magnesium
  movements of frog skeletal muscle, *J. Pharmacol. Exp. Ther.*
  188: 536.
Bianchi, C. P., Narayan, S., and Lakshminarayanaiah, N., 1975,
  Mobilization of muscle calcium and oxygen uptake in skeletal
  muscle, *in* "Calcium Transport in Contraction and Secretion"
  (E. Carafoli, F. Clementi, W. Drobikowski, and A. Margreth,
  eds.), pp. 503-515, North-Holland Publishing Company, Amsterdam.
Chirandini, D. J., and Stefani, E., 1974, Twitch potentiation by
  potassium contractures in single muscle of the frog, *J. Physiol.
  (London)* 240: 1.
Dawson, M. J., and Bianchi, C. P., 1975, Restoration of potassium
  stimulated respiration of glycerol treated muscle, *Eur. J.
  Pharmacol.* 30: 288.
Ebashi, S., 1976, Excitation-contraction coupling, *Annu. Rev.
  Physiol.* 38: 293.
Eberstein, A., and Sandow, A., 1961, Fatigue in phasic and tonic
  fibers of frog muscle, *Science* 134: 383.
Endo, M., 1975, Mechanism of caffeine on the sarcoplasmic reti-
  culum of skeletal muscle, *Proc. Japan Acad.* 51: 479.
Giese, A. C., 1973, Cell Physiology, 4th Edition, W. B. Saunders
  Company, Philadelphia.
Jenden, D., and Fairhurst, A. S., 1969, The pharmacology of
  ryanodine, *Pharmacol. Rev.* 21: 1.
Kuffler, S. W., and Williams, E. M. V., 1953a, Small nerve junctional potentials. The distribution of small motor nerves to
  frog skeletal muscle, and the membrane characteristics of the
  fibers they innervate, *J. Physiol. (London)* 121: 289.
Kuffler, S. W., and Williams, E. M. V., 1953b, Properties of the
  "slow" skeletal muscle fibers of the frog, *J. Physiol. (London)*
  121: 318.
Orentlicher, M., Reuben, J. P., Grundfest, H., and Brandt, P. W.,
  1974, Calcium binding and tension development in detergent-
  treated muscle fibers, *J. gen. Physiol.* 63: 168.
Page, S. G., 1965, A comparison of the fine structures of the
  frog slow and twitch fibers, *J. Cell Biol.* 26: 477.
Peachey, L. D., 1965, The sarcoplasmic reticulum and transverse
  tubules of the frog's sartorius, *J. Cell Biol.* 25: 209.
Sandow, A., 1973, Electromechanical transforms and the mechanism
  of excitation-contraction coupling, *J. Mechanochem. Cell Mobil.*
  2: 193.
Sandow, A., and Brust, M., 1966, Caffeine potentiation of twitch
  tension in frog sartorius muscle, *Biochem. Zeit.* 345: 232.
Taylor, S. R., Rüdel, R., and Blinks, J. W., 1975, Calcium
  transients in amphibian muscles, *Fed. Proc.* 34: 1379.
Thorens, S., and Endo, M., 1975, Calcium induced calcium release
  their physiological significance, *Proc. Japan. Acad.* 51: 473.

Van der Kloot, W., 1969, The steps between depolarization and the
    increase in the respiration of frog skeletal muscle, *J. Physiol.
    (London)* 204: 551.
Vos, E. C., and Frank, G. B., 1972, The threshold for potassium
    induced contractures of frog skeletal muscle. Potentiation
    of potassium induced contractures by pre-exposure to sub-
    threshold potassium concentrations, *Can. J. Physiol. Pharmacol.*
    50: 37.
Winegrad, S., 1970, The intracellular site of calcium activation
    of contraction in frog skeletal muscle, *J. gen. Physiol.* 55: 77.

CHAPTER 14

CALCIUM RELATED BASIS OF ACTION OF VASCULAR

AGENTS: CELLULAR APPROACHES

Frank R. Goodman

Department of Pharmacology
Dow Chemical Company
Indianapolis, Indiana 46268

INTRODUCTION

It is well established in vascular smooth muscle (Bohr, 1973; Weiss, 1977) as well as in cardiac (Fozzard, 1977; Fleckenstein, 1977) and other types of muscle (Bianchi, 1975; Ebashi, 1977) that calcium serves as a link in the events leading from membrane depolarization to muscle contraction. However, the degree of dependence on the extracellular Ca^{2+} level varies greatly among the different types of muscle. For example, contractile responsiveness in skeletal muscle is less sensitive to changes in the extracellular Ca^{2+} concentration than are contractions obtained with cardiac muscle. These differences in the degree of dependence on extracellular Ca^{2+} have been related to the volume of sarcoplasmic reticulum (SR) in the tissue (Devine et al., 1972). Skeletal muscle has a large amount of SR (Lüllmann and Peters, 1977) in relation to the amount found in cardiac or smooth muscle. In skeletal muscle, depolarization of the transverse tubular element initiates a coupling step between the transverse tubular element and the SR, which, in turn, causes the release of Ca^{2+} important for contraction. In contrast, Ca^{2+} important for initiation of contraction in cardiac muscle originates from superficial sites which are in equilibrium with interstitial space Ca^{2+} (Langer, 1976). Thus, in skeletal muscle and, to some degree, in cardiac muscle both the manner in which Ca^{2+} is utilized for the initiation of the contractile response and the mechanism(s) by which drugs interfere with this process are well characterized (Fuchs, 1974; Bianchi, 1975).

In smooth muscle the mechanisms by which Ca^{2+} becomes available to the contractile element are not as clearly defined. A wide variety of pharmacological agents are capable of interfering with either the resting tone or the contractile responsiveness of smooth muscle by interacting with tissue Ca^{2+} in several ways (Hurwitz and Suria, 1971; Prosser, 1974; Fleisch, 1974). In addition, different types of vascular smooth muscle vary in the manner in which Ca^{2+} becomes available to the contractile protein. Thus, differences observed in contractile responses of smooth muscle preparations have been attributed to variations in the utilization of Ca^{2+} from differing sites or stores. This Ca^{2+} which is known as the "activator calcium" may originate from several sources. It may come directly from the extracellular solution, from subcellular structures (e.g., sarcoplasmic reticulum, mitochondria), or from the plasma membrane (Bohr, 1973; Ford, 1976). In guinea pig ileal longitudinal smooth muscle, Hurwitz and co-workers (Hurwitz *et al.*, 1967 a,b) demonstrated that high extracellular concentrations of Ca^{2+} appear to depress membrane excitability and, under appropriate conditions, extracellular Ca^{2+} also inhibited contractile responses. On this basis it was postulated that Ca^{2+} located at surface binding sites controlled the release of Ca^{2+} from other less superficial membrane sites. Thus, agents which alter or remove superficial Ca^{2+} can initiate an inward release of Ca^{2+} which results in contraction, whereas agents which inhibit the removal of this Ca^{2+} fraction or replace it can prevent contractile responses. However, delineation of the relationship between specific Ca^{2+} pools and drug-induced alterations in Ca^{2+} movements in a variety of smooth muscle preparations is complicated due to nonspecific Ca^{2+} movements (Hudgins and Weiss, 1969; Krejci and Daniel, 1970; Weiss, 1972).

Also, in smooth muscle preparations there are functional differences in the manner in which Ca^{2+} is bound and subsequently released. The purpose of this chapter is to consider isolated vascular smooth muscle systems and the cellular basis of the drug-Ca^{2+} interaction. Initially, a brief description of some of the approaches employed for delineating how Ca^{2+} is affected by different ions or drugs will be covered. The remainder of the chapter will deal with responses to specific agents that interact with Ca^{2+} and, in turn, alter vascular responsiveness.

BASIC CELLULAR APPROACHES

In the past, several approaches have been employed to analyze how various types of vascular smooth muscle and other smooth muscle preparations sequester and subsequently utilize Ca^{2+}. The significance of this type of research is based on the idea that both the qualitative and quantitative response(s) obtained with stimulatory and inhibitory agents are a function of the manner in which Ca^{2+} is handled by different tissues.

Since it has been demonstrated that Ca^{2+} is the important link which serves as the coupler between membrane excitation and contraction in vascular smooth muscle, tension experiments have been valuable in ascertaining how different types of vascular smooth muscle respond to pharmacological agents. Previous studies have shown that alteration of tissue Ca^{2+} (by changing the concentration of Ca^{2+} in the bathing solution) helps to delineate the primary source of Ca^{2+} utilized to initiate a contractile response by different vasoactive agents. For example, lowering the Ca^{2+} concentration of the bathing solution decreases (Hinke, 1965), whereas increasing the Ca^{2+} concentration augments (Hurwitz *et al.*, 1962) K^+-induced responses. In rabbit aorta, Hudgins and Weiss (1968) demonstrated that the contractile responses to K^+, norepinephrine and histamine exhibit a differential dependence upon Ca^{2+}. Apparently, norepinephrine affected Ca^{2+} transport systems or firmly bound Ca^{2+}, whereas histamine also utilized loosely bound membrane Ca^{2+} and K^+-induced responses were dependent upon extracellular Ca^{2+} or Ca^{2+} located at superficial sites. Studies by Bohr and his associates (Bohr *et al.*, 1971) further demonstrated that agents such as caffeine can induce a selective effect on vascular smooth muscle tension responses by altering the availability of Ca^{2+}. Furthermore, the contractile response of isolated vascular smooth muscle could be divided into two separable components, a fast (initial) and a slow (maintained) component (Bohr, 1964; van Breeman, 1969). The fact that these two components can be differentially influenced by changes in the extracellular Ca^{2+} concentration has also aided in the characterization of the different mechanisms involved in excitation of smooth muscle. For example, the fast component of high K^+-induced contractile responses is known to be more related to the inward movement of Ca^{2+} across the cell membrane than to depolarization (Somlyo and Somlyo, 1968; Weiss, 1975), whereas norepinephrine and other agents appear to utilize bound cellular Ca^{2+} during the fast phase (Hinke, 1965). Low extracellular Ca^{2+} and some of the Ca^{2+}-antagonists eliminate or markedly reduce the fast component of K^+-induced contractile responses and have little, if any, effect in altering the fast component response induced by agonists such as norepinephrine, angiotensin or histamine. These observations are in accord with the concept that Ca^{2+} important for the initiation of the contractile response can originate from different Ca^{2+} sites or stores. As a result, a number of approaches have been employed in attempts to characterize the various Ca^{2+} sites or stores.

As mentioned, the effects of stimulatory or inhibitory agents on contractile responses have been shown to vary from one vascular

preparation to another. Based on several studies, it appears
that the mechanical responsiveness of small resistance vessels
is more sensitive than that of larger vessels to (a) changes in
extracellular Ca^{2+} concentration and (b) pharmacological agents
which inhibit mobilization of Ca^{2+} from the membrane (Bohr *et al.*,
1971; Goodman *et al.*, 1975). The dog terminal mesenteric artery,
for example, is more sensitive to the inhibitory effects of the
aminoglycoside antibiotic, neomycin, than is the aorta (Adams and
Goodman, 1975) and the coronary artery is very sensitive to Ca^{2+}
antagonistic compounds which interfere with transmembrane Ca^{2+}
fluxes (Fleckenstein, 1977). This differential dependence on
extracellular Ca^{2+} exhibited between large and small vessels may
be due to a lower sarcoplasmic reticulum content in small resistance
vessels (Devine *et al.*, 1972).

Thus, agents that either antagonize or effectively decrease
extracellular Ca^{2+} fluxes have contributed significantly to
delineation of the sources of Ca^{2+} important in drug-induced
contractile responses. Examples of agents of this type which
have been employed extensively in tension studies include SKF-525A
(Kalsner *et al.*, 1970), verapamil and some of its derivatives
(Haeusler, 1972) and rare earth ions such as La^{3+} and Lu^{3+} (Weiss,
1974; Weiss and Goodman, 1975). For example, use of La^{3+} (an
antagonist of Ca^{2+}) has provided valuable information about different Ca^{2+} dependent coupling mechanisms and Ca^{2+} binding sites
in muscle and nerve (Weiss, 1974). Lanthanum ion, by displacing
a portion of the surface bound (superficially located) Ca^{2+} in
cardiac tissue inhibits further exchange of Ca^{2+} and thus acts
as an uncoupler of excitation and contraction (Langer and Frank,
1972). The success obtained with La^{3+} as a Ca^{2+}-antagonist
indicated that other rare earth ions could also be of value in
the delineation of important cellular differences in Ca^{2+} dependence
and utilization. In rabbit aortic smooth muscle, it was found that
some of the other rare earth ions appeared to have qualitatively
similar effects on Ca^{2+}-dependent actions; the differences observed
were attributed to variations in their affinity for superficial
binding sites at which Ca^{2+} is normally bound (Weiss and Goodman,
1975). In contrast to the rare earth ions, verapamil and D-600
inhibit excitation-contraction coupling by specifically blocking
the slow Ca^{2+} channel in the membrane (Kohlhardt *et al.*, 1972;
Tritthardt *et al.*, 1973).

Parallel to this is the concept that other agents or ions
which alter Ca^{2+} binding at superficially-located sites would
affect the manner in which a muscle responds to other agents.
Agents capable of displacing Ca^{2+} or replacing Ca^{2+} at these sites
and not being readily removed (e.g., La^{3+}) would inhibit contraction of vascular smooth muscle. On the other hand, agents which
facilitate inward Ca^{2+} movements or increase the availability of

Ca^{2+} at membrane sites would be expected to potentiate contractile responses. Thus, tension experiments are useful not only in determining whether certain pharmacological agents are agonists or antagonists but they also can provide some insight into the possible mechanism(s) of action.

Another approach to understanding the cellular basis of excitation-contraction coupling in vascular smooth muscle involves elucidation of the Ca^{2+}-binding properties of the various vascular preparations. Studies of this type provide additional information concerning the relationship between the mobilization of bound Ca^{2+} and the induction of the contractile response. In addition to yielding information concerning the binding of Ca^{2+}, isotopic studies also provide information about the release and exchange-ability of Ca^{2+}. Perhaps more importantly, the flux studies (in combination with the tension data) help delineate complex mechanisms in a manner which cannot be obtained solely from tension studies. As previously mentioned, La^{3+} inhibits tension responses to various constrictor agents. The initial tension studies in ileal longitudinal smooth muscle demonstrated that La^{3+} was equally effective in inhibiting contractions induced by either acetylcholine or K^+ (Weiss and Goodman, 1969). Additional ^{45}Ca studies indicated that La^{3+} induced an increase in ^{45}Ca release and decreased ^{45}Ca uptake. Based on data from this and other studies with La^{3+}, it was concluded that La^{3+} altered excitation-contraction coupling primarily by preventing the rebinding of Ca^{2+} at superficial cellular sites or stores.

As with tension studies, altering the extracellular Ca^{2+} concentration of the incubation solution has been a useful approach in characterizing Ca^{2+}-binding in different tissues. Lowering the Ca^{2+} concentration increases the specific activity of ^{45}Ca in the incubation solution. Since the ^{45}Ca tissue to medium ratio represents an estimation of the amount of ^{45}Ca in the tissue relative to the amount of ^{45}Ca in the incubation solution, this value (due to ^{40}Ca-^{45}Ca competition) is a function of the concentration of nonradioactive Ca^{2+} in the bathing solution. Thus, lowering the concentration of extracellular Ca^{2+} makes it possible to increase the uptake of ^{45}Ca at depleted Ca^{2+}-binding sites because there is no competitive ^{40}Ca-^{45}Ca exchange. Therefore, when ^{45}Ca tissue to medium ratios are determined in Ca^{2+}-deficient solutions, there is a marked increase in the ratio. For example, in rabbit aortic smooth muscle (media-intimal layer) the ^{45}Ca tissue to medium ratio in a 1.5 mM Ca^{2+} solution is approximately 2.4 ml/g (Goodman and Weiss, 1971), in a 0.1 mM Ca^{2+} solution the ratio ranges from 9.5-11.5 ml/g (Goodman *et al.*, 1972; Adams *et al.*, 1974), and in a Ca^{2+}-free solution the value is approximately 30-40 ml/g (Hudgins and Weiss, 1969). The change that occurs in the tissue to medium ratio is not only a function of the extracellular Ca^{2+} concentration but also depends on the tissue being investigated. Studies in canine terminal mesenteric, carotid and aortic arteries show that the ^{45}Ca tissue to medium ratios obtained in the carotid and terminal mesenteric arteries were larger than corresponding values obtained with the aorta (Goodman et al., 1975); these results suggested that there may be less retention of ^{45}Ca in the aorta than in the other arteries. This idea was further supported by the shift of ^{45}Ca into the slow component in mesenteric arteries incubated in a Ca^{2+}-free solution (no added extracellular Ca^{2+}), whereas the aorta showed little difference resulting from changing the nonradioactive Ca^{2+} concentration in the incubation solution. In smooth muscle this gain in ^{45}Ca ratios probably represents a relative increase in bound ^{45}Ca at several tissue sites.

The question as to what are the potential sites or stores for Ca^{2+} in vascular as well as other smooth muscles has been the subject of many investigations (Prosser, 1974; Somlyo and Somlyo, 1975). Histological and histochemical studies in many smooth muscle systems have indicated the presence of subcellular structures (Somlyo and Somlyo, 1971; Devine et al., 1972; Gabella, 1973; Debbas et al., 1975) where significant quantities of Ca^{2+} may be bound. Furthermore, the isolation of sarcoplasmic reticulum has led to the suggestion that this structure might serve as a depot for cellular Ca^{2+} and, in this manner, have a role in regulating Ca^{2+} important for initiation and maintenance of mechanical responsiveness in smooth muscle (Somlyo and Somlyo, 1971; Devine et al., 1972; Somlyo et al., 1974). Although the volume of sarcoplasmic reticulum in different smooth muscles varies and suggests the presence of other sites in smooth muscle which may release Ca^{2+} (Somlyo and Somlyo, 1970), contractile responses in the absence of extracellular Ca^{2+} do appear to be correlated with the volume of sarcoplasmic reticulum.

It should be noted, however, that changing the extracellular Ca^{2+} concentration to alter ^{45}Ca tissue to medium ratios is essentially a tool for delineating the binding of ^{45}Ca in smooth muscle. In this context, both the limitations and interpretations of this type of an approach must be recognized. This procedure does not define the anatomical location of these Ca^{2+}-binding sites. Though the ^{45}Ca tissue to medium ratios are increased by lowering the extracellular Ca^{2+} concentration, this increase is a relative increase for radioactive Ca^{2+} only. The total Ca^{2+} uptake or content in a Ca^{2+}-deficient solution is, of course, decreased compared with that occurring in Ca^{2+}-containing solution. Also, this conventional technique does not detect changes in slowly exchangeable Ca^{2+} stores.

Another problem is that ^{45}Ca may be bound to superficial sites which behave as reservoirs for Ca^{2+}. An example of this is monkey ileum. The whole ileal segment and ileum with the mucosal layer removed were found to be much more resistant to Ca^{2+} depletion than was the isolated longitudinal smooth muscle (Goodman and Weiss, 1974). Furthermore, it has been suggested that the adventitial layer of vascular smooth muscle might function as a Ca^{2+} reservoir in a similar manner (Hudgins and Weiss, 1969; Goodman et al., 1975; Turlapaty et al., 1976). In order to ascertain if there is any relationship between the extracellular Ca^{2+} concentration and the rate of ^{45}Ca uptake, steady-state ^{45}Ca tissue to medium ratios also have to be determined. Lüllmann and Siegfriedt (1968) demonstrated with longitudinal muscle of guinea pig small intestine that the lower the external Ca^{2+} concentration the slower the ^{45}Ca uptake. Similarly, Hudgins and Weiss (1969), employing rabbit aortic smooth muscle, have shown that there is a rapid equilibration (10 min) of ^{45}Ca in solutions containing 1.5 to 2.5 mM Ca^{2+}, whereas it takes approximately 40 minutes in Ca^{2+}-free solution.

Further clarification of the basis of this increase in ^{45}Ca binding can be obtained from either desaturation or rate coefficient plots. These two plots have been successfully applied to vascular smooth muscle preparations. Desaturation curves, which illustrate the decline of tissue ^{45}Ca concentration as a function of time, are useful for determining both the relative size and the half-times $(T\frac{1}{2})$ of washout components. Rate coefficient curves, on the other hand, which express the decline of tissue ^{45}Ca content as a percentage of the ^{45}Ca present in the tissue during a specific time interval are more sensitive to rapid changes that occur in the loss of ^{45}Ca from the tissue. Examples of these types of plots are given in Figures 1 and 2. Generally, when ^{45}Ca loss from vascular smooth muscle is plotted as a desaturation curve, there are two or more ^{45}Ca washout components. In rabbit aorta, Hudgins and Weiss (1969) characterized a fast component with a $T\frac{1}{2}$ of 8 min and a slow component with a $T\frac{1}{2}$ of approximately 105 min. In contrast, rat aorta appears to have three washout components (DeFelice and Joiner, 1975). Although the rate of loss of ^{45}Ca from vascular smooth muscle is much greater when the sample collection intervals are shortened (Figure 1A vs Figure 1B), abbreviating the collection periods does not alter the distribution of ^{45}Ca between the slow and fast components (Goodman and Weiss, 1971). The important thing to remember, however, is that the $T\frac{1}{2}$ and the rate constants calculated from desaturation curves represent net ^{45}Ca loss rather than the true rate of ^{45}Ca loss from specific tissue compartments or sites.

Though there are limitations to the usage of these plots, they have been very helpful in delineating the effects of both ions and drugs on ^{45}Ca fluxes. Referring back to figure 1A, it

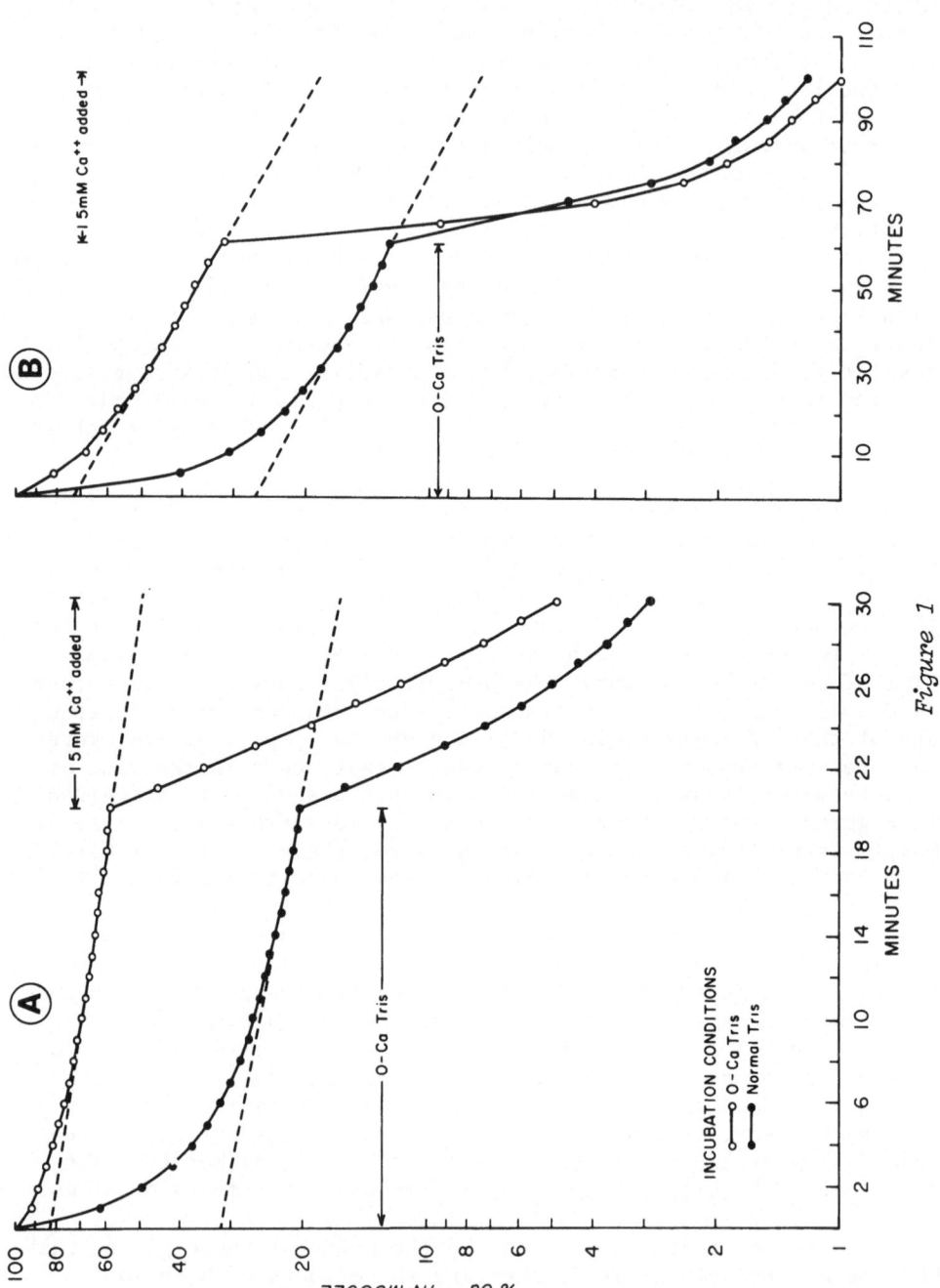

Figure 1

Figure 1.   Effect of 1.5 mM Ca²⁺ on ⁴⁵Ca efflux from rabbit aorta. Muscles were incubated for 60 min prior to washout in the desired solution plus ⁴⁵Ca.   Washout sample collection times were one minute (A) or five minutes (B).   Arrows indicate the duration of exposure to 1.5 mM Ca²⁺ during the washout (From Goodman and Weiss, 1971).

can be seen that the addition of nonradioactive Ca^{2+} during the washout results in a large displacement of the bound self-exchangeable ^{45}Ca fraction. A closer examination of this phenomenon indicates that the addition of nonradioactive Ca^{2+} induces a transient as well as a sustained increase in ^{45}Ca efflux (Figure 2B), whereas addition of La^{3+} induces only a sustained increase in the ^{45}Ca efflux rate (Figure 2A). The transient increase in ^{45}Ca efflux indicates either the presence of a limited readily depletable self-exchangeable ^{45}Ca fraction or a temporal change in membrane permeability to Ca^{2+}; a sustained increase indicates a decrease in the rate of ^{45}Ca uptake or rebinding or, alternatively, a maintained increase in membrane permeability. Thus, a considerable amount of information about the manner in which various pharmacological agents effect Ca^{2+} distribution and release can be obtained from ^{45}Ca flux studies; this topic has been adequately discussed and evaluated in a recent review (Weiss, 1977).

Brief mention should also be made of another technique which has been of some value in delineating the effects of drugs on Ca^{2+} binding and distribution in vascular smooth muscle. Studies of Ca^{2+} movements in subcellular fractions isolated from several vascular smooth muscle preparations have been reported (Fitzpatrick *et al.*, 1972; Baudouin-Legros and Meyer, 1973; Hess and Ford, 1974). On the basis of these investigations, it has been suggested that the microsomal vesicles (which consist of both plasma membrane and sarcoplasmic reticulum) could be both the storage site and the source of Ca^{2+} important for the initiation of the contractile response. Further support for this idea is that Ca^{2+} uptake by this microsomal fraction is analogous to that observed in skeletal muscle (Hurwitz *et al.*, 1973). In addition, mitochondria might function in some way as a regulator of intracellular free Ca^{2+} since it has been shown that mitochondria both contain (Debbas *et al.*, 1975) and accumulate Ca^{2+} (Vallieres *et al.*, 1975). Consequently, it is possible that pharmacological agents which alter the rate at which these subcellular structures release or sequester Ca^{2+} can induce changes in the intracellular free Ca^{2+} concentration and, in turn, alter the contractile tone of vascular smooth muscle. For example, based on subcellular data, it has been suggested that, in addition to its receptor effect, angiotensin might alter vasomotor tone by decreasing calcium binding and

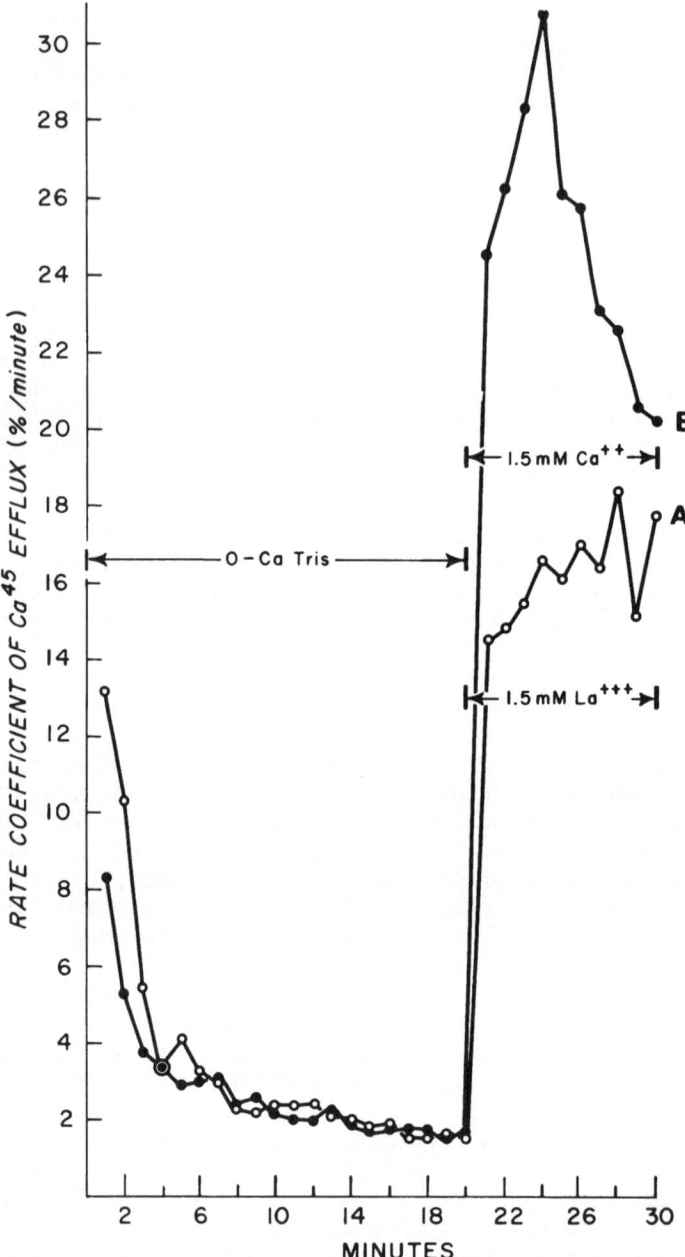

Figure 2.   Effect of 1.5 mM La^{3+} (A) or Ca^{2+} (B) on the rate at which ^{45}Ca is removed from rabbit aortic smooth muscle.   Muscles were incubated with added ^{45}Ca in Ca^{2+}-free solution for 60 min prior to washout.   (From Goodman and Weiss, 1971)

increasing the release of bound Ca^{2+} (Baudouin et al., 1972; Baudouin-Legros and Meyer, 1973). Use of subcellular preparations has also provided new information concerning the mechanism of action of phosphatidyl serine (Kutsky and Goodman, 1978). However, it is possible that isolated portions of the plasma membrane might be inverted and the microsomes obtained may be present in the form of closed vesicles (Hurwitz et al., 1975). If this is so, direct extrapolations from microsomal preparations to isolated smooth muscle preparations may not be fully justified.

CELLULAR BASIS OF ACTION OF AMINOGLYCOSIDE ANTIBIOTICS

A good example of how these cellular techniques can be employed to resolve a mechanism-related problem is the aminoglycoside antibiotics. The original studies were based on the observations by several investigators (Elmqvist and Josefsson, 1962; Vital Brazil and Prado-Franceschi, 1969) that neomycin and streptomycin inhibit Ca^{2+}-dependent reactions important in axonal membrane excitation. It was thought that these antibiotics may exert their effects by altering Ca^{2+} distribution and movements in vascular smooth muscle. Initial investigations in rabbit aortic smooth muscle with neomycin (2.1 mM and 7.0 mM), a representative aminoglycoside antibiotic, demonstrated that this antibiotic decreased the uptake of ^{45}Ca and increased ^{45}Ca efflux in a sustained manner. The mechanism for this interaction between neomycin and cellular Ca^{2+} was postulated to result from an alteration in the ability of the membrane to accumulate and bind Ca^{2+} (Adams et al., 1973).

Further examination (Goodman et al., 1974) of the actions of this antibiotic demonstrated that prior exposure of aortic strips to neomycin affected K^+-induced contractions more than those responses obtained with other unrelated vasoactive agents (e.g., norepinephrine, histamine, angiotensin). In contrast, addition of neomycin subsequent to induction of contraction decreased the contractile responses obtained with the other agents and had no effect on K^+-induced responses. Exposure of aortic strips to neomycin during ^{45}Ca washout resulted in a maintained increase in ^{45}Ca efflux which was inhibited by prior exposure to 0.05 mM ethylenediamine tetracetic acid (EDTA) but not by prior exposure to 1.5 mM Sr^{2+}. Furthermore, neomycin inhibited ^{45}Ca uptake by similar amounts at all incubation time intervals (which indicated that neomycin was not inhibiting the rate of ^{45}Ca uptake). Thus, it appeared that neomycin differentially altered tension responses to a variety of vasoactive agents by preventing Ca^{2+} uptake at those sites important for the actions of these agents. Furthermore, it was found that the effects observed with neomycin on tension responses as well as on ^{45}Ca distribution and movements could also be elicited with gentamicin, streptomycin and kanamycin (Adams et al., 1974).

Small peripheral resistance vessels might respond differently to agents than did larger conduit arteries such as the aorta (Uchida and Bohr, 1969a, b). Therefore, the comparative effects of neomycin on a variety of isolated canine vascular tissues were examined (Adams and Goodman, 1975). To determine if neomycin altered the initial contractile response or the maintained portion of the contractile response, arteries were exposed to neomycin either prior to or subsequent to the initiation of contractions. Preexposure of the vascular strips to neomycin decreased tension responses induced by norepinephrine and potassium in aorta, femoral, carotid, renal, mesenteric and coronary arteries. In contrast, when neomycin was added to the maintained portion of K^+-induced responses, coronary and terminal mesenteric arteries showed a decrease in tension, whereas responses of aortic, renal, femoral or carotid arteries were not altered. With norepinephrine-contracted strips, neomycin relaxed contractile responses in femoral, carotid, renal and terminal mesenteric arteries, but had little if any effect on the aorta. Furthermore, in perfused arteries, the inhibitory action of neomycin on K^+-induced responses was found to be inversely related to the concentration of Ca^{2+} in the perfusion fluid. On the other hand, the Ca^{2+} concentration of the perfusion fluid had no influence on the degree of inhibition by neomycin of norepinephrine responses. Thus, the manner in which neomycin altered tension responsiveness in peripheral resistance and conduit vessels of dogs could be related to the degree of dependence of each tissue on superficially bound Ca^{2+}. Further support for this view was obtained from a comparative characterization of the effects of neomycin on ^{45}Ca movements in the carotid, terminal mesenteric (as a resistance artery) and the aorta (as a conduit artery) of the dog (Goodman et al., 1975). The ^{45}Ca tissue to medium ratio in the carotid and terminal mesenteric arteries were 2-4 times greater than were the corresponding values obtained in aorta. Desaturation curves obtained from the carotid and terminal mesenteric arteries as well as from the aorta indicate that the addition of 7.0 mM neomycin increased ^{45}Ca efflux in a maintained manner; the effects on the terminal mesenteric were greater than the effects observed in either the carotid or aorta. These results are illustrated in Figure 3. These findings were interpreted to indicate that either the terminal mesenteric arteries have a relatively larger fraction of removable Ca^{2+} than does the aorta or that neomycin has a greater affinity for Ca^{2+}-binding sites in the terminal mesenteric arteries than in the aorta. In either case, the terminal mesenteric arteries would be more susceptible to the inhibitory effects of neomycin. The studies with the aminoglycoside antibiotics were then extended to arterial preparations isolated from nonhuman primates (squirrel monkeys, capuchin monkeys and baboons). The results demonstrated that

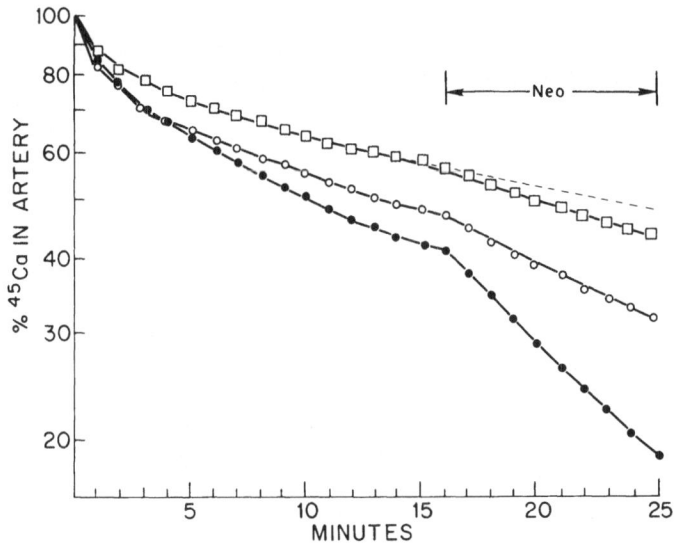

Figure 3. Effects of addition of neomycin on ^{45}Ca efflux from dog aorta (□), and carotid (○) and terminal mesenteric arteries (●). Muscles were incubated for 60 min with added ^{45}Ca prior to washout in Ca^{2+}-free solution. Arrows indicate the interval of exposure to 7.0 mM neomycin. (From Goodman et al., 1975)

neomycin, kanamycin and gentamicin inhibit contractile responses and alter ^{45}Ca movements in a manner which does not differ qualitatively from effects of these agents in canine and rabbit vascular preparations (Goodman and Adams, 1976).

In addition, the distribution of ^{14}C-labeled gentamicin was examined in rabbit aortic smooth muscle under a variety of conditions (Goodman, 1978). The uptake of ^{14}C-gentamicin reached a maximum value within 20 minutes and, as the Ca^{2+} concentration in the incubation solution was increased to 10 mM, ^{14}C-gentamicin tissue uptake was decreased significantly. The uptake of labeled gentamicin was also inhibited by 1.5 mM La^{3+} and 80 mM K^+. However, pretreatment with metabolic inhibitors (iodoacetic acid and dinitrophenol) did not alter either uptake or efflux of ^{14}C-gentamicin, and lowering the temperature of the incubation solution (to 0^oC) did not alter ^{14}C-gentamicin uptake. The loss of ^{14}C-gentamicin from the aorta was increased in a maintained manner by exposure to nonradioactive gentamicin. Furthermore, in the presence of high concentrations of nonradioactive gentamicin, the accumulation of ^{14}C-gentamicin decreased, whereas the total tissue binding of gentamicin continued to increase. A Scatchard-type plot (Figure 4) of these results indicates that, in addition to the high affinity site which binds approximately 3.25 μmol of gentamicin per gram wet weight and appears to be Ca^{2+}-specific, there are nonspecific (low affinity) binding sites on the cell membrane which do not appear to be readily saturable. Thus, these findings further support the idea that aminoglycoside antibiotics appear to be limited to surface accessible sites and consequently inhibit vascular responsiveness by affecting superficially-bound Ca^{2+} by interacting at or with sites important for Ca^{2+} binding.

The antagonistic interaction between the aminoglycoside antibiotics and Ca^{2+} has also been described in other preparations. In cardiac muscle, which is much more sensitive to the membrane effects of the aminoglycoside antibiotics than are vascular tissues, the negative inotropic effect of gentamicin has been related to an interference with Ca^{2+}-dependent functions (Adams, 1975). As shown in Table I, gentamicin also decreases ^{45}Ca uptake in a guinea pig left atrial preparation. This decrease occurred in beating but not in nonbeating (nb) atria, and it was not observed when the atrial preparations were incubated in bathing solutions containing higher concentrations of Ca^{2+}. This supports the idea of a competitive rather than a physiological (indirect) antagonism. Thus, comparison of results obtained in isolated vascular muscle with isolated cardiac muscle could possibly facilitate characterization of the manner in which certain drugs interact with Ca^{2+} and, also, the manner in which these drugs might interact with each other.

CELLULAR BASIS OF ACTION OF MANNITOL

A more recent example which (in contrast to the aminoglycoside antibiotics) is not a specific Ca^{2+}-antagonist, is mannitol. Although mannitol is widely recognized as an osmotic diuretic, the finding that increases in osmolarity can also have a vasodilatory effect suggested the possibility of another interesting drug-Ca^{2+} interaction. As previously mentioned, it is generally accepted that increases or decreases in the concentration of free Ca^{2+} in the myoplasm directly precede respective contractile or relaxant responses in vascular smooth muscle. Pretreatment with hypertonic mannitol has been shown to partially protect muscle from the effects of ischemia and hypoxia by increasing total blood flow (Willerson *et al.*, 1974). However, in isolated rat aorta (Altura *et al.*, 1975) and dog saphenous veins (McGrath and Shepherd, 1976) hyperosmolarity induces contractions rather than relaxations. Therefore, the interest in the cellular effects of mannitol was derived to a large degree from the speculation that Ca^{2+} may be involved directly or indirectly in the loss of coronary responsiveness and that mannitol might have an effect on the utilization of

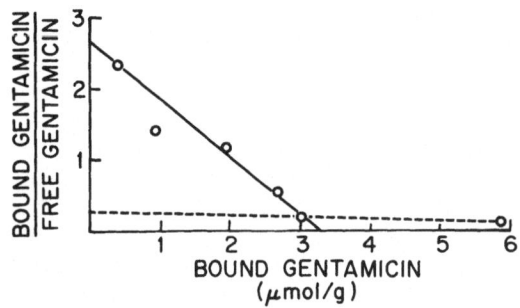

Figure 4. Scatchard plot of ^{14}C*-gentamicin binding. Muscles were exposed to* ^{14}C*-gentamicin for a 60 min period. The dashed line represents extrapolation of the low affinity binding site component. (From Goodman, 1978)*

TABLE I. ^{45}Ca TISSUE ACCUMULATION IN GUINEA PIG LEFT ATRIAL PREPARATIONS[a]

$Ca^{2+}(mM)$	^{45}Ca Accumulation $(ml/g \pm S.E.)$		P
	Control	Gentamicin-Treated	
1.0	0.666 ± 0.049	0.348 ± 0.074	< 0.005
1.0 (nb)[b]	0.352 ± 0.018	0.368 ± 0.054	> 0.7
2.5	0.575 ± 0.045	0.514 ± 0.017	> 0.15
10.0	0.460 ± 0.026	0.425 ± 0.017	> 0.15

[a]$N = 6$

[b]*non-beating*

Ca^{2+}. In preliminary studies employing canine terminal mesenteric arteries (F. R. Goodman, unpublished experiments), prior exposure to 50 mM mannitol was found to decrease contractile responses elicited with dopamine. whereas norepinephrine-induced responses were not altered. In contrast, addition of mannitol to muscles already contracted caused a decrease in tone induced by either norepinephrine or doapmine. The amount of relaxation induced by mannitol was dependent on the concentration of mannitol employed and on the concentration of the agonists. The uptake of ^{45}Ca was increased in the presence of mannitol; increasing the concentration of mannitol from 50-100 mM did not result in any further increases in ^{45}Ca uptake. Exposure of the terminal mesenteric arteries to mannitol during the washout of ^{45}Ca resulted in a significant decrease in ^{45}Ca efflux. The slow component $T_{1/2}$ increased 30% after exposure to mannitol. The question of whether these effects were specific for terminal mesenteric arteries or occurred in other vascular preparations was answered by also determining the effects of mannitol in isolated left anterior descending coronary artery (LAD), circumflex coronary artery (Circ) and branches of the LAD. Prior exposure to mannitol decreased contractile responses elicited with K^+ in the LAD and circumflex, whereas subsequent exposure to mannitol resulted in a slight relaxation. As observed in the mesenteric arteries, mannitol decreased the loss of ^{45}Ca from the coronary artery. Thus, it appears that mannitol increases the binding of ^{45}Ca rather than increasing the rate of uptake of ^{45}Ca in vascular smooth muscle. Since increasing the Ca^{2+} concentration of the incubation solution decreases the magnitude of the mannitol-induced increase in ^{45}Ca uptake, it is tempting to speculate that mannitol increases the affinity of the Ca^{2+}-binding sites for ^{45}Ca. Furthermore, the observation (Figure 5) that mannitol decreased the loss of ^{45}Ca in the presence of EDTA, whereas prior exposure to mannitol blocks the sustained increase in ^{45}Ca efflux normally induced by EDTA (Bianchi, 1965; Goodman and Weiss, 1971) suggests that mannitol may cause its vasodilatory actions by affecting the level of free Ca^{2+} important for the maintenance of vascular tone.

The basic mechanism for the manner in which mannitol alters vascular tone is still not clear. Hyperosmotic sucrose affects ^{45}Ca uptake and efflux in coronary arteries in a manner similar to mannitol, therefore this action is not specific for mannitol. On the other hand, it has been suggested that mannitol induces its vasodilatory effect in vascular smooth muscles by a mechanism unrelated to the mechanism of nitroglycerin and other vasodilating agents (Krishnamurty et al., 1977). Possibly, hyperosmotic conditions interfere with the spread of excitation in smooth muscle (Gurevich et al., 1976). In this regard, further studies are needed to delineate the mechanism of action of hyperosmotic agents

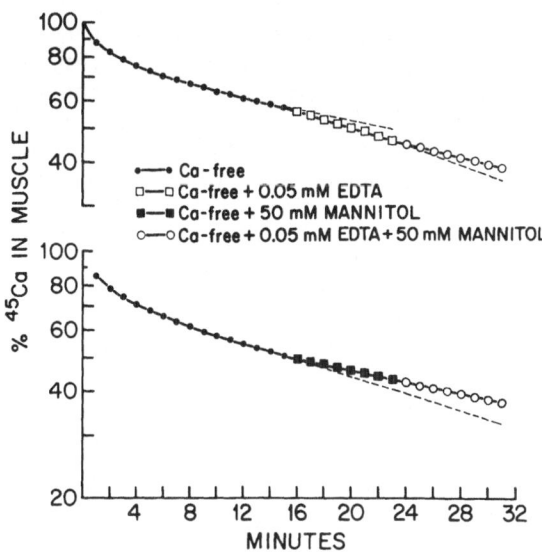

Figure 5. Effects of addition of either mannitol or EDTA on ^{45}Ca
efflux from LAD coronary smooth muscle. Muscles were incubated in
Ca^{2+}-*free solution containing* ^{45}Ca *for 60 min prior to washout.*
The dashed lines indicate extrapolation of the slow component
prior to the addition of either mannitol, EDTA or both.

and to determine whether these agents have any therapeutic usefulness in the treatment of cardiovascular disorders.

CONCLUSION

Although our knowledge about the binding and subsequent utilization of Ca^{2+} by vascular smooth muscle has increased greatly
over the past several years, information concerning the manner
in which many pharmacological agents or conditions act to alter
Ca^{2+} translocation and, in turn, induce their stimulatory or inhibitory effects is not completely resolved. Although the emphasis
in this chapter was placed upon cellular approaches, it should
not be interpreted as implying that only these give the definitive
answers. Indeed, newer techniques would definitely increase
knowledge of poorly understood mechanisms. Furthermore, not only
Ca^{2+} is affected by pharmacological agents during the excitation-
contraction coupling process. It is well known that few, if any,
pharmacological agents have only one site of action or effect.
However, the cellular importance of Ca^{2+} in the initiation of

contraction, maintenance of tone and relaxation of vascular smooth muscle is obvious. Utilization of these cellular approaches would be helpful in delineating the manner in which pharmacological agents or physiological conditions alter vascular reactivity. In addition, similar cellular approaches can be employed for characterizing (a) the mechanism(s) of action of new therapeutic agents, (b) the mechanisms by which apparently unrelated drugs interact to exert stimulatory or inhibitory effects and (c) the basis for both the mechanisms of pathological conditions on vascular function and the therapeutic control of these conditions. For example, during ischemia there is a decrease in both the magnitude and rate of Ca^{2+} uptake by the SR isolated from ischemic heart tissue (Lee et al., 1967). Thus, loss of intracellular Ca^{2+} occurs and this leads to an impairment of the contractile force. Similar events might occur in coronary arteries during ischemia. However, at the present time, there is no evidence for or against this possibility. If the cellular basis of action of the ischemic process (which results in irreversible damage to coronary arteries) was more clearly understood, the development of protective agents would be facilitated.

In general, all types of vascular smooth muscle have the property of excitability which, in turn, results in contractility. Furthermore, it can be assumed that these two processes are coupled by Ca^{2+}. However, it should be obvious from this brief review and work by others (see Weiss, 1977) that, prior to interpreting the action(s) of any particular agent on Ca^{2+} movements, the manner in which Ca^{2+} is utilized by the particular tissue must be understood. This, in combination with comparative studies (e.g., other tissues, species differences), will more precisely define the quantitative details of the influence of pharmacological agents on the contraction and relaxation of vascular smooth muscle. For example, the manner in which some agents mentioned in this chapter alter Ca^{2+} movements is schematically summarized in Figure 6. Mechanisms by which the free intracellular Ca^{2+} concentration can be elevated are illustrated as dark, thick arrows, whereas the thin arrows indicate processes which decrease the free intracellular Ca^{2+} level. According to this scheme, inhibition of contractile responses by aminoglycoside antibiotics, D-600 and rare earth ions is largely due to an inhibition of the uptake of Ca^{2+}, whereas mannitol appears to alter the loss of Ca^{2+}. In addition to inhibiting the uptake of Ca^{2+}, rare earth ions may bind on the surface membrane and replace superficial Ca^{2+}. However, this mechanism is speculative at this time and more research is needed to confirm or reject this hypothesis. Phosphatidyl serine, a natural constituent of the membrane, appears to alter responsiveness to selected stimulatory agents by removing Ca^{2+}. The chemical properties of phospholipids and their physiological role in membrane structure and function has been the

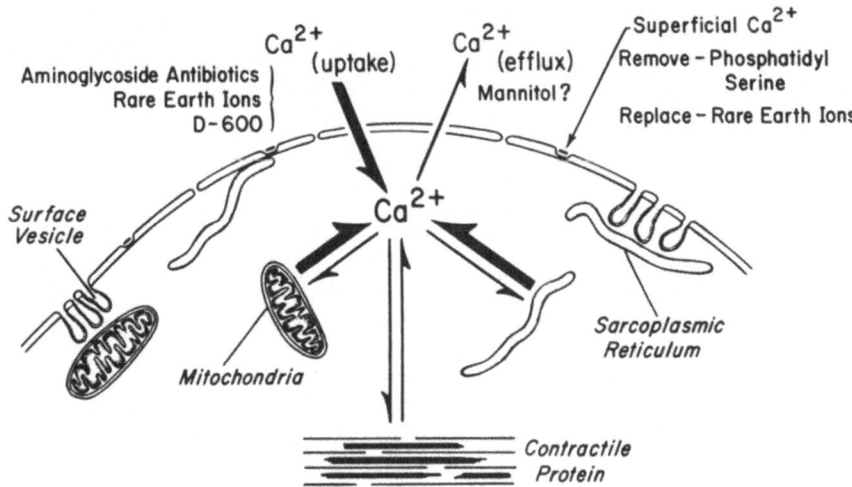

Figure 6. Diagrammatic sketch of both the structural elements and the pathways that may be involved in regulating intracellular free Ca^{2+} levels. This scheme is speculative and is drawn to show the possible mechanism(s) by which selected pharmacological agents alter Ca^{2+} movements and, in turn, influence contractile responsiveness and/or tone.

focal point of considerable research (Triggle, 1972). It has been suggested that phosphatidyl serine might function as a binding site for drug-Ca^{2+} interactions (Seeman *et al.*, 1974). Hopefully, in the future, use of microsomal and other subcellular procedures will provide more information concerning the involvement of this phospholipid in Ca^{2+}-related processes such as excitation-contraction coupling in vascular smooth muscle.

Acknowledgements

The experimental work described in this chapter was supported by National Institutes of Health Grant HL 14775 and an American Heart Association, Texas Affiliate research grant.

REFERENCES

Adams, H. R., 1975, Direct myocardial depressant effects of
  gentamicin, *Eur. J. Pharmacol.* 30: 272.
Adams, H. R. and Goodman, F. R., 1975, Differential inhibitory
  effect of neomycin on contractile responses of various canine
  arteries, *J. Pharmacol. Exp. Ther.* 193: 393.
Adams, H. R., Goodman, F. R., Lupean, V. A., and Weiss, G. B., 1973,
  Effects of neomycin on tension and ^{45}Ca movements in rabbit
  aortic smooth muscle, *Life Sci.* 12: 279.
Adams, H. R., Goodman, F. R., and Weiss, G. B., 1974, Alteration
  of contractile function and calcium ion movement in vascular
  smooth muscle by gentamicin and other aminoglycoside antibiotics,
  Antimicrob. Agents Chemother. 5: 640.
Altura, B. M., Edgarian, H., and Altura, B. T., 1975, Differential
  effects of ethanol and mannitol on contraction of arterial smooth
  muscle, *J. Pharmacol. Exp. Ther.* 193: 393.
Baudouin, M., Meyer, P., Fermandjian, S., and Morgat, J. L., 1972,
  Calcium release induced by interaction of angiotensin with its
  receptors in smooth muscle cell microsomes, *Nature* 235: 336.
Baudouin-Legros, M., and Meyer, P., 1973, Effects of angiotensin,
  catecholamines and cyclic AMP on calcium storage in aortic
  microsomes, *Brit. J. Pharmacol.* 47: 377.
Bianchi, C. P., 1965, Effect of EDTA and SCN on radiocalcium move-
  ment in frog rectus abdominis muscle during contractures induced
  by calcium removal, *J. Pharmacol. Exp. Ther.* 147: 360.
Bianchi, C. P., 1975, Cellular pharmacology of contraction of
  skeletal muscle, *in* "Cellular Pharmacology of Excitable Tissues"
  (T. Narahashi, ed.) pp. 485-519, Charles C. Thomas, Springfield,
  Illinois.
Bohr, D. F., 1964, Electrolytes and smooth muscle contraction,
  Pharmacol. Rev. 16: 85.
Bohr, D. F., 1973, Vascular smooth muscle updated, *Circ. Res.*
  32: 665.
Bohr, D. F., Sitrin, M. D., and Sobieski, J., 1971, Heterogeneity
  among vascular smooth muscles in the regulation of activator
  calcium, *in* "Vascular Neuroeffector Systems" (J. A. Bevan, R. F.
  Furchgott, R. A. Maxwell, and A. P. Somlyo, eds.) pp. 72-85, S.
  Karger, Basel.
Debbas, G., Hoffman, L., Landon, E. J., and Hurwitz, L., 1975,
  Electron microscopic localization of calcium in vascular smooth
  muscle, *Anat. Rec.* 182: 447.
DeFelice, A. F., and Joiner, P. D., 1975, Comparison of aortic
  calcium and contractility in male, female, and lactating female
  rats, *J. Pharmacol. Exp. Ther.* 194: 191.
Devine, C. E., Somlyo, A. V., and Somlyo, A. P., 1972, Sarcoplasmic
  reticulum and excitation-contraction coupling in mammalian
  smooth muscles, *J. Cell Biol.* 52: 690.

Ebashi, S., 1976, Excitation-contraction coupling, *Annu. Rev. Physiol.* 38: 293.

Elmqvist, D., and Josefsson, J. O., 1962, The nature of the neuro-muscular block produced by neomycin, *Acta Physiol. Scand.* 54: 105.

Fitzpatrick, D. F., Landon, E. J., Debbas, G., and Hurwitz, L., 1972, A calcium pump in vascular smooth muscle, *Science* 176: 305.

Fleckenstein, A., 1977, Specific pharmacology of calcium in myo-cardium, cardiac pacemakers, and vascular smooth muscle, *Annu. Rev. Pharmacol. Toxicol.* 17: 149.

Fleisch, J. H., 1974, Pharmacology of the aorta, *Blood Vessels* 11: 193.

Ford, G. D., 1976, Subcellular fractions of vascular smooth muscle exhibiting calcium transport properties, *Fed. Proc.* 35: 1298.

Fozzard, H. A., 1977, Heart: Excitation-contraction coupling, *Annu. Rev. Physiol.* 39: 201.

Fuchs, F., 1974, Striated muscle, *Annu. Rev. Physiol.* 36: 461.

Gabella, J., 1973, I. Cellular structures and electrophysiological behavior. Fine structure of smooth muscle, *Phil. Trans. R. Soc. London, Ser.* B 265: 7.

Goodman, F. R., 1978, Distribution of ^{14}C-gentamicin in vascular smooth muscle, *Pharmacology* 16: 17.

Goodman, F. R., and Adams, H. R., 1976, Negative ionotropic effects of gentamicin in guinea pig left atria, *Fed. Proc.* 35: 613.

Goodman, F. R., and Weiss, G. B., 1971, Effects of lanthanum on ^{45}Ca movements and on contractions induced by norepinephrine, histamine and potassium in vascular smooth muscle, *J. Pharmacol. Exp. Ther.* 177: 415.

Goodman, F. R., and Weiss, G. B., 1974, Contractile responses and ^{45}Ca movements in monkey ileal smooth muscle, *Arch. Int. Pharmacodyn. Ther.* 209: 14.

Goodman, F. R., Weiss, G. B., Weinberg, M. N., and Pomarantz, S. D., 1972, Effects of added or substituted potassium ion on ^{45}Ca movements in rabbit aortic smooth muscle, *Circ. Res.* 31: 672.

Goodman, F. R., Weiss, G. B., and Adams, H. R., 1974, Alterations by neomycin of ^{45}Ca movements and contractile responses in vascular smooth muscle, *J. Pharmacol. Exp. Ther.* 188: 472.

Goodman, F. R., Adams, H. R., and Weiss, G. B., 1975, Effects of neomycin on ^{45}Ca binding and distribution in canine arteries, *Blood Vessels* 12: 248.

Gurevich, M. I., Bershtein, S. A., and Evdokimov, 1976, *in* "Phys-iology of Smooth Muscle" (E. Bulbring, and M. F. Shuba, eds.) pp. 153-161, Raven Press, New York.

Haeusler, G., 1972, Differential effect of verapamil on excitation-contraction coupling in smooth muscle and on excitation-secretion coupling in adrenergic nerve terminals, *J. Pharmacol. Exp. Ther.* 180: 672.

Hess, M. L., and Ford, G. D., 1974, Calcium accumulation by subcellular fractions from vascular smooth muscle, *J. Molec. Cell.
Cardiol.* 6: 275.

Hinke, J. A. M., 1965, Calcium requirements for noradrenaline and
high potassium ion contraction in arterial smooth muscle, *in*
"Muscle" (W. M. Paul, E. E. Daniel, C. M. Kay, and G. Monckton,
eds.) pp. 269-284, Pergamon Press, New York.

Hudgins, P. M., and Weiss, G. B., 1968, Differential effects of
calcium removal upon vascular smooth muscle contraction induced
by norepinephrine, histamine and potassium, *J. Pharmacol. Exp.
Ther.* 159: 91.

Hudgins, P. M., and Weiss, G. B., 1969, Characteristics of ^{45}Ca
binding in vascular smooth muscle, *Amer. J. Physiol.* 217: 1310.

Hurwitz, L., and Suria, A., 1971, The link between agonist action
and response in smooth muscle, *Annu. Rev. Pharmacol.* 11: 303.

Hurwitz, L., Battle, F., and Weiss, G. B., 1962, Action of the
calcium antagonists cocaine and ethanol on contraction and
potassium efflux of smooth muscle, *J. gen. Physiol.* 46: 315.

Hurwitz, L., Joiner, P. D., and Von Hagen, S., 1967a, Mechanical
responses of intestinal smooth muscle in a calcium-free medium,
Proc. Soc. Exp. Biol. Med. 125: 518.

Hurwitz, L., Joiner, P. D., and Von Hagen, S., 1967b, Calcium
pools utilized for contraction in smooth muscle, *Amer. J. Physiol.*
213: 1299.

Hurwitz, L., Fitzpatrick, D. F., Debbas, G., and Landon, E. J.,
1973, Localization of calcium pump activity in smooth muscle,
Science 179: 384.

Hurwitz, L., Debbas, G., and Little, S., 1975, Effects of temperature and inorganic ions on calcium accumulation in microsomes
from intestinal smooth muscle, *Mol. Cell. Biochem.* 8: 31.

Kalsner, S., Nickerson, M., and Boyd, G. N., 1970, Selective blockade of potassium-induced contractions of aortic strips by β-
diethylaminoethyl-diphenylpropylacetate (SKF 525A), *J. Pharmacol.
Exp. Ther.* 174: 500.

Kohlhardt, M., Bauer, P., Krause, H., and Fleckenstein, A., 1972,
Differentiation of the transmembrane Na and Ca channel in
mammalian cardiac fibres by the use of specific inhibitors,
Pflügers Arch. 335: 309.

Krejci, J., and Daniel, E. E., 1970, Effect of contraction on movements of calcium 45 into and out of rat myometrium, *Amer. J.
Physiol.* 219: 256.

Krishnamurty, V. S. R., Adams, H. R., Smitherman, T. C., Templeton,
G. H., and Willerson, J. T., 1977, Influence of mannitol on
contractile responses of isolated perfused arteries, *Amer. J.
Physiol.* 232: H59.

Kutsky, P., and Goodman, F. R., 1978, Calcium incorporation by
canine aortic smooth muscle microsomes, *Arch. Int. Pharmacodyn.
Thér.,* In Press.

Langer, G. A., 1976, Events at the cardiac sarcolemma: localization and movement of contractile dependent calcium, *Fed. Proc.* 35: 1274.

Langer, G. A., and Frank, J. S., 1972, Lanthanum in heart cell culture: Effect on calcium exchange correlated with its localization, *J. Cell Biol.* 54: 441.

Lee, K. S., Ladinsky, H., and Stuckey, J. H., 1967, Decreased Ca^{2+}-uptake by sarcoplasmic reticulum after coronary artery occlusion for 60 and 90 minutes, *Circ. Res.* 21: 439.

Lüllmann, H., and Peters, T., 1977, Plasmalemmal calcium in cardiac excitation-contraction coupling, *Clin. Exp. Pharm. Physiol.* 4: 49.

Lüllmann, H., and Siegfriedt, A., 1968, Über den Calcium-Gehalt und den ^{45}Calcium-Austausch in Längsmuskulatur des Meerschweinchendünndarms, *Pflügers Arch.* 300: 108.

McGrath, M. A., and Shepherd, J. T., 1976, Hyperosmolarity: effects on nerves and smooth muscle of cutaneous veins, *Amer. J. Physiol.* 231: 141.

Prosser, C. L., 1974, Smooth muscle, *Annu. Rev. Pharmacol.* 36: 503.

Seeman, P., Chen, S. S., Chau-Wong, M., and Staiman, A., 1974, Calcium reversal of nerve blockade by alcohols, anesthetics, tranquilizers, and barbiturates, *Can. J. Physiol. Pharmacol.* 52: 526.

Somlyo, A. P., and Somlyo, A. V., 1968, Vascular smooth muscle. I. Normal structure, pathology, biochemistry, and biophysics, *Pharmacol. Rev.* 20: 197.

Somlyo, A. P., and Somlyo, A. V., 1970, Vascular smooth muscle. II. Pharmacology of normal and hypertensive vessels, *Pharmacol. Rev.* 22: 249.

Somlyo, A. V., and Somlyo, A. P., 1971, Strontium accumulation by sarcoplasmic reticulum and mitochondria in vascular smooth muscle, *Science* 174: 955.

Somlyo, A. P., and Somlyo, A. V., 1975, Ultrastructure of smooth muscle, *in* "Methods in Pharmacology, Vol. 3, Smooth Muscle" (E. E. Daniel and D. M. Paton, eds.) pp. 3-45, Plenum Press, New York.

Somlyo, A. P., Somlyo, A. V., Devine, C. E., Peters, P. D., and Hall, T. A., 1974, Electron microscopy and electron probe analysis of mitochondrial cation accumulation in smooth muscle, *J. Cell Biol.* 61: 723.

Triggle, D. J., 1972, Effects of calcium on excitable membranes and neurotransmitter action, *Progr. Surface and Memb. Sci.* 5: 267.

Tritthardt, H., Volkmann, R., Weiss, R., and Fleckenstein, A., 1973, Calcium mediated action potentials in mammalian myocardium: Alterations of membrane responses induced by changes of Ca or by promoters and inhibitors of transmembrane Ca inflow, *Naunyn-Schmied. Arch. Pharmacol.* 280: 239.

Turlapaty, D. M. V., Hester, R. K., and Carrier, O., 1976, Role of calcium in different layers of vascular smooth muscle in norepinephrine contraction, *Blood Vessels* 13: 193.

Uchida, E., and Bohr, D. F., 1969a, Myogenic tone in isolated perfused vessels, *Circ. Res.* 25: 549.

Uchida, E., and Bohr, D. F., 1969b, Myogenic tone in isolated perfused resistance vessels from rats, *Amer. J. Physiol.* 216: 1343.

Vallières, J., Scarpa, A., and Somlyo, A. P., 1975, Subcellular fractions of smooth muscle. I. Isolation, substrate utilization and Ca^{++} transport by main pulmonary artery and mesenteric vein mitochondria, *Arch. Biochem. Biophys.* 170: 659.

Van Breemen, C., 1969, Blockade of membrane calcium fluxes by lanthanum in relation to vascular smooth muscle contractility, *Arch. Int. Physiol. Biochim.* 77: 710.

Vital Brazil, O., and Prado-Franceschi, J., 1969, The neuromuscular blocking action of gentamicin, *Arch. Int. Pharmacodyn. Thér.* 179: 65.

Weiss, G. B., 1972, Alterations in ^{45}Ca distribution and movements in ileal longitudinal smooth muscle, *Agents and Actions* 2: 246.

Weiss, G. B., 1974, Cellular pharmacology of lanthanum, *Annu. Rev. Pharmacol.* 14: 343.

Weiss, G. B., 1975, Stimulation with high potassium, *in* "Methods in Pharmacology, Vol. 3, Smooth Muscle" (E. E. Daniel and D. M. Paton, eds.) pp. 339-345, Plenum Press, New York.

Weiss, G. B., 1977, Calcium and contractility in vascular smooth muscle, *in* "Advances in General and Cellular Pharmacology", (T. Narahashi and C. P. Bianchi, eds.) Vol. 2, pp. 71-154, Plenum Press, New York.

CONTRIBUTORS

Julius C. Allen
Section of Cardiovascular
  Sciences
Department of Internal Medicine
Baylor College of Medicine
Houston, Texas 77030

C. Paul Bianchi
Department of Pharmacology
Jefferson Medical College
Thomas Jefferson University
Philadelphia, Pennsylvania 19107

Maurice B. Feinstein
Department of Pharmacology
University of Connecticut
  Health Center
Farmington, Connecticut 06032

Joy S. Frank
Department of Physiology and
  Cardiovascular Research
  Laboratory
UCLA Center for the Health
  Sciences
Los Angeles, California 90024

Frank R. Goodman
Department of Pharmacology
Dow Chemical Company
Indianapolis, Indiana 46268

Leon Hurwitz
Department of Pharmacology
University of New Mexico
  School of Medicine
Albuquerque, New Mexico 87131

Suzanne G. Laychock
Department of Pharmacology
Vanderbilt University
  School of Medicine
Nashville, Tennessee 37232

Linda J. McGuffee
Department of Pharmacology
University of New Mexico
  School of Medicine
Albuquerque, New Mexico 87131

Rodney L. Parsons
Department of Physiology and
  Biophysics
University of Vermont
Burlington, Vermont 05401

James W. Putney, Jr.
Department of Pharmacology
Wayne State University
  School of Medicine
Detroit, Michigan 48201

Gideon A. Rodan
Department of Oral Biology
School of Medicine and
  Dental Medicine
University of Connecticut
Farmington, Connecticut 06032

L. Rosenberger
Department of Biochemical
  Pharmacology
State University of New York
Buffalo, New York 14214

David H. Ross
Departments of Pharmacology
  and Psychiatry
University of Texas
  Health Sciences Center
San Antonio, Texas 78284

Ronald P. Rubin
Department of Pharmacology
Medical College of Virginia
Virginia Commonwealth University
Richmond, Virginia 23298

D. J. Triggle
Department of Biochemical
  Pharmacology
State University of New York
Buffalo, New York 14214

William Van der Kloot
Department of Physiology and
  Biophysics
Health Sciences Center
  State University of New York
Stony Brook, New York 11794

George B. Weiss
Department of Pharmacology
University of Texas
  Health Sciences Center
Dallas, Texas 75235

INDEX